Oxidative Stress: Mechanisms and Disease Pathogenesis

Edited by Edwin Reynolds

hayle
medical

New York

Hayle Medical,
750 Third Avenue, 9th Floor,
New York, NY 10017, USA

Visit us on the World Wide Web at:
www.haylemedical.com

ISBN: 978-1-63241-858-6

Cataloging-in-Publication Data

Oxidative stress : mechanisms and disease pathogenesis / edited by Edwin Reynolds.
    p. cm.
Includes bibliographical references and index.
ISBN 978-1-63241-858-6
1. Oxidative stress. 2. Oxidative stress--Pathophysiology. 3. Oxidation-reduction reaction.
4. Stress (Physiology). I. Reynolds, Edwin.
RB170 .O95 2020
616.39--dc21

Table of Contents

Preface

The purpose of the book is to provide a glimpse into the dynamics and to present opinions and studies of some of the scientists engaged in the development of new ideas in the field from very different standpoints. This book will prove useful to students and researchers owing to its high content quality.

Oxidative stress is an imbalance in the production of free radicals and the body's inability to counteract their harmful effects or detoxify. This imbalance can cause disruptions in cellular signaling. Oxidative stress implies an increased production of oxidizing species and decrease in the effectiveness of antioxidant defenses. Moderate oxidation can trigger apoptosis, while more severe cases cause necrosis. Oxidative stress is considered to be an important element in the pathogenesis of neurodegenerative diseases, such as Alzheimer's disease, Huntington's disease, Lou Gehrig's disease, multiple sclerosis, autism, etc. Oxidative stress has been implicated in the incidence of cardiovascular diseases, as oxidation of LDL is a precursor to plaque formation. This book elucidates the concepts and innovative models around prospective developments with respect to oxidative stress. It unravels the recent studies in the mechanisms and disease pathogenesis of oxidative stress. Coherent flow of topics, student-friendly language and extensive use of examples make this book an invaluable source of knowledge.

At the end, I would like to appreciate all the efforts made by the authors in completing their chapters professionally. I express my deepest gratitude to all of them for contributing to this book by sharing their valuable works. A special thanks to my family and friends for their constant support in this journey.

Editor

Metallothionein-I+II Reduces Oxidative Damage and Apoptosis after Traumatic Spinal Cord Injury in Rats

Camilo Rios,[1] **Iván Santander,**[2] **Marisela Méndez-Armenta** ⓘ,[3] **Concepción Nava-Ruiz,**[3] **Sandra Orozco-Suárez,**[4] **Marcela Islas,**[2] **Verónica Barón-Flores,**[1] **and Araceli Diaz-Ruiz** ⓘ[2]

[1]*Departamento de Sistemas Biológicos, Universidad Autónoma Metropolitana Unidad Xochimilco Ciudad de México, Mexico*
[2]*Departamento de Neuroquímica, Instituto Nacional de Neurología y Neurocirugía Manuel Velasco Suárez,*
  Ciudad de México, Mexico
[3]*Laboratorio de Patología Experimental, Instituto Nacional de Neurología y Neurocirugía Manuel Velasco Suárez,*
  Ciudad de México, Mexico
[4]*Unidad de Investigación Médica en Enfermedades Neurológicas, Hospital de Especialidades, Centro Médico Nacional Siglo XXI,*
  Ciudad de México, Mexico

Correspondence should be addressed to Araceli Diaz-Ruiz; adiaz@innn.edu.mx

Guest Editor: Min-Cheol Kang

After spinal cord injury (SCI), some self-destructive mechanisms start leading to irreversible neurological deficits. It is known that oxidative stress and apoptosis play a major role in increasing damage after SCI. Metallothioneins I and II (MT) are endogenous peptides with known antioxidant, neuroprotective capacities. Taking advantage of those capacities, we administered exogenous MT to rats after SCI in order to evaluate the protective effects of MT on the production of reactive oxygen species (ROS) and lipid peroxidation (LP), as markers of oxidative stress. The activities of caspases-9 and -3 and the number of annexin V and TUNEL-positive cells in the spinal cord tissue were also measured as markers of apoptosis. Rats were subjected to either sham surgery or SCI and received vehicle or two doses of MT ($10 \, \mu g$ per rat) at 2 and 8 h after surgical procedure. The results showed a significant increase in levels of MT protein by effect of SCI and SCI plus treatment at 12 h, while at 24 h an increase of MT was observed only in the injury plus treatment group ($p < 0.05$). ROS production was decreased by effect of MT in lesioned tissue; likewise, we observed diminished LP levels by MT effect both in the sham group and in the group with SCI. Also, the results showed an increase in the activity of caspase-9 due to SCI, without changes by effect of MT, as compared to the sham group. Caspase-3 activity was increased by SCI, and again, MT treatment reduced this effect only at 24 h after injury. Finally, the results of the number of cells positive to annexin V and TUNEL showed a reduction due to MT treatment both at 24 and 72 h after the injury. With the findings of this work, we conclude that exogenously administered MT has antioxidant and antiapoptotic effects after SCI.

1. Introduction

After spinal cord injury (SCI), a series of self-destructive mechanisms initiate to produce irreversible damage to the surrounding tissue, with consequent motor and sensitive deficits [1]. Among those damaging mechanisms, the ischemia after trauma with subsequent energy failure and ATP deficit [2] produces depolarization of the plasma membrane leading, in turn, to increased intracellular calcium by opening calcium voltage-activated channels. Excessive calcium entry to cells produces reactive oxygen and nitrogen species (ROS and RNS, respectively). The ROS include superoxide anion ($O_2 \bullet^-$), hydrogen peroxide (H_2O_2), and hydroxyl radical ($\bullet OH$). $O_2 \bullet^-$ is produced through several pathways during normal metabolism, and superoxide dismutase (SOD) enzymes convert $O_2 \bullet^-$ into H_2O_2. H_2O_2 is reduced to H_2O by catalase, glutathione peroxidase (GPx), and thioredoxin [3]. Likewise, nitric oxide ($\bullet NO$) synthesized by the activation of constitutive and inducible nitric oxide synthases after SCI [4, 5] can react with $O_2^{\bullet-}$ to form the highly reactive oxidizing agent, peroxynitrite (ONOO–). The increased production of ROS and RNS after SCI cause oxidative damage to proteins, DNA, and cellular lipids, polyunsaturated fatty acids in cell membranes, triggering free radical chain reactions to cause lipid peroxidation (LP) [6]. Furthermore, damage to proteins and DNA activates the mechanisms of cell death by apoptosis [7]. Apoptosis occurs through intrinsic and extrinsic apoptotic pathways. The intrinsic one starts when mitochondria are exposed to a pathological overload of calcium; opening of the mitochondrial permeability transition pore (mPTP) is triggered, activating the initiator caspase-9 and subsequently activating the effector caspase-3 [8]. Based on this information, it has been proposed that the prevention of apoptosis after damage could be a key target to preventing spinal cord tissue damage and to promoting improved motor function after SCI. On the other hand, we have reported that metallothioneins (MTs) could play an important role in regulating oxidative damage [9]. They are known to be nonenzymatic intracellular proteins of low molecular weight, consisting of 61–62 amino acid residues, and high content of cysteines (25–30%). They form disulfide bridges and have high affinity for metals, binding 5–7 zinc atoms, 12 copper atoms, or 7 atoms of cadmium per mole of protein [9]. Three protein isoforms (MT-I, MT-II, and MT-III) have been identified in the central nervous system [9]; from these, MT-I and MT-II are located in the central nervous system and peripheral tissues; MT-III isoform is expressed specifically in the brain and spinal cord [10] neurons. A common feature observed in numerous studies is the remarkable ability of MT-I and II to reduce cell death and oxidative brain damage [11]. MTs are known to have high antioxidant capacity, even greater than that of glutathione, and this antioxidant mechanism has been proposed as responsible for its neuroprotective effect [12]. MT easily reacts with •OH, O2•⁻, and •NO radicals, and thiol groups can bind ONOO– and peroxynitrous acid (ONOOH), making this protein a highly efficient antioxidant defense [12–14]. Likewise, the neuroprotective effect of MT has been reported to reduce apoptosis in transgenic mice overexpressing MT. They showed reduced cell death and oxidative tissue damage after traumatic brain injury [15]. Finally, it has been reported that MT-III attenuated the apoptosis of neurons in the CA1 region of the hippocampus in a model of Alzheimer's disease in mice [16]. In the present study, we evaluated the antioxidant and antiapoptotic effects of MT in a model of SCI contusion in rats.

2. Materials and Methods

2.1. Animals. We used female Wistar rats weighing 200 to 250 g of body weight; they were maintained under standard laboratory conditions and had free access to food and water, following the guidelines established internationally and nationally by the Mexican Official Standard NOM-062-ZOO-1999 (which observes technical specifications for the production, care, and use of laboratory animals) and the guidelines for Care and Use of Laboratory Animals of the National Institutes of Health (USA). API MT-I + II with a zinc content about 6%, from rabbit liver, purity ≥95%, was purchased from Creative BioMart.

2.2. Surgical Procedure. All animals were subjected to either a sham procedure (laminectomy only) or spinal cord injury (SCI) by contusion according to the report of Basso et al. [17], under pentobarbital (50 mg/kg i.p.) anesthesia. An incision was made by extending from the mid to low thoracic regions, followed by a laminectomy, including the caudal portion of T9 and all of T10, to expose the spinal cord. The NYU weight-drop device was used in order to produce the SCI by contusion. Then, the SCI was produced by dropping the 10 g rod from a distance of 25 mm. The surgical site was sutured in layers. Rats were allowed to recover from anesthetic and surgical procedures in an intensive care unit for small animals (Schroer Manufacturing Co., Kansas City, MO, USA), and the animals received food and water *ad libitum*. Their intestine and bladder were manually expressed twice a day, and they were routinely inspected visually for skin irritation and decubitus ulcers.

2.3. Experimental Design and Treatment with MT-I + II. The rats were randomly assigned to either one of the following four groups: group 1, sham surgery plus vehicle i.p. (saline solution, 0.9% NaCl); group 2, sham surgery plus MT i.p. (metallothionein); group 3, animals with SCI plus vehicle; and group 4, rats with SCI plus treatment with MT. The MT was exogenously i.p. administered at doses of 10 μg per rat, dissolved in saline solution, according to the previous reports by Penkowa and Hidalgo [18], starting two and eight hours after SCI, following the schedule reported previously (Diaz-Ruiz et al. [19]). According to that report, a dose of 10 μg is enough to produce therapeutic benefits, while a higher dose showed no further neuroprotective effect.

2.4. Metallothionein Protein Assay. Seventy-three animals were sacrificed at two different times (12 and 24) after surgical procedure. The content of MT was estimated by the silver-saturation method as described by Scheuhammer and Cherian [20] and modified by Rojas and Ríos [21]. Briefly, fresh tissue samples of about 0.02 g were homogenized in 300 μl of a 0.05 M phosphate buffer (pH = 7) and 0.375 M NaCl mixture (1.5 : 1 *v/v*). Then, 250 μl of silver nitrate solution (20 ppm) and 400 μl of glycine buffer (0.5 M, pH 8.5) were added. After standing at room temperature for 5 min, 100 μl of rat hemolyzed erythrocytes was added and the mixture was boiled for 2 min, then centrifuged at 4000 x/g for 5 min. The latter step was repeated twice. MT content was estimated by measuring the silver content of the supernatant fractions (diluted 1 : 10 with 3% HNO_3 *v/v*) using an atomic absorption spectrophotometer (Perkin-Elmer 3110) equipped with an HGA-600 furnace and AS60 autosampler. The results were expressed as nmol of metallothionein per gram of wet tissue.

2.5. Reactive Oxygen Species Assay. To evaluate the amount of reactive oxygen species (ROS) in the spinal cord tissue, thirty-one animals were sacrificed (prior anesthesia) at 4 h after surgery procedure, as reported by Liu et al. [22], as the time for increased production of hydrogen peroxide and superoxide radical. ROS were assayed following the method previously reported by Pérez-Severiano et al. [23]. The samples of fresh tissue were taken at the level of the ninth thoracic vertebra (a single sample from each rat), 2 mm from the caudal area and 2 mm from the rostral area, covering only the epicenter of the lesion or laminectomy. Tissue was homogenized in 20 volumes of saline solution (0.9% NaCl), and aliquots of $100 \mu l$ were incubated in the presence of $5 \mu M$ $2',7'$-dichlorodihydrofluorescein diacetate (DCF) at 37°C for 60 min. Fluorescent signals were recorded at the end of the incubation time at an excitation wavelength of 488 nm and an emission wavelength of 525 nm in a Perkin-Elmer LS50B luminescence spectrometer. A standard curve was constructed using increasing concentrations of DCF incubated in parallel. Results were expressed as nmol of $2',7'$-dichlorodihydrofluorescein diacetate (DCF) per gram of wet tissue per hour of incubation.

2.6. Lipid Peroxidation Assay. The LP was assessed as a marker of oxidative damage, using lipid-fluorescence product formation as a marker. Forty-two animals were killed by decapitation 24 h after either SCI or sham surgery, when the peak of LP levels is reached, according to Diaz-Ruiz et al. [6]. The samples of wet tissue were taken in the same way as described above. Lipid-soluble fluorescent products (LFP), an index of LP, were measured according to the technique described by Triggs and Willmore [24] and modified by Santamaría et al. [25]. Briefly, each sample of spinal cord tissue was homogenized in 3 ml of saline solution (0.9% NaCl). One-milliliter aliquots of the homogenate were added to 4 ml of a chloroform-methanol mixture (2:1, *v/v*). After stirring, the mixture was ice-cooled for 30 min to allow phase separation and the fluorescence of the chloroform layer was measured in a Perkin-Elmer LS50B luminescence spectrophotometer at 370 nm (excitation) and 430 nm (emission). The sensitivity of the spectrophotometer was adjusted to 150 fluorescence units with a quinine standard solution (0.1 g/ml). The values were expressed as fluorescent units per gram of wet tissue.

2.7. Activities of Caspases-9 and -3. To characterize the antiapoptotic effect of MT, the activities of caspases 9 and 3 were measured. Ninety-four rats were killed at 24 and 72 hours according to reports by Ríos et al. [7] as the times for maximal activity of the caspases after SCI. Animals were killed by decapitation, and one centimeter (5 mm from the caudal area and 5 mm from the rostral area) of spinal cord wet tissue was obtained from each rat. Caspase-9 activity was measured by using a caspase-9 fluorometric protease ELISA Kit that recognizes the sequence LEHD (Chemicon MCH6 kit) [7]. The assay detects the cleavage of LEHD-AFC (7-amino-4-trifluoromethyl coumarin), as a substrate. LEHD-AFC emits blue light that was detected at 400 nm; upon cleavage of the substrate by MCH-6 or related caspases, free AFC emits a yellow-green fluorescence at 505 nm, which was quantified by using a fluorescence plate reader (BioTek model FLX 800TB). Comparison of the fluorescence of AFC from an apoptotic sample with an uninduced control allowed us to determine the increase in caspase-9 activity.

Caspase-3 activity was measured by using a Calbiochem Caspase-3 Activity Assay Kit. The enzyme cleaves specifically after aspartate residues in a different peptide sequence (DEVD). The DEVD substrate is also labeled with the fluorescent molecule AFC, so the reaction can be monitored by a blue to green shift in fluorescence upon cleavage of the AFC fluorophore [26]. The results were expressed in arbitrary fluorescence units per milligram of protein (measured according to Lowry, 1951) of 5 to 8 animals per groups.

2.8. Annexin V and TUNEL Immunodetection. Thirty-five animals were killed at either 24 and 72 h after SCI to assess the antiapoptotic effect of MT by immunohistochemical technique. Approximately 1 cm (5 mm from the caudal area and 5 mm from the rostral area) of the spinal cord at the T9 level was removed immediately after cardiac perfusion with 0.1 M phosphate buffered saline (PBS) and 4% paraformaldehyde solution in PBS and post-fixed for one week at 4°C and processed for embedding in paraffin. Longitudinal sections were then cut (12 μm thickness) with the aid of a microtome (Leica RM2125 RT, Germany) and mounted onto poly-l-lysine-coated slides. To have a comparable area for evaluation, the ependymus was taken as the point of reference, and the area with the most tissue destruction was considered to be the epicenter of the injury. Only this section was considered for the analysis. Then, the sections were washed in 0.12 M phosphate buffer saline (PBS, pH 7.2–7.6) and incubated for 30 min at room temperature with blocking solution, 1% normal horse serum (Vector Lab) in PBS 0.12 M. Later, the sections were incubated with anti-annexin V (Santa Cruz Labs, SC-8300) antibody diluted in PBS (1:200) and neurofilament (Santa Cruz Labs, SC-32273) for 24 h at 4°C. After that, the sections were washed with PBS 0.12 M for 15 min and incubated for 2 h at room temperature with the goat anti-mouse IgG Alexa 488 and Alexa 546 (Molecular Probes, Invitrogen Lab, A21121, A11030) diluted in PBS. In the next step, the sections were counterstained with Hoechst (Invitrogen) or propidium iodide (Sigma) for 1 min and a final washing was performed in PBS 0.12 M for 10 min, gently dried, and cover-slipped with Vectashield (Vector Lab) mounting medium. The samples were observed in a fluorescence microscope (Carl Zeiss), with refrigerated camera (Evolution) and an image analyzer Image-Pro Plus 7 (Media Cybernetics).

2.9. Analysis of the Number of Annexin V- and TUNEL-Positive Cells. Annexin V- and TUNEL-positive cells were counted in the cross-longitudinal sections of the spinal cord at the lesion site. All images were digitized using an Evolution MP freeze camera (Media Cybernetics, USA) connected to an Axio Lab microscope (Zeiss, Germany) and Image-Pro Plus 7 software to analyze the images and count the cells. The average cell density per unit volume was determined with the optical fractionator method [27]. This procedure allowed the determination of the fraction of tissue in which neurons were counted. Every third section was sampled (for a total of 10 sections). Then, the first sampling fraction was 1/3; this is called the section sampling fraction. A volume fraction of each tissue was taken, and the

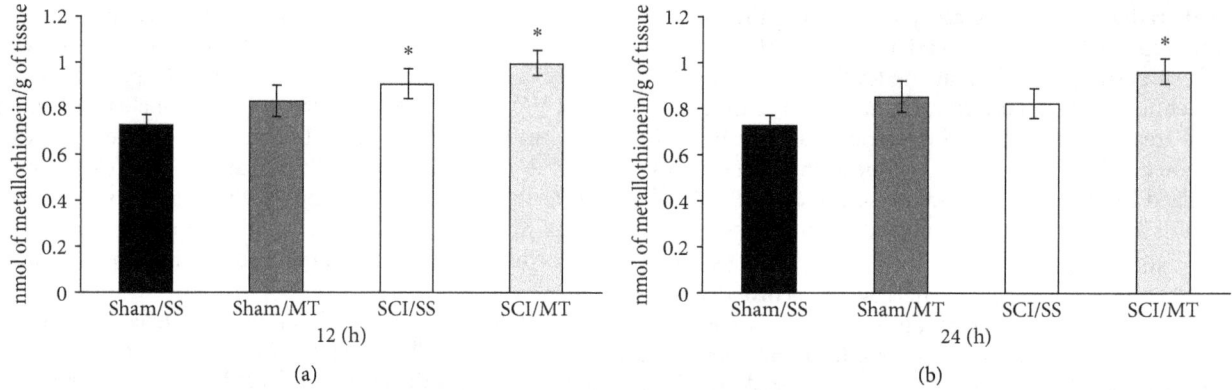

FIGURE 1: Spinal cord tissue metallothionein (MT) levels of rats submitted to either spinal cord injury or sham operation and evaluated at 12 (a) and 24 h (b) after surgery and treated with saline solution (SS) or MT (10 μg/rat). Sham: rats without spinal cord injury; SCI: rats at two times after spinal cord injury. The results are expressed as mean ± SEM of 8 to 11 animals per group, *different from the sham/SS group ($p < 0.05$). One-way ANOVA followed by Tukey's test.

area sampling fraction (asf) = area (frame)/area ($x \cdot y$) was the area of counting frame ($220 \times 180\,\mu$m), relative to the area associated with each field in the computer monitor. The third sampling fraction reflected that cells were not counted in the entire thickness of the tissue at each sampling location. Instead, a three-dimensional probe of a known height was placed in the tissue. The thickness of the tissue ($6\,\mu$m) divided by the height of the dissector was the third sampling fraction. This is called the tissue sampling fraction or tsf. The estimate of the total cell number was therefore the sum of cells counted ($\Sigma Q-$), multiplied by the reciprocal of the three fractions of the brain region sampled as represented by

$$N \frac{1}{4}\sum Q - \left(\frac{1}{\text{ssf}}\right)\left(\frac{1}{\text{asf}}\right)(\text{tsf}), \qquad (1)$$

where N is the estimate of the total cell number and $\Sigma Q-$ is the number of counted cells on all sections. In order to standardize the counting, the same volume fraction was used for each experimental group. This method was standardized and validated by West [27] and modified by Besio et al. [28].

2.10. Statistical Analysis. An exploratory analysis of the data was performed to determine normal distribution (Kolmogorov-Smirnov's test) and homogeneity of variances, applying Levene's test. The results of MT protein levels, amount of ROS, and activities of caspases-9 and -3 were analyzed applying one-way ANOVA, followed by Tukey's test for multiple comparisons. Data of annexin V (24 and 72 h) and TUNEL-positive cells (24 h) were analyzed using Student's t-test. The results of the LP- and TUNEL-positive cell (only 72 h) counting were analyzed using the Kruskal-Wallis test, followed by Mann-Whitney's U test for multiple comparisons, due to lack of normal distribution and homogeneity of variances of data. All analyses were performed with an SPSS 22.0 software. Differences were considered statistically significant when $p < 0.05$.

3. Results

3.1. Both the Lesion and Treatment with MT Increased the Concentration of Metallothionein Proteins after SCI. The content of metallothionein proteins present in the spinal cord tissue was assessed at 12 (Figure 1(a)) and 24 h (Figure 1(b)) following either laminectomy (sham) or SCI from animals receiving either vehicle (saline solution) or MT (10 μg/rat) at 2 and 8 h after surgical procedure. The results are shown as mean values ± SEM and are expressed as nmol of metallothionein per gram of tissue. Figure 1(a) shows an average baseline value of 0.723 ± 0.042 ($n = 8$) of metallothionein in intact animals that received vehicle (sham/SS) while the mean values for sham injury and MT was 0.831 ± 0.066 ($n = 9$); no significant differences were observed ($p = 0.23$). Likewise, the mean value of rats with SCI and vehicle (SCI/SS) was 0.911 ± 0.063 ($n = 10$) and the value from rats with lesion plus MT (SCI/MT) was of 0.999 ± 0.055 ($n = 8$); both values were statistically significant as compared to the sham/SS group. Also, Figure 1(b) shows the mean values ± S.E.M. of MT content in animals without lesion with vehicle or MT (0.727 ± 0.049 ($n = 11$) and 0.852 ± 0.053 ($n = 9$), respectively) while average values ± S.E.M. of injury groups treated with either vehicle or MT were 0.826 ± 0.040 ($n = 10$) and 0.96 ± 0.064 ($n = 8$), respectively; only the sham/SS vs. SCI/MT group showed statistically significant differences ($p = 0.004$).

3.2. Exogenous Metallothionein Reduces the Production of Reactive Oxygen Species after SCI. Shown in Figure 2 are the results of the amount of reactive oxygen species (ROS) present in the spinal cord tissue of animals either treated or not with MT. The values are expressed as mean ± SEM of $n = 28$ animals. The results are given as nmol of $2',7'$-dichlorofluorescein (DCF) formed per gram of wet tissue per hour. As observed, the values of ROS in group sham/SS was 0.76 ± 0.06 ($n = 6$), while the sham/MT group was 0.42 ± 0.11 ($n = 8$); likewise, the value in the SCI/SS group was 1.49 ± 0.27 ($n = 6$) and 0.86 ± 0.11 for the SCI/MT group ($n = 8$). The results show an increase in the

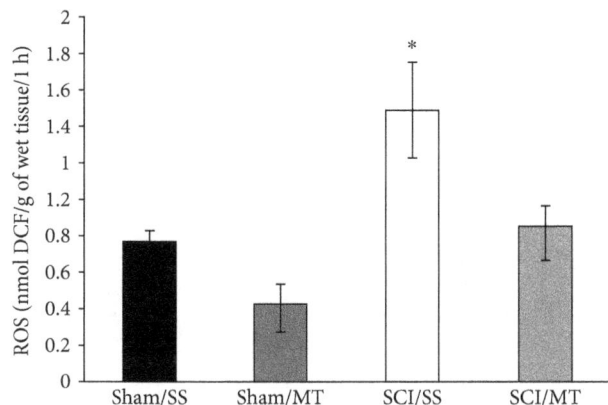

FIGURE 2: Formation of reactive oxygen species (ROS) spinal cord tissue, 4 h after surgery procedure. The results are expressed as me an ± SEM of nmol of $2',7'$-dichlorofluorescein diacetate (DCF) formed per grams of wet tissue per hour of 6 to 8 animals per group. Sham/SS: animals with laminectomy only plus saline solution and Sham/MT: rats with laminectomy with metallothionein (10 μg per rat) at 2 and 8 h surgical procedure. SCI/SS: spinal cord injury and treatment with saline solution; SCI/MT: spinal cord contusion and treatment with metallothionein. One-way ANOVA following Tukey's test, $^*p < 0.05$, different from all groups.

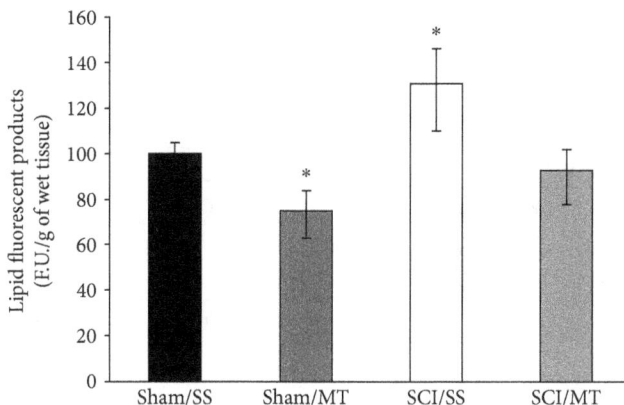

FIGURE 3: Effect of metallothionein (MT) upon lipid peroxidation (LP) levels evaluated 4 h after surgical procedure in rats. The results are expressed as means ± SEM of florescence units per gram of wet tissue of 9 to 14 animals per group. Sham/SS: animals with laminectomy only plus saline solution; Sham/MT: rats with laminectomy with MT (10 μg per rat) at 2 and 8 h after surgery; SCI/SS: spinal cord injury and treatment with saline solution; SCI/ MT: spinal cord contusion and treatment with metallothionein. Kruskal-Wallis following Mann-Whitney's U test, $^*p < 0.05$, different of all groups; $^{**}p < 0.05$ different vs. SCI/SS.

amount of ROS due to the damage, which is reversed by MT treatment ($p < 0.05$). Finally, we did not find statistically significant differences due to the effect of MT on the noninjured tissue. One-way ANOVA followed Tukey's test.

3.3. Metallothionein Reduces Tissue Lipid Peroxidation in Both Healthy and Damaged Tissue.
The results of LP levels after sham and SCI procedure are shown in Figure 3. The values are expressed as mean ± SEM of $n = 42$ animals and are expressed in fluorescence units per gram of wet tissue. The average values observed in group sham/SS was 99.58 ± 7.4 ($n = 14$), while in the sham group treated with MT, the mean value was reduced to 75.02 ± 5.47 ($n = 9$); this reduction was statistically significant ($p < 0.05$). Likewise, in the groups with SCI without treatment (SCI/SS), there was an increase in the LP of 132.50 ± 8.47 ($n = 9$) and the group treated with MT (SCI/MT) showed a statistically significant reduction to 94.96 ± 5.33 ($n = 10$). The results show that the treatment with MT has an antioxidant effect, since it was able to reduce the LP in both tissues submitted only to the surgical procedure and after damage. The Kruskal-Wallis test was used following Mann-Whitney's U test.

3.4. Exogenous Metallothionein Did Not Change Caspase-9 Activity after Spinal Cord Injury.
To assess the intrinsic apoptotic pathway, we measured the activity of caspase-9 at 24 (Figure 4(a)) and 72 h (Figure 4(b)) following laminectomy (sham) or SCI.

The results are shown as mean values ± S.E.M. and are expressed as florescence units per mg of protein per 1-hour incubation. Figure 4(a) shows a mean of 190.67 ± 21.02 ($n = 6$) of caspase-9 activity in sham-injury animals receiving vehicle (sham/SS), while the mean value for sham-injury plus

MT was 143.40 ± 11.00 ($n = 5$). No significant differences were observed. Likewise, rats with SCI and vehicle (SCI/SS) showed a mean of 250.94 ± 28.35 ($n = 8$) and the value from rats with lesion plus MT (SCI/MT) was 325.50 ± 32.72 ($n = 5$); both values were statistically significant as compared to the sham/SS group.

Figure 4(b) shows the mean values ± S.E.M. of caspase-9 activity 72 h after the surgical procedure. Animals without lesion, with vehicle or MT treatment, showed values of 178.80 ± 14.12 ($n = 5$) and 244.50 ± 26.67 ($n = 5$), respectively, while average values ± SEM of injury groups treated with vehicle or MT were of 451.42 ± 61.35 ($n = 6$) and 485.58 ± 54.09 ($n = 6$), respectively. No differences were found among groups by effect of MT treatment.

3.5. Treatment with Exogenous MT Diminished Caspase-3 Activity Only 24 h after Surgical Procedure.
The results of the activity of caspase-3 assessed at 24 and 72 h following laminectomy (sham) or spinal cord contusion injury model (SCI) are shown in Figures 5(a) and 5(b). The results are shown as mean values ± SEM and are expressed as florescence units per mg of protein per 1 hour. Figure 5(a) shows an average value of 580.29 ± 56.03 ($n = 7$) of caspase-3 activity from animals without injury receiving vehicle (sham/SS), while the mean value for sham-injury plus MT was 270.71 ± 41.18 ($n = 7$) observing a statistically significant reduction of due to MT treatment ($p < 0.05$). Likewise, rats with SCI plus vehicle (SCI/SS) showed a mean of 1048.94 ± 101.22 ($n = 8$); this increase was different vs. the sham/SS group ($p < 0.05$). Likewise, the value from rats with SCI plus MT (SCI/MT) was 678.44 ± 64.64 ($n = 9$), a reduction vs. SCI/SS. Also, Figure 5(b) shows the mean values ± S.E.M. of caspase-3 activity, 72 h after surgical procedure. Animals without lesion plus vehicle or MT

(a)

(b)

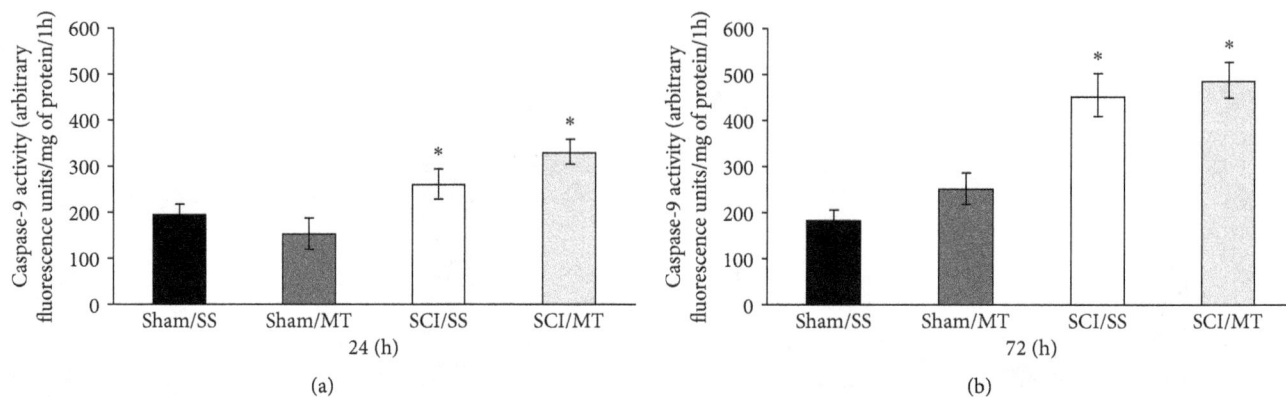

FIGURE 4: Caspase-9 activity measured in spinal cord tissue at 24 (a) and 72 h (b) after surgery procedure. Sham/SS: animals with laminectomy only plus saline solution; Sham/MT: rats with laminectomy with MT (10 μg per rat) at 2 and 8 h after surgery; SCI/SS: spinal cord injury and treatment with saline solution; SCI/MT; spinal cord contusion and treatment with metallothionein at 2 and 8 h after damage. The results are expressed in arbitrary fluorescence units per mg of protein per 1 h and correspond to the average value $\pm$ SEM of 5 to 8 animals per group, *different from the Sham/SS group ($p < 0.05$). One-way ANOVA followed by Tukey's test.

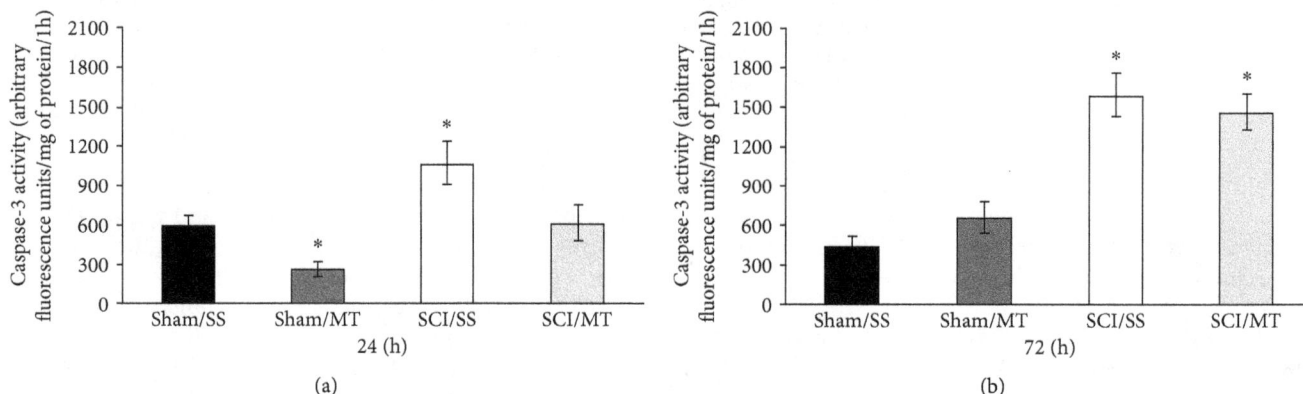

(a)

(b)

FIGURE 5: Caspase-3 activity measured in spinal cord tissue at 24 (a) and 72 h (b) after surgery procedure. Sham/SS: animals with laminectomy only plus saline solution; Sham/MT: rats with laminectomy with MT (10 μg per rat) at 2 and 8 h after surgery; SCI/SS: spinal cord injury and treatment with saline solution; SCI/MT: spinal cord contusion and treatment with metallothionein at 2 and 8 h after damage. The results are expressed in arbitrary fluorescence units per mg of protein per 1 h and correspond to the average value $\pm$ SEM of 4 to 9 animals per group, *different from the Sham/SS group ($p < 0.05$). One-way ANOVA followed by Tukey's test.

showed values of 418.38 ± 56.81 ($n = 4$) and 625.10 ± 60.03 ($n = 5$), respectively. Meanwhile, average values $\pm$ S.E.M. of injury groups treated with either vehicle or MT were 1573.75 ± 204.75 ($n = 4$) and 1473.25 ± 213.91 ($n = 4$), respectively, with a statistical reduction in caspase-3 activity ($p < 0.05$) as compared to the sham/SS group.

3.6. Metallothionein Reduces the Number of Annexin V-Positive Cells after Spinal Cord Injury.

Figures 6(a)–6(d) show representative images of annexin V-positive cells analyzed at 24 and 72 h after injury of animals with SCI treated with vehicle or MT. Likewise, Figures 6(e) and 6(f) show the number of cells positive to Annexin V from rats with SCI and treated either with vehicle or with MT and evaluated at 24 or 72 h after damage. The results are expressed as the number of cells positive to Annexin V per mm^3 and are expressed as the average value $\pm$ SEM of 3 to 6 animals per group. As can be observed, there is a decrease in the number of annexin V-positive cells in animals both killed at 24 h and at 72 and treated with MT (548 ± 16.68 and 809 ± 37.31,

respectively) as compared to SCI plus vehicle evaluated at those times (747 ± 46.11 and 1069 ± 46.41); these reductions were 26.64 and 25.32%, respectively, and were statistically significant ($p < 0.05$).

3.7. Metallothionein Reduces the Number of TUNEL-Positive Cells after Spinal Cord Injury, at 72 h after SCI.

Figures 7(a)–7(d) show representative images of TUNEL-positive cells observed at 24 and 72 h after injury. Representative images from animals with SCI plus vehicle and rats lesioned plus MT are shown. Likewise, Figures 7(e) and 7(f) show the counting of TUNEL-positive cells evaluated 24 and 72 h after lesion, respectively. As observed, a nonsignificant decrease in the number of TUNEL-positive cells was found in the animals treated with SCI plus MT as compared SCI/SS, evaluated at 24 h after the damage. Meanwhile, animals killed 72 h after injury showed a mean of 612 ± 40.56 in SCI animals treated with vehicle, while TUNEL-positive cells were 389 ± 11.88 in animals treated with SCI plus MT.

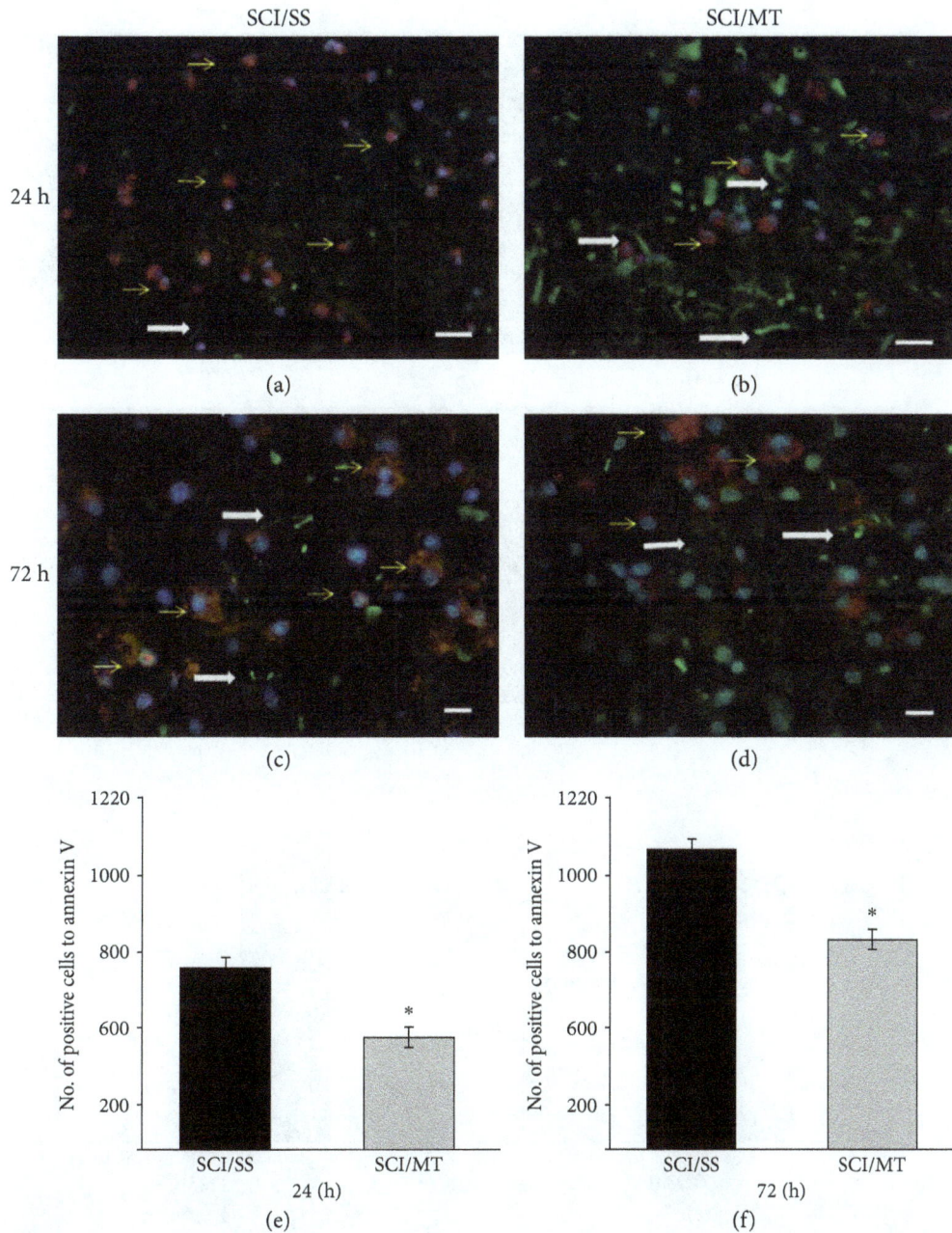

FIGURE 6: Representative microphotographs of annexin V-positive cells (red, Alexa 546) and neurofilaments (green, Alexa 488) in the injury area after spinal cord contusion and sacrificed at 24 or 72 hours after damage. (a, c) Animals with spinal cord injury (SCI) plus saline solution (SS); (b, d) rats with SCI and treated with two doses of metallothionein (MT) starting at 2 and 8 h after the lesion; all animals were sacrificed at 24 h after SCI. (a, b) Animals with similar conditions described above for SS and (c) and SCI plus MT but sacrificed 72 hours after injury. Yellow arrows showed annexin V-reactive cells, as well as some immunoreactive fibers to NF (white arrows); the MT reduced neuronal damage and preserved a greater number of fibers, Scale bar 20 μm. (e, f): Number of annexin V-positive cells per mm^3 measured at 24 or 72 h, respectively, after damage. The results are shown as average values ± SEM of 3–6 animals per group. Student's T test, $^*p < 0.05$.

This difference reached significance ($p < 0.05$) and represents a 36.44% reduction.

4. Discussion

The results of the present work showed that MT increased in the injured tissue of rats treated or not with MT, only at short times (12 h) after injury. At 24 h, only animals treated with

exogenously administered MT continue with increased levels of MT protein. This increase in MT proteins by exogenously administered MT seems to reduce the amount of ROS (only in damage tissue) while this antioxidant effect is also observed as a reduction of LP both in animals from the sham group and in the lesioned group (SCI/SS). As the effect of exogenously administered MT is observed both in the sham-injury and SCI animals, we can conclude that MT is

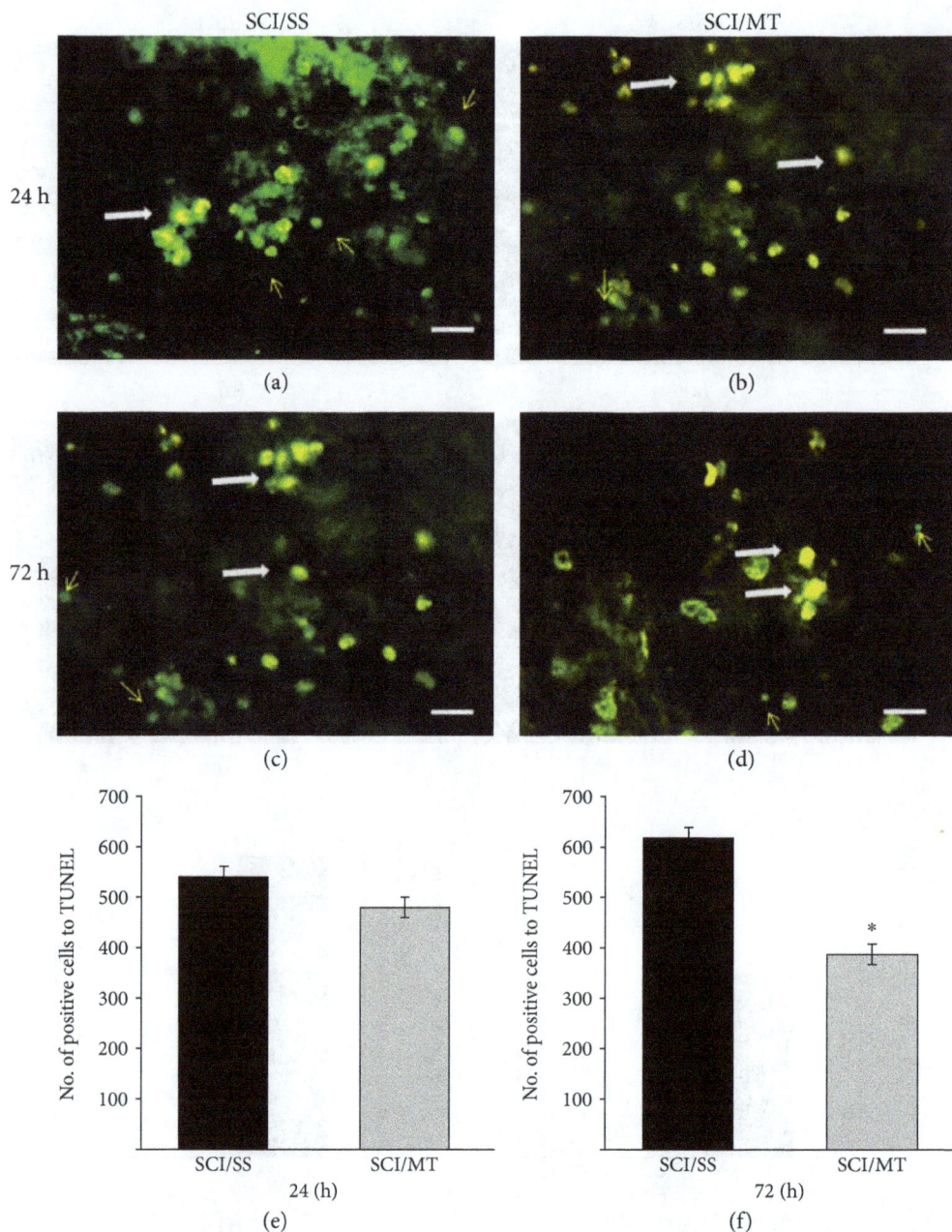

FIGURE 7: Representative microphotographs of TUNEL-positive cells in the injury area after spinal cord contusion and sacrificed at 24 or 72 hours after damage. (a, c) Animals with spinal cord injury (SCI) plus saline solution (SS); (b, d) rats with SCI and treated with two doses of metallothionein (MT) starting at 2 and 8 h after the lesion; all animals were sacrificed at 24 h after SCI. (a, b) Animals with similar condition described above for SS and panels: SCI plus MT but sacrificed 72 hours after injury. Arrows showed TUNEL-positive cells (bright green), and orange cells showed TUNEL and propidium iodide which means that they die by necrosis (white arrow). Scale bar 20 μm. (e, f) Number of TUNEL-positive cells per mm^3 measured at 24 or 72 h, respectively, after damage. The results are shown as average values $\pm$ SEM of 3–6 animals per group. Mann-Whitney's U test, $^*p < 0.05$.

exerting a direct antioxidant effect on tissue, even in the basal conditions of the cells, but only in the LP biomarker. The antioxidant effect of MT may be due to the large number of thiol groups present in the MT molecule. Cai and Cherian [12] showed that MT exerts a greater antioxidant effect than glutathione, accompanied by a cytoprotective effect. Likewise, it has been described that MT reacts easily with hydroxyl radical, superoxide radical, and nitric oxide, while thiol groups from MT clusters A and B can bind anion

peroxynitrite and peroxynitric acid, making MT a highly efficient antioxidant defense molecule [13, 14]. In studies carried out in cultures of modified cells overexpressing MT-I and II, it is possible to observe a clear protection against oxidative stress conditions, in opposition to what happens if those proteins are not expressed [29, 30]. In addition, the antioxidant capacity of MT has been tested in models of damage to the central nervous system, where MT reduced lipoperoxidation and nitration of tyrosine generated by peroxynitrite formation [9] Recently, Duan et al. [31] showed that MT treatment protected against Cd-induced hepatotoxicity, as a result of the antioxidant effect of the protein.

On the other hand, this study demonstrated that MT has no effect on the activity of caspase-9 at all times evaluated, suggesting that the intrinsic pathway is not involved in the antiapoptotic effect of MT, observed both as a reduction of caspase-3 and as a diminution in the number of TUNEL- and annexin V-positive cells. This suggests that MT may be acting through the extrinsic pathway or regulating the inflammatory response [32], which in turn may reduce the death receptor-induced apoptosis [33]. This explanation remains speculative, until the effects of MT on inflammatory response after SCI might be characterized in future experiments.

On the other hand, this study demonstrated that MT reduces the activity of caspase-3 only in the early stage of apoptosis (24 h). It is known that this protease is involved in the two pathways that lead to cell death by apoptosis, the intrinsic or mitochondrial glutamate receptors activated by quinolinic (QUIN) and kainic (KA) acids [34]. The extrinsic pathway is activated by death receptors, where TNF acts as an effector of the processes of chromatin condensation and DNA fragmentation [35]. Reduction of caspase-3 activity may be the result of the ability of MT to diminish microglial activation and QUIN production, as demonstrated by Chung et al. [36] in a brain trauma model. They found that the neurotoxic kynurenine pathway intermediate QUIN is rapidly produced, within 24 h, by reactive microglia after trauma, and exogenously administered MT attenuates this effect. Recently, Leung et al. [37] showed that exogenous MT-II acts via the LRP1 receptor to alter the inflammatory response of microglia following TNFα stimulation, providing a more supportive environment for axon growth. Similarly, we observed that MT decreases the activity of caspase-3 in the sham group, suggesting that this protein can cross the blood-brain barrier to induce a cytoprotective effect. The exact mechanism by which it could be transported through this barrier has not yet been elucidated; however, it is thought that it could be transported through the low-density lipoprotein megalin receptor [38].

In this study, we observe that several cells were colocalizing TUNEL (green color, figure) and propidium iodide (orange color, figure), indicating the coincidence of necrotic cell death; based on the classical definition and the morphological criteria of necrosis, this is the most frequent mechanism by which nerve cells die by excitotoxicity. Under certain conditions, necrotic cells might also show fragmentation of DNA [33] and TUNEL-positive staining. In those cases, both cell death processes may be occurring simultaneously. In our study, it was not possible to rule out that positivity to the TUNEL found in the lesion area is related to both death processes [39]. The classic division between apoptosis and necrosis has been discussed, and a model that proposed a continuity is suggested, between the classical pathway of apoptosis mediated by caspases and necrosis or cell lysis [40]. The intermediate steps that pose would be the following: (a) programmed cell death similar to apoptosis, (b) cell death independent of caspases, and

(c) similar programmed cell death to necrosis. Especially this criterion is important in the analysis of cell death that occurs in neurological processes as well as spinal cord injury.

In this study, we observed a reduction of positive cells to annexin V and TUNEL due to the effect of MT in both early and late stages of apoptosis. Previous research has shown the presence of cell death by apoptosis in neurons, oligodendrocytes, microglia, and astrocytes after an SCI [1, 41, 42]. Liu et al. [43], using specific markers to differentiate between neurons and glia, demonstrated the presence of TUNEL-positive cells from 4 h to 14 days in groups of both neurons and glial cells after an SCI. Likewise, they observed that the number of positive cells increases with time in the periphery of the lesion, concluding that cell death by apoptosis contributes to neuronal and glial death, after an SCI, and that the process promotes the expansion of the damage from the epicenter towards the periphery. In the same way, our results agree with those obtained by Penkowa et al. [44], in a model of brain damage induced by kainic acid (KA). In that study, the authors used a transgenic mouse overexpressing MT, and they found a decreased number of positive cells to TUNEL, three days after treatment with KA, as compared to the group without MT overexpression. In the same direction, they observed a lower neurodegeneration of CA3 cells of the hippocampus, confirming a neuroprotective effect of the MT in that model. Recently, Prado et al. [45] demonstrated an increase of TUNEL-positive cells in animals deficient to MT in a cryolesion model of the cerebral cortex.

Despite being different models of damage, those results confirm an antiapoptotic function of MT-II in various models of cell death. Likewise, when the rats were administered with MT, a better preservation of neuronal prolongations was observed, which were visible using the antibody against neurofilament [46], in according with the present work, a greater number of immunoreactive neurofilament fibers in the groups treated with MT are shown qualitatively (Figure 6). This finding is in addition to those previously observed by various groups in which they propose MTs as possible neuroprotective proteins in models of damage to the nervous system including focal brain injury [15], focal cerebral ischemia [47], and spinal cord injury [48]. Regarding neural regeneration, it has been proposed that MT promotes neuritic elongation and increases the axonal size in the cortex of damaged adult rats [46] and promotes neuritic growth in retinal ganglion cells [49]. The antiapoptotic mechanism of MT is unknown; however, it can be hypothesized that, after a mechanical or cytotoxic damage to neurons, several factors are activated that induce the expression of MT-I/-II, mainly in adjacent astrocytes. MT-I/-II is released, both actively and passively by astrocytes into the extracellular space near the lesion. Those MT deposits can interact with low-density lipoprotein receptors, LRP1 and LRP2 (megalin), and activate signal transduction involving both the MAPK and PI3k/Akt pathways and the CREB growth factor, which acts to promote neuronal survival and neuritic growth. Interestingly, dual activation of those signaling pathways is generally associated to the activation of growth factor receptors [50] and it has been observed that the expression of

MT-I/-II increases rapidly (up to 8 times) after an SCI [51], and the total expression of MT proteins increases in a biphasic manner at 4 and 24 h after an SCI in rats [19], making those proteins an early line of defense against spinal cord damage. Finally, the findings of this work are important in understanding what mechanisms are acting after MT induction by lesion that can improve motor function and increase the amount of tissue preserved after an SCI, as demonstrated previously by our group [48].

5. Conclusion

Our findings demonstrate that exogenously administered metallothionein is an effective antioxidant and antiapoptotic treatment decreasing the extrinsic pathway (initiated by inflammation) and resulting in a diminished cell death after a traumatic spinal cord injury.

Acknowledgments

This study was supported by PRODEP/SEP and CONACYT grant 183667. The authors thank Ricardo Gaxiola for his technical assistance.

References

[1] N. A. Silva, N. Sousa, R. L. Reis, and A. J. Salgado, "From basics to clinical: a comprehensive review on spinal cord injury," *Progress in Neurobiology*, vol. 114, pp. 25–57, 2014.

[2] S. Torres, H. Salgado-Ceballos, J. L. Torres et al., "Early metabolic reactivation versus antioxidant therapy after a traumatic spinal cord injury in adult rats," *Neuropathology*, vol. 30, no. 1, pp. 36–43, 2010.

[3] E. D. Hall, J. A. Wang, J. M. Bosken, and I. N. Singh, "Lipid peroxidation in brain or spinal cord mitochondria after injury," *Journal of Bioenergetics and Biomembranes*, vol. 48, no. 2, pp. 169–174, 2016.

[4] A. Díaz-Ruiz, A. Ibarra, F. Pérez-Severiano, G. Guízar-Sahagún, I. Grijalva, and C. Ríos, "Constitutive and inducible nitric oxide synthase activities after spinal cord contusion in rats," *Neuroscience Letters*, vol. 319, no. 3, pp. 129–132, 2002.

[5] A. Diaz-Ruiz, P. Vergara, F. Perez-Severiano et al., "Cyclosporin-A inhibits inducible nitric oxide synthase activity and expression after spinal cord injury in rats," *Neuroscience Letters*, vol. 357, no. 1, pp. 49–52, 2004.

[6] A. Diaz-Ruiz, C. Rios, I. Duarte et al., "Cyclosporin-A inhibits lipid peroxidation after spinal cord injury in rats," *Neuroscience Letters*, vol. 266, no. 1, pp. 61–64, 1999.

[7] C. Ríos, S. Orozco-Suarez, H. Salgado-Ceballos et al., "Antiapoptotic effects of dapsone after spinal cord injury in rats," *Neurochemical Research*, vol. 40, no. 6, pp. 1243–1251, 2015.

[8] T. A. Precht, R. A. Phelps, D. A. Linseman et al., "The permeability transition pore triggers Bax translocation to mitochondria during neuronal apoptosis," *Cell Death & Differentiation*, vol. 12, no. 3, pp. 255–265, 2005.

[9] D. Juárez-Rebollar, C. Rios, C. Nava-Ruíz, and M. Méndez-Armenta, "Metallothionein in brain disorders," *Oxidative Medicine and Cellular Longevity*, vol. 2017, Article ID 5828056, 12 pages, 2017.

[10] I. Hozumi, "Roles and therapeutic potential of metallothioneins in neurodegenerative diseases," *Current Pharmaceutical Biotechnology*, vol. 14, no. 4, pp. 408–413, 2013.

[11] R. K. Stankovic, R. S. Chung, and M. Penkowa, "Metallothioneins I and II: neuroprotective significance during CNS pathology," *The International Journal of Biochemistry & Cell Biology*, vol. 39, no. 3, pp. 484–489, 2007.

[12] L. Cai and M. G. Cherian, "Zinc-metallothionein protects from DNA damage induced by radiation better than glutathione and copper- or cadmium-metallothioneins," *Toxicology Letters*, vol. 136, no. 3, pp. 193–198, 2003.

[13] M. Aschner and A. K. West, "The role of MT in neurological disorders," *Journal of Alzheimer's Disease*, vol. 8, no. 2, pp. 139–145, 2005.

[14] N. Romero-Isart and M. Vasák, "Advances in the structure and chemistry of metallothioneins," *Journal of Inorganic Biochemistry*, vol. 88, no. 3-4, pp. 388–396, 2002.

[15] M. Giralt, M. Penkowa, N. Lago, A. Molinero, and J. Hidalgo, "Metallothionein-1+2 protect the CNS after a focal brain injury," *Experimental Neurology*, vol. 173, no. 1, pp. 114–128, 2002.

[16] F. Ma, H. Wang, B. Chen, F. Wang, and H. Xu, "Metallothionein 3 attenuated the apoptosis of neurons in the CA1 region of the hippocampus in the senescence-accelerated mouse/PRONE8 (SAMP8)," *Arquivos de Neuro-Psiquiatria*, vol. 69, no. 1, pp. 105–111, 2011.

[17] D. M. Basso, M. S. Beattie, and J. C. Bresnahan, "Graded histological and locomotor outcomes after spinal cord contusion using the NYU weight-drop device versus transection," *Experimental Neurology*, vol. 139, no. 2, pp. 244–256, 1996.

[18] M. Penkowa and J. Hidalgo, "Metallothionein treatment reduces proinflammatory cytokines IL-6 and TNF-α and apoptotic cell death during experimental autoimmune encephalomyelitis (EAE)," *Experimental Neurology*, vol. 170, no. 1, pp. 1–14, 2001.

[19] A. Diaz-Ruiz, M. Alcaraz-Zubeldia, V. Maldonado, H. Salgado-Ceballos, M. Mendez-Armenta, and C. Rios, "Differential time-course of the increase of antioxidant thiol-defenses in the acute phase after spinal cord injury in rats," *Neuroscience Letters*, vol. 452, no. 1, pp. 56–59, 2009.

[20] A. M. Scheuhammer and M. G. Cherian, "Quantification of metallothioneins by a silver-saturation method," *Toxicology and Applied Pharmacology*, vol. 82, no. 3, pp. 417–425, 1986.

[21] P. Rojas and C. Ríos, "Metallothionein inducers protect against 1-methyl-4-phenyl-1,2,3,6-tetrahydropyridine neurotoxicity in mice," *Neurochemical Research*, vol. 22, no. 1, pp. 17–22, 1997.

[22] D. Liu, Y. Shan, L. Valluru, and F. Bao, "Mn (III) tetrakis (4-benzoic acid) porphyrin scavenges reactive species, reduces oxidative stress, and improves functional recovery after experimental spinal cord injury in rats: comparison with methylprednisolone," *BMC Neuroscience*, vol. 14, no. 1, p. 23, 2013.

[23] F. Pérez-Severiano, A. Santamaría, J. Pedraza-Chaverri, O. N. Medina-Campos, C. Ríos, and J. Segovia, "Increased formation of reactive oxygen species, but no changes in glutathione peroxidase activity, in striata of mice transgenic for the Huntington's disease mutation," *Neurochemical Research*, vol. 29, no. 4, pp. 729–733, 2004.

[24] W. J. Triggs and L. J. Willmore, "In vivo lipid peroxidation in rat brain following intracortical Fe2+ injection," *Journal of Neurochemistry*, vol. 42, no. 4, pp. 976–980, 1984.

[25] A. Santamaría and C. Ríos, "MK-801, an N-methyl-D-aspartate receptor antagonist, blocks quinolinic acid-induced lipid peroxidation in rat corpus striatum," *Neuroscience Letters*, vol. 159, no. 1-2, pp. 51–54, 1993.

[26] A. Diaz-Ruiz, C. Zavala, S. Montes et al., "Antioxidant, antiinflammatory and antiapoptotic effects of dapsone in a model of brain ischemia/reperfusion in rats," *Journal of Neuroscience Research*, vol. 86, no. 15, pp. 3410–3419, 2008.

[27] M. J. West, "New stereological methods for counting neurons," *Neurobiology of Aging*, vol. 14, no. 4, pp. 275–285, 1993.

[28] W. Besio, M. Cuellar-Herrera, H. Luna-Munguia, S. Orozco-Suárez, and L. Rocha, "Effects of transcranial focal electrical stimulation alone and associated with a sub-effective dose of diazepam on pilocarpine-induced status epilepticus and subsequent neuronal damage in rats," *Epilepsy & Behavior*, vol. 28, no. 3, pp. 432–436, 2013.

[29] S. Wanpen, P. Govitrapong, S. Shavali, P. Sangchot, and M. Ebadi, "Salsolinol, a dopamine-derived tetrahydroisoquinoline, induces cell death by causing oxidative stress in dopaminergic SH-SY5Y cells, and the said effect is attenuated by metallothionein," *Brain Research*, vol. 1005, no. 1-2, pp. 67–76, 2004.

[30] Y. Kondo, J. M. Rusnak, D. G. Hoyt, C. E. Settineri, B. R. Pitt, and J. S. Lazo, "Enhanced apoptosis in metallothionein null cells," *Molecular Pharmacology*, vol. 52, no. 2, pp. 195–201, 1997.

[31] Y. Duan, J. Duan, Y. Feng et al., "Hepatoprotective activity of vitamin E and metallothionein in cadmium-induced liver injury in *Ctenopharyngodon idellus*," *Oxidative Medicine and Cellular Longevity*, vol. 2018, Article ID 9506543, 12 pages, 2018.

[32] M. Ø. Pedersen, R. Jensen, D. S. Pedersen et al., "Metallothionein-I+II in neuroprotection," *BioFactors*, vol. 35, no. 4, pp. 315–325, 2009.

[33] S. Elmore, "Apoptosis: a review of programmed cell death," *Toxicologic Pathology*, vol. 35, no. 4, pp. 495–516, 2007.

[34] E. Pérez-Navarro, N. Gavaldà, E. Gratacòs, and J. Alberch, "Brain-derived neurotrophic factor prevents changes in Bcl-2 family members and caspase-3 activation induced by excitotoxicity in the striatum," *Journal of Neurochemistry*, vol. 92, no. 3, pp. 678–691, 2005.

[35] A. G. Porter and R. U. Jänicke, "Emerging roles of caspase-3 in apoptosis," *Cell Death & Differentiation*, vol. 6, no. 2, pp. 99–104, 1999.

[36] R. S. Chung, Y. K. Leung, C. W. Butler et al., "Metallothionein treatment attenuates microglial activation and expression of neurotoxic quinolinic acid following traumatic brain injury," *Neurotoxicity Research*, vol. 15, no. 4, pp. 381–389, 2009.

[37] J. Y. K. Leung, W. R. Bennett, A. E. King, and R. S. Chung, "The impact of metallothionein-II on microglial response to tumor necrosis factor-alpha (TNFα) and downstream effects on neuronal regeneration," *Journal of Neuroinflammation*, vol. 15, no. 1, p. 56, 2018.

[38] J. Y. K. Leung, W. R. Bennett, R. P. Herbert et al., "Metallothionein promotes regenerative axonal sprouting of dorsal root ganglion neurons after physical axotomy," *Cellular and Molecular Life Sciences*, vol. 69, no. 5, pp. 809–817, 2012.

[39] C. Portera-Cailliau, D. L. Price, and L. J. Martin, "Excitotoxic neuronal death in the immature brain is an apoptosis-necrosis morphological continuum," *The Journal of Comparative Neurology*, vol. 378, no. 1, pp. 10–87, 1997.

[40] D. E. Schmechel, "Apoptosis in neurodegenerative disorders," in *Apoptosis in Neurobiology*, Y. A. Hannum and R. M. Boustany, Eds., pp. 23–48, CRC Press, Washington, DC, USA, 1999.

[41] J. E. Springer, R. D. Azbill, and P. E. Knapp, "Activation of the caspase-3 apoptotic cascade in traumatic spinal cord injury," *Nature Medicine*, vol. 5, no. 8, pp. 943–946, 1999.

[42] M. S. Beattie, A. A. Farooqui, and J. C. Bresnahan, "Review of current evidence for apoptosis after spinal cord injury," *Journal of Neurotrauma*, vol. 17, no. 10, pp. 915–925, 2000.

[43] X. Z. Liu, X. M. Xu, R. Hu et al., "Neuronal and glial apoptosis after traumatic spinal cord injury," *The Journal of Neuroscience*, vol. 17, no. 14, pp. 5395–5406, 1997.

[44] M. Penkowa, S. Florit, M. Giralt et al., "Metallothionein reduces central nervous system inflammation, neurodegeneration, and cell death following kainic acid-induced epileptic seizures," *Journal of Neuroscience Research*, vol. 79, no. 4, pp. 522–534, 2005.

[45] J. Prado, P. Pifarré, M. Giralt, J. Hidalgo, and A. García, "Metallothioneins I/II are involved in the neuroprotective effect of sildenafil in focal brain injury," *Neurochemistry International*, vol. 62, no. 1, pp. 70–78, 2013.

[46] R. S. Chung, J. C. Vickers, M. I. Chuah, and A. K. West, "Metallothionein-IIA promotes initial neurite elongation and postinjury reactive neurite growth and facilitates healing after focal cortical brain injury," *The Journal of Neuroscience*, vol. 23, no. 8, pp. 3336–3342, 2003.

[47] G. Trendelenburg, K. Prass, J. Priller et al., "Serial analysis of gene expression identifies metallothionein-II as major neuroprotective gene in mouse focal cerebral ischemia," *The Journal of Neuroscience*, vol. 22, no. 14, pp. 5879–5888, 2002.

[48] S. Arellano-Ruiz, C. Rios, H. Salgado-Ceballos et al., "Metallothionein-II improves motor function recovery and increases spared tissue after spinal cord injury in rats," *Neuroscience Letters*, vol. 514, no. 1, pp. 102–105, 2012.

[49] M. Fitzgerald, P. Nairn, C. A. Bartlett, R. S. Chung, A. K. West, and L. D. Beazley, "Metallothionein-IIA promotes neurite growth via the megalin receptor," *Experimental Brain Research*, vol. 183, no. 2, pp. 171–180, 2007.

[50] R. S. Chung, J. Hidalgo, and A. K. West, "New insight into the molecular pathways of metallothionein-mediated neuroprotection and regeneration," *Journal of Neurochemistry*, vol. 104, no. 1, pp. 14–20, 2008.

[51] J. B. Carmel, A. Galante, P. Soteropoulos et al., "Gene expression profiling of acute spinal cord injury reveals spreading inflammatory signals and neuron loss," *Physiological Genomics*, vol. 7, no. 2, pp. 201–213, 2001.

2

Terminalia bellirica (Gaertn.) Roxb. Extract and Gallic Acid Attenuate LPS-Induced Inflammation and Oxidative Stress via MAPK/NF-κB and Akt/AMPK/Nrf2 Pathways

Miori Tanaka,[1] Yoshimi Kishimoto,[2] Mizuho Sasaki,[1] Akari Sato,[1] Tomoyasu Kamiya,[3] Kazuo Kondo,[2,4] and Kaoruko Iida ⓘ[1,5]

[1]Department of Food and Nutritional Sciences, Graduate School of Humanities and Sciences, Ochanomizu University, 2-1-1 Otsuka, Bunkyo-ku, Tokyo 112-8610, Japan
[2]Endowed Research Department "Food for Health", Ochanomizu University, 2-1-1 Otsuka, Bunkyo-ku, Tokyo 112-8610, Japan
[3]Research and Development Division, Toyo Shinyaku Co Ltd, 7-28 Yayoigaoka, Tosu-shi, Saga 841-0005, Japan
[4]Institute of Life Innovation Studies, Toyo University, 1-1-1 Izumino, Itakura-machi, Ora-gun, Gunma 374-0193, Japan
[5]Institute for Human Life Innovation, Ochanomizu University, 2-1-1 Otsuka, Bunkyo-ku, Tokyo 112-8610, Japan

Correspondence should be addressed to Kaoruko Iida; iida.kaoruko@ocha.ac.jp

Academic Editor: Silvana Hrelia

Excessive oxidative stress plays a critical role in the progression of various diseases. Recently, we showed that *Terminalia bellirica* (Gaertn.) Roxb. extract (TBE) inhibits inflammatory response and reactive oxygen species (ROS) production in THP-1 macrophages. However, molecular mechanisms underlying anti-inflammatory and antioxidant activities of TBE and its major polyphenolic compounds gallic acid (GA) and ellagic acid (EA) remain unclear. We found that TBE and GA attenuated LPS-induced inflammatory mediator expression, ROS production, and activation of mitogen-activated protein kinase (MAPK) and nuclear factor-kappa B (NF-κB) in RAW 264 macrophages. Furthermore, TBE and GA increased antioxidant enzyme expression along with upstream mediators nuclear factor erythroid-2-related factor 2 (Nrf2), Akt, and AMP-activated protein kinase (AMPK). Importantly, knockdown of Nrf2 by siRNA and specific inhibition of Akt and AMPK significantly reduced antioxidant enzyme expression induced by TBE and GA. Finally, *in vivo* effects on histopathology and gene expression were assessed in tissues collected after intraperitoneal injection of LPS with or without TBE treatment. TBE enhanced antioxidant enzyme expression and improved acute kidney injury in LPS-shock model mice. In conclusion, TBE and GA exert protective effects against inflammation and oxidative stress by suppressing MAPK/NF-κB pathway and by activating Akt/AMPK/Nrf2 pathway. These results suggest that TBE and GA might be effective for the treatment of inflammation-related diseases.

1. Introduction

Inflammation is an innate defense system of the human body against environmental injuries and pathogens. However, excessive inflammation contributes to serious tissue damage and the development of human diseases such as atherosclerosis, diabetes, and cancer [1]. Many investigations have suggested a relationship between activation of macrophages, which are pivotal immune cells for regulating inflammation, and human inflammatory disorders [2]. Macrophage-mediated inflammatory responses are typically triggered by pathogen-associated molecular patterns (PAMPs) recognized by toll-like receptors (TLRs) [3, 4]. Lipopolysaccharide (LPS), the most representative PAMPs produced by gram-negative bacteria, is a ligand of TLR4 that can activate downstream signaling pathways such as mitogen-activated protein kinase (MAPK) and nuclear factor-kappa B (NF-κB), eventually leading to the generation of proinflammatory cytokines, chemokines, nitric oxide (NO), and reactive oxygen species (ROS) [5, 6]. ROS have been shown to activate MAPK and NF-κB pathways and result in inflammation [7, 8]. Indeed, inhibiting ROS production was reported to suppress inflammatory mediator expression in macrophages [9]. Therefore, the modulation of cellular redox status is a key regulator of inflammatory response and important for providing a therapeutic strategy against inflammation-related diseases.

Oxidative stress results from an imbalance between excessive amounts of ROS and the antioxidant defense system. The human body has the ability to protect cells against oxidative damage with endogenous antioxidant enzymes (e.g., heme oxygenase-1 (HO-1), catalase, NADPH quinone oxidoreductase 1 (NQO1), and glutamate-cysteine ligase modifier subunit (GCLM)). In addition, exogenous antioxidants such as polyphenol, and vitamins C and E are obtained through diet. The consumption of some polyphenols has been reported to induce antioxidant enzyme expression and activity [10, 11]. Nuclear factor erythroid-2-related factor 2 (Nrf2) is a primary transcription factor that regulates antioxidant enzyme expression. Nrf2 plays an imperative role in cellular defense against oxidative stress and inflammation by activating antioxidant cascades [12–14]. The transcriptional activity of Nrf2 protein is suppressed by its negative regulator Kelch-like ECH-associated protein 1 (Keap1) under homeostatic conditions; however, upon oxidative stress, Nrf2 translocates to the nucleus where it binds to the antioxidant responsive element (ARE) [15]. In addition to the Keap1/Nrf2 pathway, phosphorylation of Nrf2 by several cytosolic kinases (e.g., protein kinase C, phosphoinositide 3-kinase (PI3K)/Akt, and MAPK) has been shown to facilitate release of Nrf2 from Keap1 and subsequent antioxidant signal cascades [16].

PI3K and its downstream mediator Akt constitute a critical signaling pathway regulating a variety of biological processes such as cell growth, proliferation, apoptosis, and protein synthesis [17]. PI3K/Akt pathway has also been implicated in Nrf2-mediated antioxidant response [16]. AMP-activated protein kinase (AMPK), a heterotrimeric serine/threonine kinase, is a crucial energy sensor of cellular metabolism in response to various metabolic stresses such as oxidative stress, inflammation, and hypoxia [18]. Previous studies suggested that AMPK can stimulate nuclear accumulation of Nrf2 [19] and protect against inflammation by inhibiting NF-κB signaling pathway [20]. Moreover, Sag et al. [21] demonstrated that AMPK deletion dramatically increased inflammatory mediator expression in LPS-stimulated macrophages. Several polyphenols (e.g., resveratrol, quercetin, and catechins) have also been shown to downregulate NF-κB signaling and inflammatory response through the activation of PI3K/Akt and AMPK [22–24]. Although mechanistic connections between both PI3K/Akt and AMPK pathways and inflammation have been frequently reported, potential roles of PI3K/Akt and AMPK in antioxidant effects induced by dietary-derived polyphenols mostly remain unclear.

Terminalia bellirica (Gaertn.) Roxb. extract (TBE) is obtained from the fruit of *T. bellirica* tree, which is distributed throughout Southeast Asia and used as a folk medicine for diabetes, rheumatism, and hypertension in traditional Indian Ayurvedic medicine [25]. Multiple studies have suggested antiobesity, hypoglycemic [26], hypolipidemic [27], and antihypertensive [28] properties of the fruit. The major polyphenolic compounds of this fruit are reported to be gallic acid (GA), ellagic acid (EA), and gallate esters [29]. GA has been shown to exert curative effects against obesity-related atherosclerosis and insulin resistance via the activation of AMPK [30, 31]. Our previous report revealed that TBE inhibited inflammatory mediator expression and ROS production in THP-1 macrophages [32], but there is little information about anti-inflammatory and antioxidant activities of TBE and underlying mechanisms in this process. This study examined protective effects of TBE and its major bioactive ingredients on inflammation and oxidative stress, as well as the underlying molecular mechanisms, by utilizing LPS-stimulated macrophages and LPS-shock model mice.

2. Materials and Methods

2.1. Reagents. TBE was provided by Toyo Shinyaku Co. Ltd. (Saga, Japan). The total polyphenol content of TBE powder was 23.1% in our previous study [32]. The powder was dissolved in deionized water at 40 mg/mL and used in experiments. GA, EA, LPS (from *Escherichia coli* O11:B4), palmitic acid, Hank's balanced salt solution (HBSS), 3-(4,5-dimethylthiazol-2-y1)-2,5-diphenyltetrazoliumbromide (MTT), L-Arginine, LY294002, and compound C were purchased from Sigma-Aldrich (St Louis, MO, USA). Dulbecco's modified eagle medium (DMEM), fetal bovine serum (FBS), and penicillin/streptomycin were obtained from Gibco (Life Technologies, Carlsbad, CA, USA). Diaminofluorescein-2 (DAF-2) was acquired from Sekisui Medical (Tokyo, Japan). 5-(And-6)-chloromethyl-2′,7′-dichlorohydrofluorescein diacetate (CM-H$_2$DCFDA), Nrf2 Stealth RNAi siRNA, and Lipofectamine RNAiMAX were purchased from Thermo Fisher Scientific (Waltham, MA, USA).

2.2. HPLC Analysis of Phenolic Compounds. HPLC analysis of phenolic components in TBE was performed. The TBE stock solution was diluted with 50% ethanol (v/v) at 1 mg/mL, filtered through a 0.45 μm PTFE filter, and injected into a UK-C18 HT (3 μm particle size, 3 × 100 mm, Imtakt Corporation) HPLC column. The mobile phases were 1% formic acid in water (v/v) as eluent A, and 99% acetonitrile, 1% formic acid (v/v) as eluent B. The gradient program was as follows: 0–3 min, 95% A, 5% B; 3–11.5 min, 75% A, 25% B; 11.5–13.5 min, 20% A, 80% B; and 13.5–17 min, 95% A, 5% B. The detection was UV absorbance at 276 nm. GA and EA were quantified by comparison with a multipoint calibration curve obtained from the corresponding standard (GA (Sigma-Aldrich) and EA (Wako Pure Chemical)).

2.3. Cell Culture and Treatment. The murine macrophage cell line RAW 264 was obtained from the RIKEN Cell Bank (Ibaraki, Japan). Cells were cultured in DMEM supplemented with 10% FBS, 100 U/mL penicillin, and 100 μg/mL streptomycin at 37°C and 5% CO$_2$. For fatty acid treatment, palmitic acid was dissolved in 100 mM NaOH for 15 min at 70°C. 100 mM palmitic acid solution was then mixed with prewarmed fatty acid-free BSA (10% in DMEM) to yield 8 mM palmitic acid stock solution. The solution was incubated for 15 min at 55°C and stored at −20°C until use.

2.4. Cell Viability. Cell viability was determined by MTT assay. RAW 264 macrophages were seeded in 24-well plates at a density of 3.5×10^5 cells/mL and incubated for 48 h at 37°C and 5% CO_2. Cells were treated with 100–400 μg/mL TBE or 11.5–46 μg/mL GA (same concentrations as the amount contained in TBE according to the HPLC analysis) for 8 h. Afterwards, fresh media containing MTT (0.5 mg/mL) was added to each well and incubated for 3 h. The culture medium was carefully removed and the resulting formazan crystals were dissolved in DMSO (250 μL/well). The absorbance was measured at 540 nm using a microplate reader (BioTek Instruments, Tokyo, Japan).

2.5. Real-Time RT-PCR. RAW 264 macrophages were seeded in 12-well plates at a density of 3.5×10^5 cells/mL and incubated for 48 h at 37°C and 5% CO_2. Cells were pretreated with 100–400 μg/mL TBE, 46 μg/mL GA, or 1.6 μg/mL EA (same concentration as the amount contained in TBE according to the HPLC analysis) for 1 h and then LPS (100 ng/mL) was added and incubation was continued for an additional 4 h. For palmitic acid treatment, cells were pretreated with 400 μg/mL TBE or 46 μg/mL GA for 1 h and then palmitic acid (400 μM) was added and incubated for 12 h. Total cellular RNA was extracted using RNAiso Plus (Takara Bio, Shiga, Japan) according to the manufacturer's instructions. We reverse transcribed first-stand complementary DNA from 2 μg of total RNA using a High Capacity cDNA Reverse Transcription Kit (Applied Biosystems, Foster City, CA, USA). Real-time PCR was performed on a StepOnePlus Real-Time PCR System (Applied Biosystems) using Power SYBR Green PCR mix (Applied Biosystems). The results are expressed as the copy number ratio of the target mRNA to GAPDH mRNA. Primers of genes encoding tumor necrosis factor-alpha (TNF-α) (*Tnf*), interleukin-1 beta (IL-1β) (*Il1b*), IL-6 (*Il6*), inducible nitric oxide synthase (iNOS) (*Nos2*), monocyte chemoattractant protein-1 (MCP-1) (*Ccl2*), class A scavenger receptor (SR-A) (*Msr1*), HO-1 (*Hmox1*), catalase (*Cat*), NQO1 (*Nqo1*), GCLM (*Gclm*), and Nrf2 (*Nfe2l2*) were obtained from Sigma-Aldrich. Primer sequences are listed in Supplementary Table S1.

2.6. Western Blot Analysis. RAW 264 macrophages were seeded in 6-well plates at a density of 3.5×10^5 cells/mL and incubated for 72 h at 37°C and 5% CO_2. Cells were pretreated with 100–400 μg/mL TBE for 1 h and then LPS (100 ng/mL) was added and incubation was continued for 0.5, 2, and 6 h. Total protein was extracted using M-PER Mammalian Protein Extraction Reagent (Thermo Fisher Scientific). Cytosolic and nuclear fractionation was performed using NE-PER Nuclear and Cytoplasmic Extraction Reagents (Thermo Fisher Scientific). Equal amounts of cellular proteins were electrophoresed on 10% sodium dodecyl sulfate-polyacrylamide gels and transferred to Immobilon-P membranes (Merck Millipore, Billerica, MA, USA). Membranes were blocked with 5% skim milk or 5% BSA and incubated with primary antibodies against iNOS (Sigma-Aldrich), SR-A, NF-κB p65, IκB-α, Nrf2, Lamin B (Santa Cruz Biotechnology, Dallas, TX, USA), HO-1 (Enzo Life Sciences, Farmingdale, NY, USA), catalase (AbFrontier, Seoul, Korea),

p38 MAPK, c-jun N-terminal kinase (JNK), extracellular signal-regulated kinase (ERK), Akt, AMPK, β-actin, and GAPDH (Cell Signaling Technology, Danvers, MA, USA). After washing with TBS-T, membranes were incubated with peroxidase-conjugated secondary antibodies: anti-rabbit (Cell Signaling Technology), anti-mouse, and anti-goat (Santa Cruz Biotechnology). Chemiluminescent detection of specific proteins was developed with ECL Select Western Blotting Detection Reagent (GE Healthcare, Little Chalfont, UK). All signals were detected by an ImageQuant LAS 4000 system (Fujifilm, Tokyo, Japan).

2.7. Measurement of NO Production. NO levels were measured using DAF-2, a sensitive fluorescent dye for the detection of NO. RAW 264 macrophages were seeded in 24-well plates at a density of 3.5×10^5 cells/mL and incubated for 48 h at 37°C and 5% CO_2. Cells were pretreated with 100–400 μg/mL TBE for 1 h and then LPS (100 ng/mL) was added and incubation was continued for 6 h. Next, 10 μM DAF-2 and 5 mM L-arginine in fresh HBSS was added and cells were incubated for an additional 2 h at 37°C. After incubation, the fluorescent intensity of culture supernatant was determined at 495 nm excitation and 515 nm emission using a microplate reader.

2.8. Measurement of Intracellular ROS Production. Intracellular ROS levels were determined by measuring the oxidative conversion of cell permeable 5-(and 6)-chloromethyl-2',7'-dichlorodihydrofluorescein diacetate (CM-H_2DCFDA) to dichlorofluorescein (DCF), a fluorescent product. RAW 264 macrophages were seeded in 24-well plates at a density of 3.5×10^5 cells/mL and incubated for 48 h at 37°C and 5% CO_2. Cells were pretreated with 100–400 μg/mL TBE or 11.5–46 μg/mL GA for 1 h and then LPS (100 ng/mL) was added and incubation was continued for 7 h. After washing cells with HBSS, 10 μM CM-H_2DCFDA/HBSS was added and incubated for further 30 min at 37°C. The fluorescent intensity was detected at 492 nm excitation and 517 nm emission with a microplate reader. DCF fluorescence images were acquired under a BZ-X710 fluorescence microscope (20x objective lens, KEYENCE, Osaka, Japan).

2.9. Small Interfering RNA Transfection. RAW 264 macrophages were transfected with 60 nM Nrf2 siRNA or negative control (NC) siRNA using Lipofectamine RNAiMAX for 48 h. After transfection, cells were pretreated with 400 μg/mL TBE or 46 μg/mL GA for 1 h and then LPS (100 ng/mL) was added and incubation was continued for 4 h. Real-time RT-PCR was performed as described above.

2.10. Animal Experiments. Male ICR mice (8 weeks, 36–43 g) were purchased from Sankyo Labo Service Corporation (Tokyo, Japan). All animal experiments were approved by the Animal Ethics Committee of Ochanomizu University (approved number; 17025R) and performed in accordance with Act on Welfare and Management of Animals. Mice were randomly divided into two groups: LPS ($n = 6$) and LPS + TBE ($n = 6$). TBE (400 mg/kg body weight, dissolved in water) was orally administered to mice once a day for 3 consecutive days. One hour after the last administration, all mice

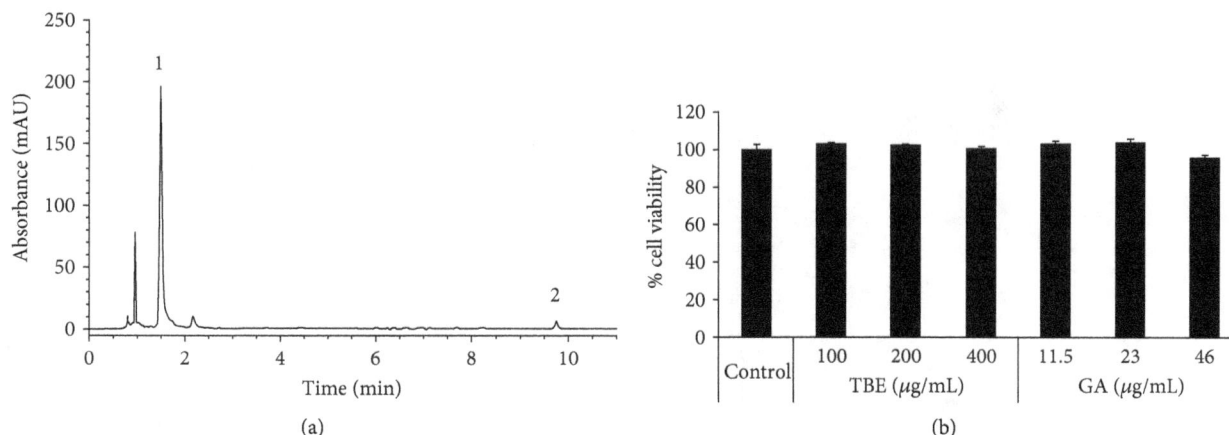

(a)

(b)

FIGURE 1: HPLC-ESI/MS chromatogram of TBE solution and effects of TBE and GA on cell viability in macrophages. (a) Peaks indicate (1) gallic acid and (2) ellagic acid. (b) RAW 264 cells were treated with 100–400 μg/mL TBE or 11.5–46 μg/mL GA for 8 h, and then cell viability was determined by MTT assay. Data represent mean ± SD, $n = 3$.

were intraperitoneally injected with LPS (2 mg/kg body weight). Kidney tissues were collected at 24 h post LPS injection and subsequently used for real-time RT-PCR and histopathological examination.

2.11. Histopathological Examination.
Kidney tissues from mice were fixed with 3.7% formaldehyde, embedded in paraffin, and cut into 5 μm sections. Sections were stained with hematoxylin and eosin (HE) and viewed under a BZ-X710 fluorescence microscope (40x objective lens). The extent of interstitial hyperemia was scored using a semiquantitative scale designed to evaluate interstitial hyperemia. The score (ranging between 1 and 4) was judged as follows: 1, normal kidney; 2, mild hyperemia; 3, moderate hyperemia; and 4, severe hyperemia by two blinded investigators. The percentage of glomerular capillary narrowing was also analyzed by two investigators.

2.12. Statistical Analysis.
Comparisons between treatment groups were performed using an unpaired t-test or one-way analysis of variance (ANOVA) followed by Tukey's post hoc test. Differences were considered statistically significant when $p < 0.05$. Statistical analyses were performed using the GraphPad Prism 5 software package (GraphPad Software, La Jolla, CA, USA).

3. Results

3.1. Polyphenol Composition of TBE by HPLC Analysis.
To determine the polyphenol composition of TBE, we performed HPLC analysis. According to the HPLC analytical plot, contents of GA and EA in TBE solution (40 mg/mL) were 4.6 mg/mL and 0.16 mg/mL, respectively (Figure 1(a)). Thus, the contents of GA and EA in TBE powder were calculated to be 115 mg/g and 4 mg/g, suggesting that gallic acid is the major polyphenolic compound of TBE.

3.2. Effects of TBE and GA on Cell Viability in RAW 264 Cells.
We first analyzed the effects of TBE and GA on the viability of RAW 264 macrophages by MTT assay. As shown in Figure 1(b), no cytotoxic effect was observed when cells were

exposed to TBE (100–400 μg/mL) or GA (11.5–46 μg/mL) for 8 h.

3.3. TBE Exerted Anti-Inflammatory Effect in LPS-Stimulated Macrophages.
As the production of inflammatory mediators is a well-known response to LPS stimulation in macrophages, we examined the effect of TBE on inflammatory mediator expression. TBE significantly reduced LPS-induced mRNA expression of TNF-α, IL-1β, IL-6, MCP-1, iNOS, and SR-A, as well as protein expression of iNOS and SR-A (Figures 2(a) and 2(b)). NO production was also examined because excessive NO production is associated with inflammatory responses. As shown in Figure 2(c), LPS caused a considerable release of NO, but TBE significantly decreased the level of NO production. To evaluate regulatory mechanisms of TBE on inflammatory signaling pathways, we analyzed its inhibitory effect on NF-κB and MAPK activation. Western blot analysis revealed that the nuclear translocation of NF-κB p65 and phosphorylation of NF-κB p65, p38, JNK, and ERK were increased by LPS. Treatment with TBE effectively inhibited the nuclear translocation of NF-κB and phosphorylation of all these proteins, whereas TBE did not affect phosphorylation of IκB (Figures 2(d) and 2(e)).

3.4. Effects of GA and EA on Inflammatory Mediator Expression in LPS- and Palmitic Acid-Stimulated Macrophages.
The present HPLC analysis showed that TBE contains GA and EA and that GA is the major polyphenolic compound of TBE. Therefore, we assessed the effects of GA and EA in TBE on inflammatory mediator expression. As shown in Figure 3(a), LPS upregulated the expression of TNF-α, IL-1β, IL-6, MCP-1, iNOS, and SR-A in macrophages. GA treatment significantly reduced LPS-induced expression of TNF-α, IL-1β, MCP-1, and iNOS as well as TBE, but EA had no effect. Similar to LPS, saturated fatty acid such as palmitic acid is known to exert proinflammatory activity in macrophages via TLR4. As shown in Figure 3(b), palmitic acid increased the mRNA expression of IL-1β and MCP-1, while TBE significantly suppressed the expression of these genes and GA reduced IL-1β expression.

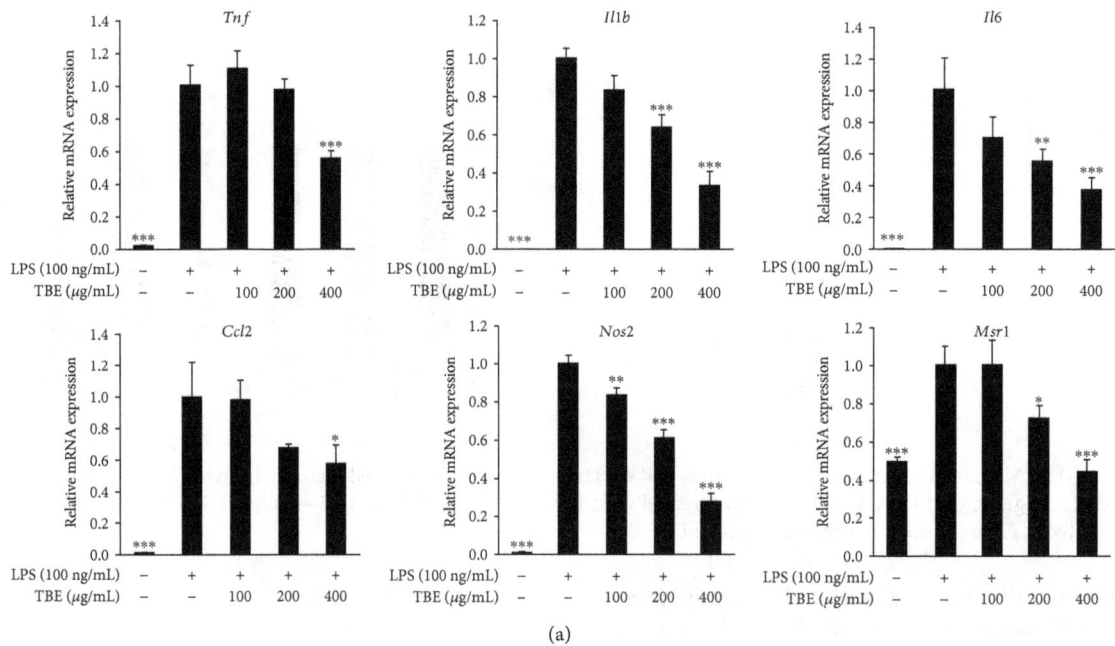

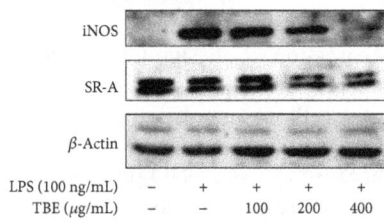

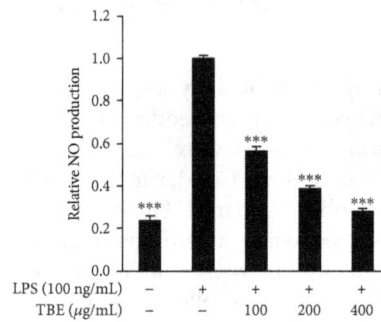

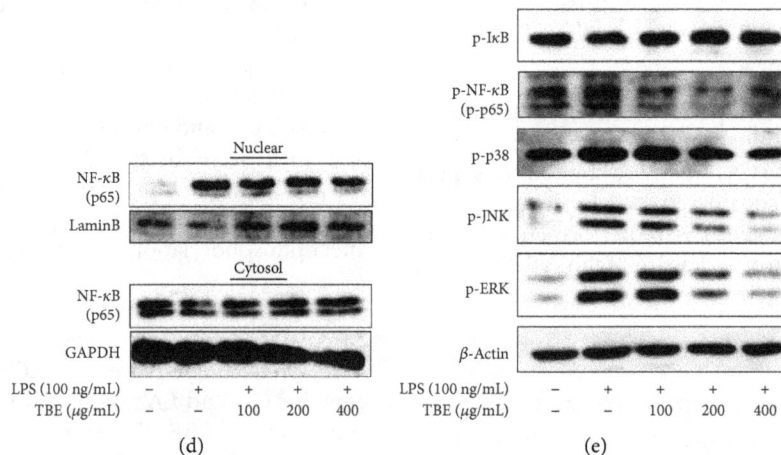

FIGURE 2: Effect of TBE on inflammatory mediator expression and inflammatory signaling pathway in LPS-stimulated macrophages. (a) RAW 264 cells were pretreated with 100–400 μg/mL TBE for 1 h, followed by treatment with 100 ng/mL LPS for 4 h. The mRNA levels of *Tnf*, *Il1b*, *Il6*, *Ccl2*, *Nos2*, and *Msr1* were detected by real-time RT-PCR. (b, c) RAW 264 cells were pretreated with 100–400 μg/mL TBE for 1 h, followed by treatment with 100 ng/mL LPS for 6 h. (b) The protein levels of iNOS and SR-A were detected by Western blotting. (c) NO levels in the culture medium were measured using DAF-2. (d) RAW 264 cells were pretreated with 100–400 μg/mL TBE for 1 h, followed by treatment with 100 ng/mL LPS for 2 h. NF-κB activation was determined by measuring cytosolic and nuclear p65 levels. (e) RAW 264 cells were pretreated with 100–400 μg/mL TBE for 1 h, followed by treatment with 100 ng/mL LPS for 0.5 h. NF-κB and MAPK activation were assessed by measuring p-IκB, P-NF-κB, p-p38, p-JNK, and p-ERK. Data represent mean $\pm$ SD, $n = 3$ ($^{*}p < 0.05$, $^{**}p < 0.01$, $^{***}p < 0.001$ compared to LPS group).

(a)

(b)

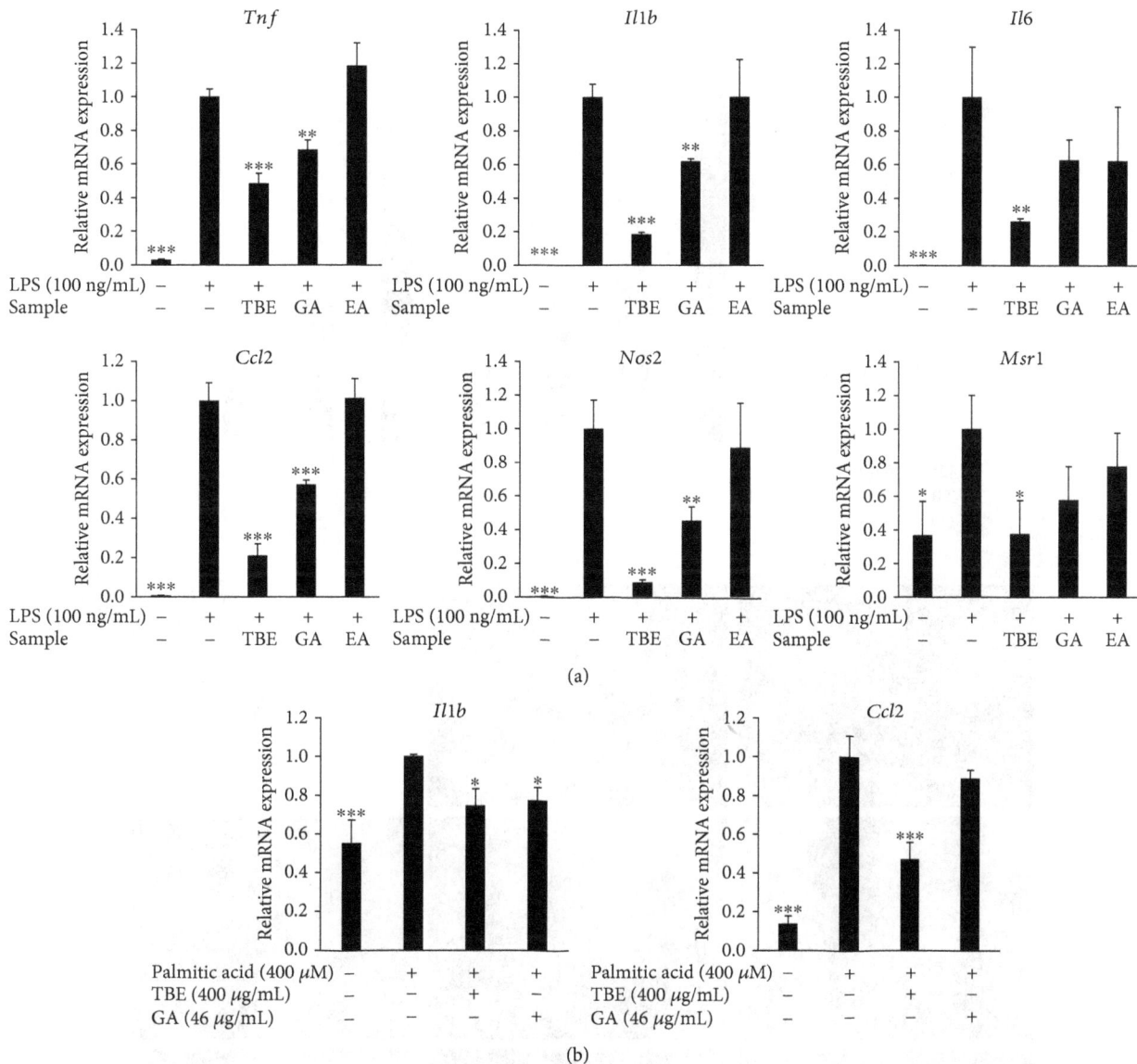

FIGURE 3: Effects of TBE, GA, and EA on inflammatory mediator expression in LPS- and palmitic acid-stimulated macrophages. (a) RAW 264 cells were pretreated with 400 μg/mL TBE, 46 μg/mL GA, or 1.6 μg/mL EA for 1 h, followed by treatment with 100 ng/mL LPS for 4 h. The mRNA levels of Tnf, Il1b, Il6, Ccl2, Nos2, and Msr1 were detected by real-time RT-PCR. (b) RAW 264 cells were pretreated with 400 μg/mL TBE or 46 μg/mL GA for 1 h, followed by treatment with 400 μM palmitic acid for 12 h. The mRNA levels of Il1b and Ccl2 were detected by real-time RT-PCR. Data represent mean ± SD, $n = 3$ ($^*p < 0.05$, $^{**}p < 0.01$, $^{***}p < 0.001$ compared to LPS or palmitic acid group).

3.5. TBE and GA Suppressed ROS Production in LPS-Stimulated Macrophages. Elimination of ROS production is important for controlling inflammatory response. To confirm the antioxidant effects of TBE and GA in LPS-stimulated macrophages, we measured intracellular ROS production using CM-H$_2$DCFDA. As shown in Figures 4(a) and 4(b), ROS production was greatly increased by LPS, showing obvious green fluorescence, while TBE and GA significantly suppressed the level of ROS production in a dose-dependent manner.

3.6. TBE Enhanced the Antioxidant Defense System in LPS-Stimulated Macrophages. The antioxidant defense system, such as antioxidant enzymes, is important for the suppression

of oxidative stress and inflammatory response. We found that LPS had almost no effect on the mRNA or protein expression of HO-1, NQO1, and GCLM and decreased the expression of catalase. Treatment with TBE significantly upregulated the expression of these genes and the protein expression of catalase in the presence of LPS (Figures 5(a) and 5(b)). Nrf2 translocation from the cytoplasm to the nucleus plays a key role in Nrf2 activation and the transcription of antioxidant enzymes. As shown in Figure 5(c), LPS had no effect on the nuclear translocation of Nrf2, while TBE increased Nrf2 protein within the nuclear fraction. In addition, as previous reports suggested that some protein kinases such as PI3K/Akt and AMPK are involved in Nrf2 translocation [16, 19], we examined the effect of TBE on Akt and AMPK pathways.

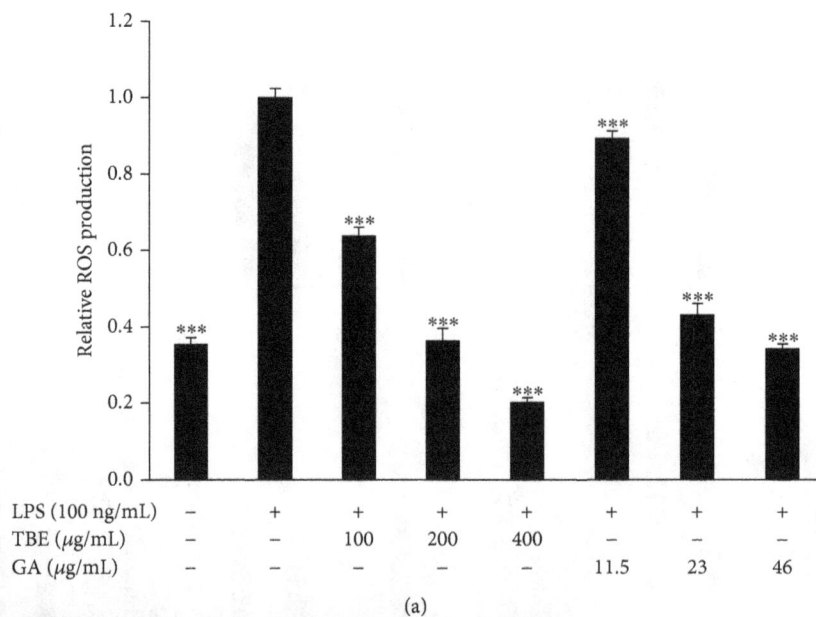

(a)

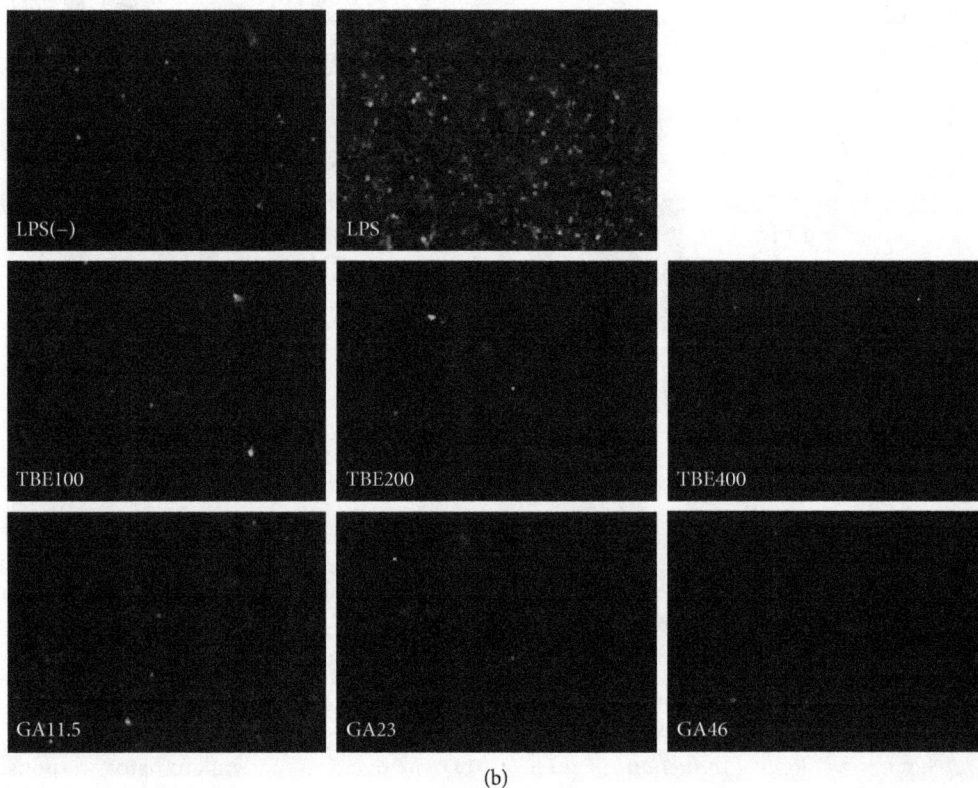

(b)

FIGURE 4: Effects of TBE and GA on ROS production in LPS-stimulated macrophages. (a, b) RAW 264 cells were pretreated with 100–400 μg/mL TBE or 11.5–46 μg/mL GA for 1 h, followed by treatment with 100 ng/mL LPS for 7 h. Intracellular ROS levels were measured using CM-H$_2$DCFDA. Data represent mean ± SD, $n = 3$ (***$p < 0.001$ compared to LPS group).

Phosphorylation of Akt and AMPK was slightly increased in LPS-treated cells, but a significant level of Akt and AMPK phosphorylation occurred in cells treated with TBE (Figure 5(d)).

3.7. Effects of GA and EA on Antioxidant Enzyme Expression in LPS-Stimulated Macrophages. We also analyzed the effects of GA and EA in TBE on antioxidant enzyme expression in LPS-stimulated macrophages. The impacts of TBE, GA, and EA on antioxidant enzyme expression is similar to the effects on inflammatory mediator expression, that is, TBE and GA significantly induced the expression of HO-1, catalase, NQO1, and GCLM, but EA did not affect the expression of these genes (Figure 6).

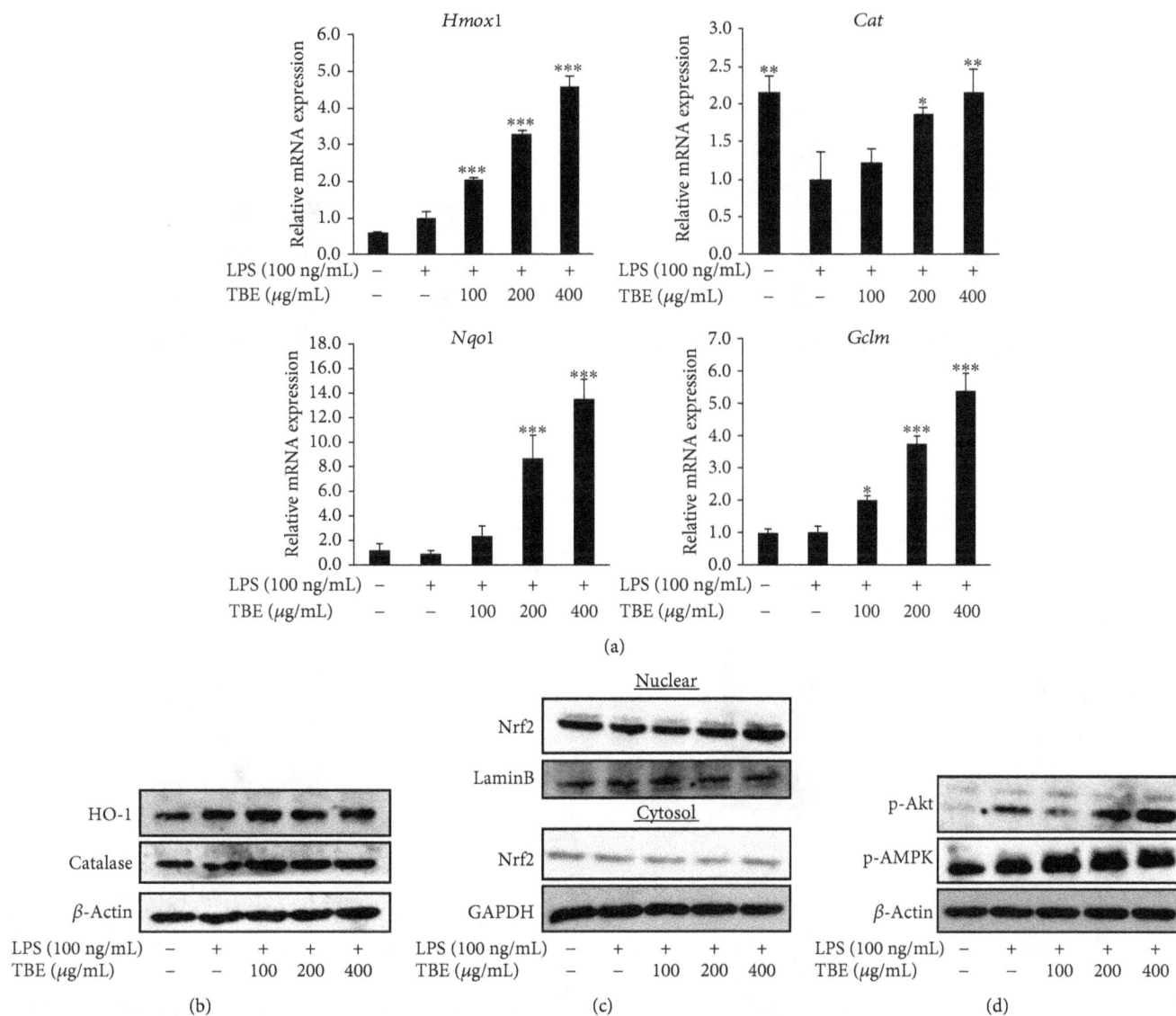

FIGURE 5: Effect of TBE on antioxidant enzyme expression and antioxidant signaling pathway in LPS-stimulated macrophages. (a) RAW 264 cells were pretreated with 100–400 μg/mL TBE for 1 h, followed by treatment with 100 ng/mL LPS for 4 h. The mRNA levels of *Hmox1*, *Cat*, *Nqo1*, and *Gclm* were detected by real-time RT-PCR. (b) RAW 264 cells were pretreated with 100–400 μg/mL TBE for 1 h, followed by treatment with 100 ng/mL LPS for 6 h. The protein levels of HO-1 and catalase were detected by Western blotting. (c) RAW 264 cells were pretreated with 100–400 μg/mL TBE for 1 h, followed by treatment with 100 ng/mL LPS for 2 h. Nrf2 activation was determined by measuring cytosolic and nuclear Nrf2 levels. (d) RAW 264 cells were pretreated with 100–400 μg/mL TBE for 1 h, followed by treatment with 100 ng/mL LPS for 0.5 h. Akt and AMPK activation was detected by Western blotting. Data represent mean ± SD, $n = 3$ ($^{*}p < 0.05$, $^{**}p < 0.01$, $^{***}p < 0.001$ compared to LPS group).

3.8. Blocking Nrf2 Signaling Attenuated the Antioxidant Effects of TBE and GA in LPS-Stimulated Macrophages.

Nrf2, a major transcriptional factor regulating the expression of antioxidant enzymes, is involved in the suppression of oxidative stress. To confirm whether the antioxidant effects of TBE and GA are mediated by Nrf2, we silenced Nrf2 gene expression in RAW 264 macrophages. When Nrf2 siRNA was transfected into cells, the level of Nrf2 expression was decreased by approximately 60% compared with cells transfected with NC siRNA (Figure 7(a)). As shown in Figure 7(b), knockdown of Nrf2 significantly inhibited the increase in mRNA expression of catalase and GCLM induced by TBE and GA, without affecting the expression of HO-1 and NQO1. These results show that Nrf2 activation accounts at least in part for the antioxidant effects of TBE and GA in our system.

3.9. Involvement of PI3K/Akt and AMPK Pathways in Antioxidant Enzyme Expression by TBE.

TBE is capable of activating Akt and AMPK in LPS-stimulated macrophages (Figure 5(d)). To determine whether Akt and AMPK are responsible for the increased expression of antioxidant enzymes induced by TBE, we used LY294002 (Akt inhibitor) and compound C (AMPK inhibitor). As shown in Figure 8,

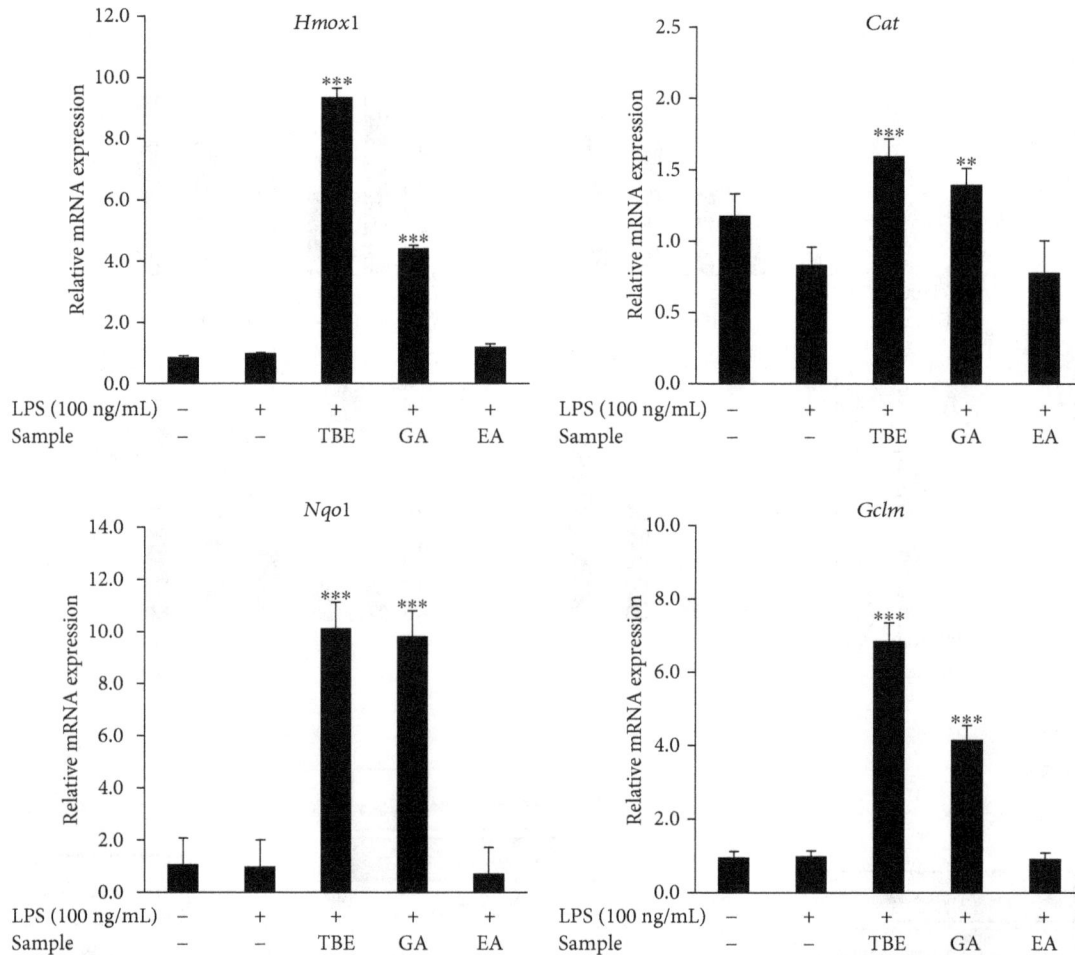

FIGURE 6: Effects of TBE, GA, and EA on antioxidant enzyme expression in LPS-stimulated macrophages. RAW 264 cells were pretreated with 400 μg/mL TBE, 46 μg/mL GA, or 1.6 μg/mL EA for 1 h, followed by treatment with 100 ng/mL LPS for 4 h. The mRNA levels of *Hmox1*, *Cat*, *Nqo1*, and *Gclm* were detected by real-time RT-PCR. Data represent mean ± SD, $n = 3$ (**$p < 0.01$, ***$p < 0.001$ compared to LPS group).

TBE significantly induced the expression of HO-1, catalase, NQO1, and GCLM. However, treatment of cells with LY294002 and compound C resulted in significant inhibition of TBE-induced antioxidant enzyme expression, indicating that the antioxidant effect of TBE is largely dependent on PI3K/Akt and AMPK signaling.

3.10. TBE Increased Antioxidant Enzyme Expression and Improved Kidney Injury in LPS-Shock Model Mice. As the present data indicate that TBE exhibits antioxidant and anti-inflammatory properties in LPS-stimulated macrophages, we assessed *in vivo* protective effects of TBE in LPS-shock model mice. As shown in Figure 9(a), TBE significantly induced the mRNA expression of antioxidant enzymes (catalase, NQO1, and GCLM) but tended to reduce the mRNA expression of inflammatory mediators (TNF-α and IL-6) in kidney tissues. As shown in Figure 9(b), histopathological examination of kidney tissues from the LPS group showed severe lesions including interstitial hyperemia, inflammatory cell infiltration in glomeruli, and glomerular capillary narrowing. In contrast, these kidney injury features were attenuated in the TBE-treated group. The score of interstitial hyperemia was 2.3 ± 0.3 in the LPS group and 1.8 ± 0.1

in the LPS + TBE group. The percentage of glomerular capillary narrowing was 33.2 ± 7.4% in the LPS group and 16.5 ± 7.1% in the LPS + TBE group. These results suggest that TBE might efficiently prevent oxidative stress and inflammation in endotoxemic mice.

4. Discussion

Owing to its high polyphenol content, the fruit of *T. bellirica* has been reported to have beneficial effects including antioxidant [33], hypoglycemic [26], and hypolipidemic [27] activities. The present study showed that TBE contains GA and EA and that approximately 50% of the polyphenolic compounds contained in TBE is GA. We demonstrated that TBE and GA attenuated LPS-induced inflammatory mediator overexpression, NO production, ROS production, and NF-κB nuclear translocation in macrophages. Huang et al. [34] reported that GA suppressed LPS-induced inflammatory cytokine production and the mRNA and protein expression of NF-κB, which is partially consistent with our results. We also found that TBE suppressed phosphorylation of not only NF-κB p65 but also p38, JNK, and ERK without altering phosphorylation of IκB. NF-κB p65 is held in its inactive

(a)

■ NC
□ Nrf2 siRNA

(b)

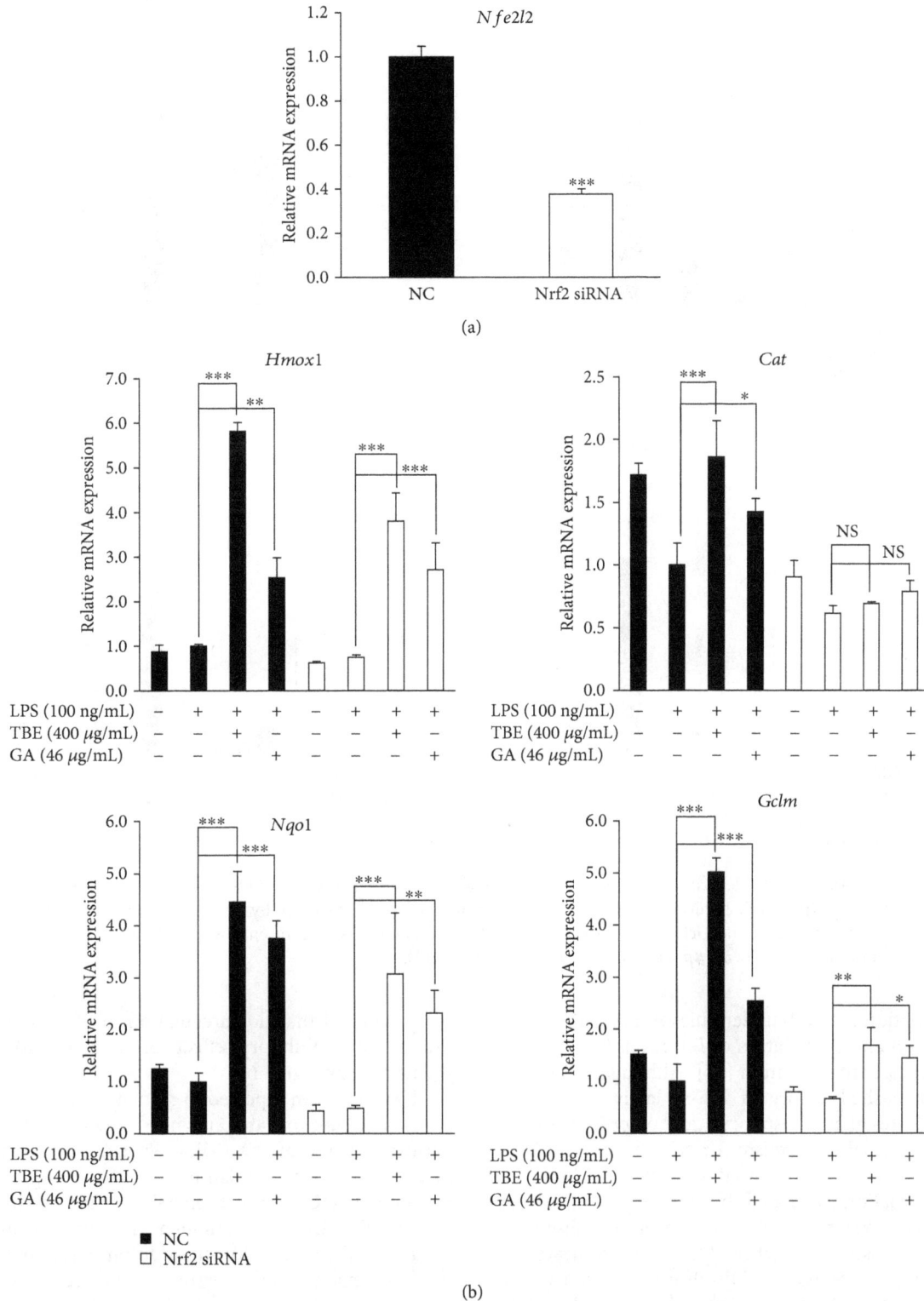

FIGURE 7: Knockdown of Nrf2 attenuated antioxidant enzyme expression induced by TBE and GA in LPS-stimulated macrophages. (a) RAW 264 cells were transfected with 60 nM Nrf2 siRNA or NC siRNA for 48 h. The mRNA levels of *Nfe2l2* were detected by real-time RT-PCR. Data represent mean ± SD, $n = 3$ (***$p < 0.001$ compared to NS group). (b) After transfection of 60 nM Nrf2 siRNA or NC siRNA for 48 h, RAW 264 cells were pretreated with 400 μg/mL TBE or 46 μg/mL GA for 1 h, followed by treatment with 100 ng/mL LPS for 4 h. The mRNA levels of *Hmox1, Cat, Nqo1,* and *Gclm* were detected by real-time RT-PCR. Data represent mean ± SD, $n = 3$ (*$p < 0.05$, **$p < 0.01$, ***$p < 0.001$; NS, no significant difference).

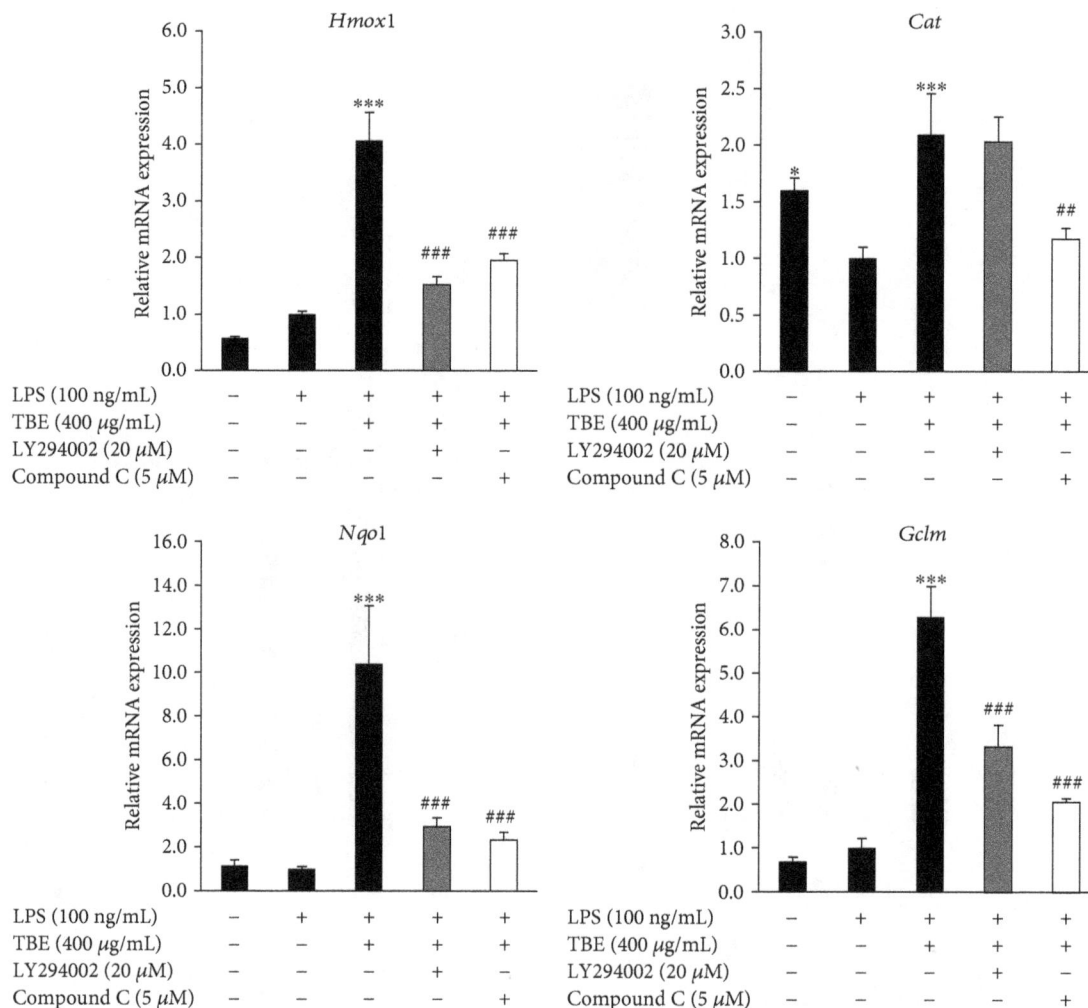

FIGURE 8: Inhibition of Akt and AMPK reduced TBE-induced antioxidant enzyme expression in LPS-stimulated macrophages. RAW 264 cells were pretreated with 400 μg/mL TBE, 20 μM LY294002, or 5 μM compound C for 1 h, followed by treatment with 100 ng/mL LPS for 4 h. The mRNA levels of *Hmox1*, *Cat*, *Nqo1*, and *Gclm* were detected by real-time RT-PCR. Data represent mean ± SD, $n = 3$ ($^*p < 0.05$, $^{***}p < 0.001$ compared to LPS group; $^{##}p < 0.01$, $^{###}p < 0.001$ compared to TBE group).

form by association with IκB under quiescent conditions, but phosphorylation and degradation of IκB result in p65 dissociation and nuclear translocation [35]. Although IκB signaling is an established theory of NF-κB activation, recent evidence indicates that phosphorylation of p65 by several kinases is a principal mechanism for NF-κB transcriptional activation. Olson et al. [36] reported that p38 MAPK induced p65 phosphorylation mediated by mitogen- and stress-activated protein kinase 1 (MSK1), as well as subsequent inflammatory cytokine production. Our results indicate that TBE may regulate LPS-induced NF-κB translocation via the suppression of NF-κB p65 phosphorylation mediated by MAPK but not via the suppression of IκB phosphorylation. Additionally, TBE decreased the mRNA and protein expression of SR-A, a major pattern recognition receptor found on macrophages that binds to modified low-density lipoprotein (LDL), as well as PAMPs including LPS [37]. Recent reports have shown that SR-A is required for LPS-induced MAPK and NF-κB activation by cooperating with TLR4 in macrophages [38, 39]. Therefore,

we speculated that downregulation of SR-A might contribute to the inhibitory effect of TBE on MAPK/NF-κB inflammatory signaling.

Nrf2 has been reported to regulate cellular redox homeostasis, and antioxidant enzyme production through Nrf2 pathway is one of the major defense mechanisms against oxidative stress and inflammation [14]. Exogenous overexpression of HO-1 and its metabolite carbon monoxide by use of HO-1 inducers inhibited LPS-induced inflammation *in vitro* and *in vivo* [40]. In addition, treatment of catalase inhibitor exacerbated liver injury and led to high lethality from microbial sepsis in mice [41]. In the present study, we found that TBE and GA increased the expression of antioxidant enzymes (HO-1, catalase, NQO1, and GCLM) and activated Nrf2 nuclear translocation in RAW 264 cells. As antioxidant enzymes are produced in response to oxidative stress itself, we assessed intracellular ROS levels. TBE and GA significantly suppressed LPS-induced ROS production, suggesting that antioxidant enzyme expression by TBE and GA might not be mediated by ROS generation. Furthermore,

(a)

(b)

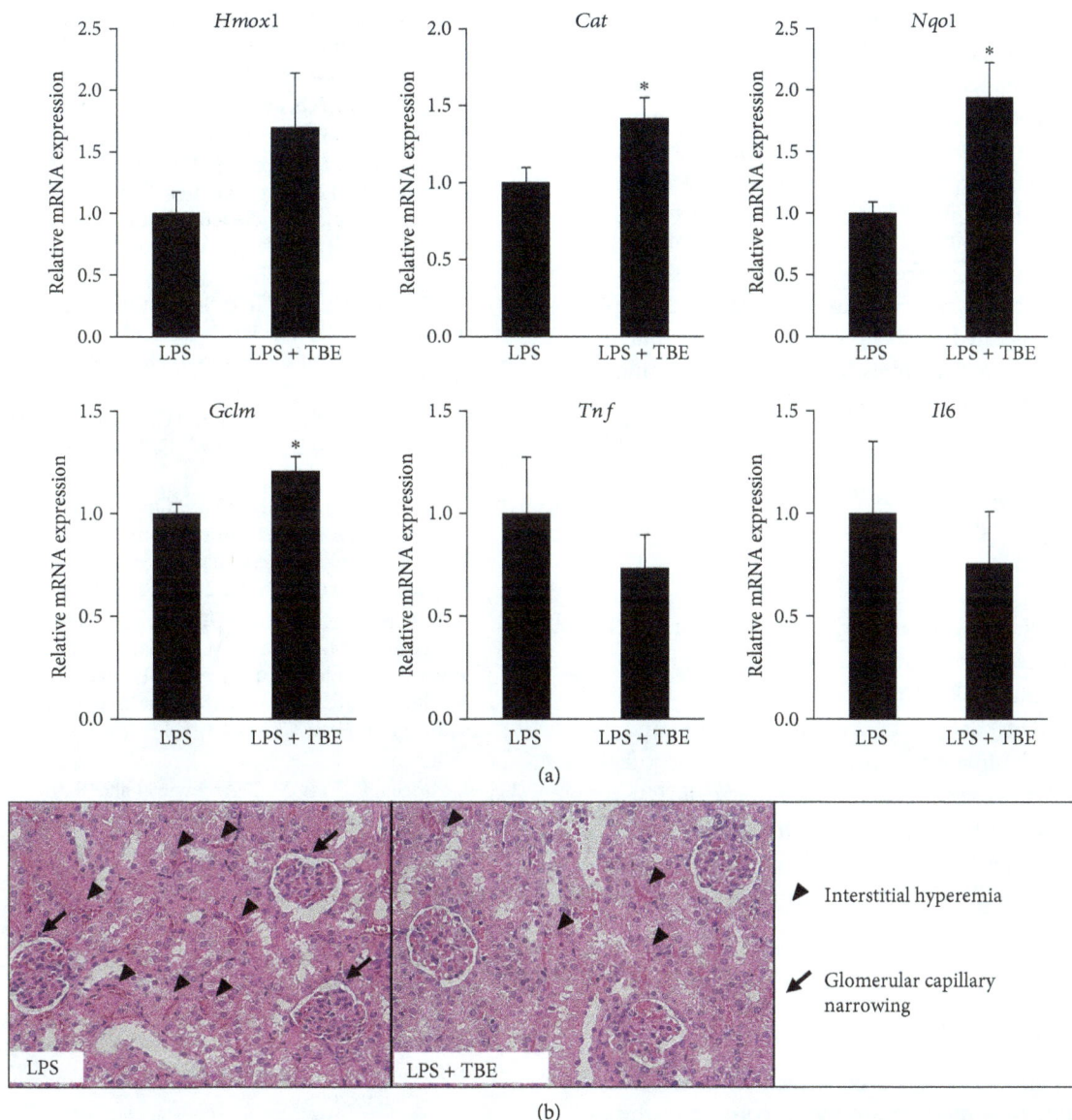

FIGURE 9: Protective effect of TBE on LPS-induced kidney injury in mice. (a, b) Mice were orally administrated 400 mg/kg TBE or water for 3 days, followed by intraperitoneal injection of 2 mg/kg LPS. Kidney tissues were collected at 24 h post LPS injection. (a) The mRNA levels of *Hmox1*, *Cat*, *Nqo1*, *Gclm*, *Tnf*, and *Il6* were detected by real-time RT-PCR. (b) Histopathological findings of kidney injury were observed by HE staining. Data represent mean ± SE, $n = 6$ ($^*p < 0.05$ compared to LPS group).

the effects of TBE and GA on catalase and GCLM expression were attenuated when Nrf2 expression was disrupted by siRNA transfection. Several kinases (e.g., PI3K/Akt, AMPK, protein kinase C, and MAPK) are implicated in Nrf2-mediated antioxidant enzyme expression [16, 19]. We also examined the role of PI3K/Akt and AMPK pathways on antioxidant enzyme expression by using specific inhibitors. The present data showed that blockage of PI3K/Akt and AMPK signaling significantly reduced TBE-induced antioxidant enzyme expression, indicating the involvement of PI3K/Akt and AMPK pathway activation in the upregulatory effect of TBE on Nrf2-targeted antioxidant genes. As not only Nrf2 but also other transcription factors such as hypoxia-

inducible factor-1α [42] and peroxisome proliferator-activated receptors [43] are known to regulate antioxidant gene expression, further research is needed to identify mechanisms underlying antioxidative effect of TBE.

Previous studies have shown that some polyphenols (e.g., resveratrol, quercetin, and catechins) suppressed LPS-induced inflammatory mediator expression via the activation of PI3K/Akt and AMPK [22-24]. However, in the present study, inhibition of PI3K/Akt and AMPK had no effect on decreasing LPS-induced mRNA expression of inflammatory mediators by TBE (data not shown). Thus, the inhibitory effect of TBE and GA on LPS-induced inflammatory response might be mediated by the suppression of MAPK/NF-κB pathway, which occurs independently of PI3K/Akt and AMPK activation.

Finally, we tested the anti-inflammatory and antioxidant properties of TBE in endotoxin-shocked mice. Intraperitoneal injection of LPS has been shown to cause excessive inflammation in whole body organs including the liver, kidney, and lung [44–46]. In the present study, TBE significantly induced antioxidant enzyme expression and improved kidney injury in LPS-shock model mice but had little effect in LPS-induced liver and lung injury (data not shown). Acute kidney injury is one of the most frequent symptoms of sepsis and increases the mortality rate compared with sepsis alone [45]. Recent study suggested that GA was mainly distributed in kidney tissue after oral administration [47], explaining the beneficial effect of TBE to ameliorate kidney injury. GA has also been shown to attenuate dextran sulfate sodium-induced colitis by upregulating Nrf2 pathway and its downstream targets [48]. Therefore, the protective effect of TBE on kidney injury might result from its antioxidant activity.

In conclusion, our present study demonstrated that TBE and GA enhance antioxidant defense capacity through the activation of Akt/AMPK/Nrf2 pathway in LPS-stimulated macrophages. Our data also showed that TBE and GA exhibit anti-inflammatory activities by downregulating MAPK/NF-κB pathway. The in vivo efficacy of TBE was partly confirmed in LPS-shock model mice. These findings provide new perspectives for novel therapeutic approaches using dietary-derived antioxidants against oxidative stress and inflammation-related diseases.

Disclosure

Part of this manuscript has been presented in *Atherosclerosis Supplements* as meeting abstract according to the following link: https://www.sciencedirect.com/science/article/pii/S156756881830388X?via%3Dihub.

Acknowledgments

This study was supported by JSPS KAKENHI Grant Nos. JP16H03033, JP15H02895, and JP18J13346.

References

[1] U. Weiss, "Inflammation," *Nature*, vol. 454, no. 7203, p. 427, 2008.

[2] I. M. Jou, C. F. Lin, K. J. Tsai, and S. J. Wei, "Macrophage-mediated inflammatory disorders," *Mediators of Inflammation*, vol. 2013, Article ID 316482, 3 pages, 2013.

[3] T. H. Mogensen, Pathogen recognition and inflammatory signaling in innate immune defenses," *Clinical Microbiology Reviews*, vol. 22, no. 2, pp. 240–273, 2009.

[4] A. Aderem and R. J. Ulevitch, "Toll-like receptors in the induction of the innate immune response," *Nature*, vol. 406, no. 6797, pp. 782–787, 2000.

[5] Y. C. Lu, W. C. Yeh, and P. S. Ohashi, "LPS/TLR4 signal transduction pathway," *Cytokine*, vol. 42, no. 2, pp. 145–151, 2008.

[6] L. F. de Souza, F. Barreto, E. G. da Silva et al., "Regulation of LPS stimulated ROS production in peritoneal macrophages from alloxan-induced diabetic rats: involvement of high glucose and PPARγ," *Life Sciences*, vol. 81, no. 2, pp. 153–159, 2007.

[7] I. T. Lee and C. M. Yang, "Role of NADPH oxidase/ROS in pro-inflammatory mediators-induced airway and pulmonary diseases," *Biochemical Pharmacology*, vol. 84, no. 5, pp. 581–590, 2012.

[8] M. J. Morgan and Z. G. Liu, "Crosstalk of reactive oxygen species and NF-κB signaling," *Cell Research*, vol. 21, no. 1, pp. 103–115, 2011.

[9] H. Y. Hsu and M. H. Wen, "Lipopolysaccharide-mediated reactive oxygen species and signal transduction in the regulation of interleukin-1 gene expression," *The Journal of Biological Chemistry*, vol. 277, no. 25, pp. 22131–22139, 2002.

[10] M. S. Fernandez-Pachon, G. Berna, E. Otaolaurruchi, A. M. Troncoso, F. Martin, and M. C. Garcia-Parrilla, "Changes in antioxidant endogenous enzymes (activity and gene expression levels) after repeated red wine intake," *Journal of Agricultural and Food Chemistry*, vol. 57, no. 15, pp. 6578–6583, 2009.

[11] R. Masella, R. Vari, M. D'Archivio et al., "Extra virgin olive oil biophenols inhibit cell-mediated oxidation of LDL by increasing the mRNA transcription of glutathione-related enzymes," *The Journal of Nutrition*, vol. 134, no. 4, pp. 785–791, 2004.

[12] M. R. de la Vega, M. Dodson, C. Gross et al., "Role of Nrf2 and autophagy in acute lung injury," *Clinical Microbiology Reviews*, vol. 2, no. 2, pp. 91–101, 2016.

[13] N. G. Innamorato, A. I. Rojo, A. J. Garcia-Yague, M. Yamamoto, M. L. de Ceballos, and A. Cuadrado, "The transcription factor Nrf2 is a therapeutic target against brain inflammation," *Journal of Immunology*, vol. 181, no. 1, pp. 680–689, 2008.

[14] B. M. Hybertson, B. Gao, S. K. Bose, and J. M. McCord, "Oxidative stress in health and disease: the therapeutic potential of Nrf2 activation," *Molecular Aspects of Medicine*, vol. 32, no. 4–6, pp. 234–246, 2011.

[15] A. Loboda, M. Damulewicz, E. Pyza, A. Jozkowicz, and J. Dulak, "Role of Nrf2/HO-1 system in development, oxidative stress response and diseases: an evolutionarily conserved mechanism," *Cellular and Molecular Life Sciences*, vol. 73, no. 17, pp. 3221–3247, 2016.

[16] H. K. Bryan, A. Olayanju, C. E. Goldring, and B. K. Park, "The Nrf2 cell defence pathway: Keap1-dependent and -independent mechanisms of regulation," *Biochemical Pharmacology*, vol. 85, no. 6, pp. 705–717, 2013.

[17] J. S. L. Yu and W. Cui, "Proliferation, survival and metabolism: the role of PI3K/AKT/mTOR signalling in pluripotency and cell fate determination," *Development*, vol. 143, no. 17, pp. 3050–3060, 2016.

[18] D. G. Hardie, F. A. Ross, and S. A. Hawley, "AMPK: a nutrient and energy sensor that maintains energy homeostasis," *Nature Reviews. Molecular Cell Biology*, vol. 13, no. 4, pp. 251–262, 2012.

[19] M. S. Joo, W. D. Kim, K. Y. Lee, J. H. Kim, J. H. Koo, and S. G.

Kim, "AMPK facilitates nuclear accumulation of Nrf2 by phosphorylating at serine 550," *Molecular and Cellular Biology*, vol. 36, no. 14, pp. 1931–1942, 2016.

[20] A. Salminen, J. M. T. Hyttinen, and K. Kaarniranta, "AMP-activated protein kinase inhibits NF-κB signaling and inflammation: impact on healthspan and lifespan," *Journal of Molecular Medicine*, vol. 89, no. 7, pp. 667–676, 2011.

[21] D. Sag, D. Carling, R. D. Stout, and J. Suttles, "Adenosine 5'-monophosphate-activated protein kinase promotes macrophage polarization to an anti-inflammatory functional phenotype," *Journal of Immunology*, vol. 181, no. 12, pp. 8633–8641, 2008.

[22] Y. Zong, L. Sun, B. Liu et al., "Resveratrol inhibits LPS-induced MAPKs activation via activation of the phosphatidylinositol 3-kinase pathway in murine RAW 264.7 macrophage cells," *PLoS One*, vol. 7, no. 8, article e44107, 2012.

[23] C. Q. Xu, B. J. Liu, J. F. Wu et al., "Icariin attenuates LPS-induced acute inflammatory responses: involvement of PI3K/Akt and NF-κB signaling pathway," *European Journal of Pharmacology*, vol. 642, no. 1–3, pp. 146–153, 2010.

[24] S. Chung, H. Yao, S. Caito, J. W. Hwang, G. Arunachalam, and I. Rahman, "Regulation of SIRT1 in cellular functions: role of polyphenols," *Archives of Biochemistry and Biophysics*, vol. 501, no. 1, pp. 79–90, 2010.

[25] M. Modak, P. Dixit, J. Londhe, S. Ghaskadbi, and T. P. A. Devasagayam, "Indian herbs and herbal drugs used for the treatment of diabetes," *Journal of Clinical Biochemistry and Nutrition*, vol. 40, no. 3, pp. 163–173, 2007.

[26] H. Makihara, T. Shimada, E. Machida et al., "Preventive effect of Terminalia bellirica on obesity and metabolic disorders in spontaneously obese type 2 diabetic model mice," *Journal of Natural Medicines*, vol. 66, no. 3, pp. 459–467, 2012.

[27] H. P. Shaila, S. L. Udupa, and A. L. Udupa, "Hypolipidemic activity of three indigenous drugs in experimentally induced atherosclerosis," *International Journal of Cardiology*, vol. 67, no. 2, pp. 119–124, 1998.

[28] A. Khan and A. Gilani, "Pharmacodynamic evaluation of Terminalia bellerica for its antihypertensive effect," *Journal of Food and Drug Analysis*, vol. 16, pp. 6–14, 2008.

[29] B. Pfundstein, S. K. El Desouky, W. E. Hull, R. Haubner, G. Erben, and R. W. Owen, "Polyphenolic compounds in the fruits of Egyptian medicinal plants (*Terminalia bellerica, Terminalia chebula* and *Terminalia horrida*): characterization, quantitation and determination of antioxidant capacities," *Phytochemistry*, vol. 71, no. 10, pp. 1132–1148, 2010.

[30] T. T. Ou, M. C. Lin, C. H. Wu, W. L. Lin, and C. J. Wang, "Gallic acid attenuates oleic acid-induced proliferation of vascular smooth muscle cell through regulation of AMPK-eNOS-FAS signaling," *Current Medicinal Chemistry*, vol. 20, no. 31, pp. 3944–3953, 2013.

[31] K. V. Doan, C. M. Ko, A. W. Kinyua et al., "Gallic acid regulates body weight and glucose homeostasis through AMPK activation," *Endocrinology*, vol. 156, no. 1, pp. 157–168, 2015.

[32] M. Tanaka, Y. Kishimoto, E. Saita et al., "*Terminalia bellirica* extract inhibits low-density lipoprotein oxidation and macrophage inflammatory response *in vitro*," *Antioxidants*, vol. 5, no. 2, 2016.

[33] S. Guleria, A. K. Tiku, and S. Rana, "Antioxidant activity of acetone extract/fractions of *Terminalia bellerica* Roxb. fruit,"

Indian Journal of Biochemistry & Biophysics, vol. 47, no. 2, pp. 110–116, 2010.

[34] L. Huang, L. Hou, H. Xue, and C. Wang, "Gallic acid inhibits inflammatory response of RAW264.7 macrophages by blocking the activation of TLR4/NF-κB induced by LPS," *Xi Bao Yu Fen Zi Mian Yi Xue Za Zhi*, vol. 32, no. 12, pp. 1610–1614, 2016.

[35] M. S. Hayden and S. Ghosh, "Shared principles in NF-κB signaling," *Cell*, vol. 132, no. 3, pp. 344–362, 2008.

[36] C. M. Olson, M. N. Hedrick, H. Izadi, T. C. Bates, E. R. Olivera, and J. Anguita, "p38 mitogen-activated protein kinase controls NF-κB transcriptional activation and tumor necrosis factor alpha production through RelA phosphorylation mediated by mitogen- and stress-activated protein kinase 1 in response to *Borrelia burgdorferi* antigens," *Infection and Immunity*, vol. 75, no. 1, pp. 270–277, 2007.

[37] M. Hollifield, E. B. Ghanem, W. J. S. de Villiers, and B. A. Garvy, "Scavenger receptor A dampens induction of inflammation in response to the fungal pathogen *Pneumocystis carinii*," *Infection and Immunity*, vol. 75, no. 8, pp. 3999–4005, 2007.

[38] H. Yu, T. Ha, L. Liu et al., "Scavenger receptor A (SR-A) is required for LPS-induced TLR4 mediated NF-κB activation in macrophages," *Biochimica et Biophysica Acta (BBA) - Molecular Cell Research*, vol. 1823, no. 7, pp. 1192–1198, 2012.

[39] T. A. Seimon, A. Obstfeld, K. J. Moore, D. T. Golenbock, and I. Tabas, "Combinatorial pattern recognition receptor signaling alters the balance of life and death in macrophages," *Proceedings of the National Academy of Sciences of the United States of America*, vol. 103, no. 52, pp. 19794–19799, 2006.

[40] K. Tsoyi, T. Y. Lee, Y. S. Lee et al., "Heme-oxygenase-1 induction and carbon monoxide-releasing molecule inhibit lipopolysaccharide (LPS)-induced high-mobility group box 1 release in vitro and improve survival of mice in LPS- and cecal ligation and puncture-induced sepsis model in vivo," *Molecular Pharmacology*, vol. 76, no. 1, pp. 173–182, 2009.

[41] M. Jia, Y. Jing, Q. Ai et al., "Potential role of catalase in mice with lipopolysaccharide/D-galactosamine-induced fulminant liver injury," *Hepatology Research*, vol. 44, no. 11, pp. 1151–1158, 2014.

[42] S. M. Yeligar, K. Machida, and V. K. Kalra, "Ethanol-induced HO-1 and NQO1 are differentially regulated by HIF-1α and Nrf2 to attenuate inflammatory cytokine expression," *The Journal of Biological Chemistry*, vol. 285, no. 46, pp. 35359–35373, 2010.

[43] G. Kronke, A. Kadl, E. Ikonomu et al., "Expression of heme oxygenase-1 in human vascular cells is regulated by peroxisome proliferator-activated receptors," *Arteriosclerosis, Thrombosis, and Vascular Biology*, vol. 27, no. 6, pp. 1276–1282, 2007.

[44] K. Hamesch, E. Borkham-Kamphorst, P. Strnad, and R. Weiskirchen, "Lipopolysaccharide-induced inflammatory liver injury in mice," *Laboratory Animals*, vol. 49, Supplement 1, pp. 37–46, 2015.

[45] A. Zarjou and A. Agarwal, "Sepsis and acute kidney injury," *Journal of the American Society of Nephrology*, vol. 22, no. 6, pp. 999–1006, 2011.

[46] G. Matute-Bello, C. W. Frevert, and T. R. Martin, "Animal models of acute lung injury," *American Journal of Physiology. Lung Cellular and Molecular Physiology*, vol. 295, no. 3, pp. L379–L399, 2008.

[47] F. W. Ma, Q. F. Deng, X. Zhou et al., "The tissue distribution and urinary excretion study of gallic acid and protocatechuic acid after oral administration of *Polygonum capitatum* extract in rats," *Molecules*, vol. 21, no. 4, p. 399, 2016.

[48] A. K. Pandurangan, M. Norhaizan, N. Mohebali, and L. C. Yeng, "Gallic acid attenuates dextran sulfate sodium-induced experimental colitis in BALB/c mice," *Drug Design, Development and Therapy*, vol. 9, pp. 3923–3934, 2015.

mTOR Modulates Methamphetamine-Induced Toxicity through Cell Clearing Systems

Gloria Lazzeri ⓘ,[1] Francesca Biagioni ⓘ,[2] Federica Fulceri ⓘ,[3] Carla L. Busceti ⓘ,[2] Maria C. Scavuzzo,[1] Chiara Ippolito,[3] Alessandra Salvetti ⓘ,[3] Paola Lenzi ⓘ,[1] and Francesco Fornai ⓘ[1,2]

[1]Department of Translational Research and New Technologies in Medicine and Surgery, Human Anatomy, University of Pisa, Via Roma 55, Pisa 56126, Italy
[2]I.R.C.C.S Neuromed, Via Atinense 18, Pozzilli 86077, Italy
[3]Department of Clinical and Experimental Medicine, University of Pisa, Via Roma 55, Pisa 56126, Italy

Correspondence should be addressed to Francesco Fornai; francesco.fornai@med.unipi.it

Academic Editor: Brian Harvey

Methamphetamine (METH) is abused worldwide, and it represents a threat for public health. METH exposure induces a variety of detrimental effects. In fact, METH produces a number of oxidative species, which lead to lipid peroxidation, protein misfolding, and nuclear damage. Cell clearing pathways such as ubiquitin-proteasome (UP) and autophagy (ATG) are involved in METH-induced oxidative damage. Although these pathways were traditionally considered to operate as separate metabolic systems, recent studies demonstrate their interconnection at the functional and biochemical level. Very recently, the convergence between UP and ATG was evidenced within a single organelle named autophagoproteasome (APP), which is suppressed by mTOR activation. In the present research study, the occurrence of APP during METH toxicity was analyzed. In fact, coimmunoprecipitation indicates a binding between LC3 and P20S particles, which also recruit p62 and alpha-synuclein. The amount of METH-induced toxicity correlates with APP levels. Specific markers for ATG and UP, such as LC3 and P20S in the cytosol, and within METH-induced vacuoles, were measured at different doses and time intervals following METH administration either alone or combined with mTOR modulators. Western blotting, coimmunoprecipitation, light microscopy, confocal microscopy, plain transmission electron microscopy, and immunogold staining were used to document the effects of mTOR modulation on METH toxicity and the merging of UP with ATG markers within APPs. METH-induced cell death is prevented by mTOR inhibition, while it is worsened by mTOR activation, which correlates with the amount of autophagoproteasomes. The present data, which apply to METH toxicity, are also relevant to provide a novel insight into cell clearing pathways to counteract several kinds of oxidative damage.

1. Introduction

Methamphetamine (METH) is a highly addictive and neuro-toxic drug, which causes a variety of neuropsychiatric alterations mainly affecting the dopamine (DA) mesostriatal and mesolimbic systems in the brain [1, 2]. Exposure to repeated doses of METH produces striatal DA depletion and loss of mesostriatal DA terminals [3–12].

In the cell body of the substantia nigra *pars compacta* (SNpc), METH produces alterations in the cytoplasm which also occur in DA-PC12 cells and extend to the cytoplasm and nucleus of striatal GABA neurons [6, 13–16]. These alterations configure as multilamellar whorl staining for ubiquitin, parkin, and alpha-synuclein [6, 15, 17]. Recent studies indicate that high METH doses may reduce the number of nigral cell bodies [8, 18]. METH toxicity against DA cell bodies and axons relates to an increase of DA release and oxidative species [19]. In fact, METH alters the vesicular storage of DA [20–22], it inhibits physiological DA metabolism, which is naturally operated by MAO-A [23, 24], and it reverts and/or inhibits the activity of the plasma membrane DA transporter (DAT), thus leading to a loss of DAT-binding sites [1, 25, 26]. All these effects contribute to rise of dramatically free DA levels within the cytosol of DA-containing cells. Since DA is no longer metabolized by MAO-A, it undergoes self-oxidation and spontaneous conversion to DA quinones, which in turn generate highly reactive oxidative species [27, 28]. In this way, a redox imbalance is generated by METH, which is detrimental for the integrity of both axon terminals and cell bodies where oxidized proteins, lipids, and nucleic acids are generated [29, 30]. A key molecular mechanism of protein oxidation consists in binding to cysteinyl residues to generate disulphuric bridges, which alter protein conformation [28, 31]. In this way, misfolded proteins such as alpha-synuclein [6, 14], ubiquitin [6, 32], prion protein [33], and parkin [6, 34] are generated. Again, METH inhibits complex II of the mitochondrial respiratory chain, which further elevates oxidative species and increases the number of altered mitochondria [35–39]. METH also oxidizes lipids to produce highly reactive by-products such as 4-hydroxynonenal [34, 40, 41]. All these oxidized substrates represent a target for cell clearing systems, which promote their removal. Thus, autophagy (ATG) and ubiquitin-proteasome (UP) represent a powerful defense to counteract redox imbalance generated by such a drug of abuse, and they are both challenged by METH administration. In detail, UP activity is inhibited by METH [13, 15, 16, 34], while UP inhibitors produce subcellular alterations which overlap with those produced by METH [6, 14, 42]. In line with this, METH toxicity is enhanced by concomitant exposure to UP inhibitors [15, 43]. ATG is quickly engaged during METH in PC12 cells [22, 44] and *in vivo*, in the SNpc and striatum [6, 15, 45]. Similarly to UP inhibitors, ATG blockers worsen METH toxicity [37]. Despite a massive engagement of ATG, which should sort neuroprotection, its activity is impaired by METH itself since the high amount of substrates (misfolded proteins and damaged mitochondria) engulfs this clearing system [16, 37, 46]. Therefore, despite being ATG overexpressed following METH [22, 44], it is not considered to be effective due to a lack of its progression [37, 46]. Such a combined defect in cell clearing systems produced by METH paves the way to deleterious effects induced by oxidative species, which are abundantly produced by such a drug of abuse.

Recently, a cell clearing organelle, which possesses both ATG and UP components, was described. This organelle appears as a multilamellar vacuole, which carries both UP and ATG key antigens [47]. This organelle corresponds to the "autophagoproteasome" (APP) as being defined in the Glossary published in the consensus manuscript "Guidelines for the Use and Interpretation of Assays for Monitoring Autophagy (3rd Edition)" by Klionsky et al. [48]. In the recent manuscript, it was demonstrated that APP is strongly activated by mTOR inhibition [47]. In fact, when the mTOR inhibitor rapamycin is administered, roughly all UP-positive puncta detected by P20S immunostaining at confocal microscopy move towards LC3-positive vacuoles, thus producing a massive switch from cytosolic to compartmentalized proteasome [47]. Despite a strong involvement of UP and ATG per se during METH toxicity, no study so far investigated what happens to this merging organelle. In the present manuscript, we dissect the ultrastructural morphometry of both UP and ATG components in different cell compartments, alone and in combination to merge within the autophagoproteasome (APP), under the effects of various METH doses at different time intervals. A variety of techniques were used to investigate these effects encompassing plain light microscopy, confocal microscopy, transmission electron microscopy, Western blotting, and coimmunoprecipitation. In detail, we aimed to assess whether (i) the autophagoproteasome was operating in the DA-containing PC12 cell line, (ii) the autophagoproteasome was modified following METH exposure, (iii) the amount of this organelle was associated with the modulation of METH toxicity, and (iv) whether these phenomena depend on mTOR activity as tested during either mTOR inhibition or activation.

2. Materials and Methods

2.1. Cell Cultures. In the current study, we chose the rat pheochromocytoma PC12 cell line, since these cells are able to synthetize and release DA and they express DA receptors on their external membrane. This is key in the case of METH, which exerts its mechanisms of action mainly by affecting molecular targets, which regulate DA transmission. In fact, the presence of DA and DA receptors, as well as DA uptake mechanisms, renders PC12 cell lines closer to DA terminals compared with their ancestors (i.e., chromaffin cells of the adrenal medulla). This concept is reinforced by the presence of the isoform of monoamine oxidase (MAO) type A, which characterizes also DA neurons, contrasting with the established prevalence of MAO type B within chromaffin cells of the adrenal medulla. Therefore, PC12 cells represent a model to predict the neurotoxicity of METH on central DA neurons with significant implications for the treatment of neuropsychiatric and neurodegenerative disorders [49].

The PC12 cell line was obtained from a cell bank (IRCCS San Martino Institute, Genova). The cells were grown in RPMI 1640 medium (Sigma-Aldrich, St. Louis, MO, USA) supplemented with heat inactivated 10% horse serum (HS, Sigma) and 5% fetal bovine serum (FBS, Sigma), penicillin (50 IU/ml)/streptomycin (50 mg/ml, Sigma), under standard culture conditions in a humidified atmosphere containing 5% CO_2 at 37°C. Experiments took place during the log phase of cell growth. At this time, cells were seeded into cell culture plates and they were incubated at 37°C in 5% CO_2 for further 24 hours. In particular, for transmission electron microscopy (TEM) and coimmunoprecipitation experiments, 1×10^6 PC12 cells were seeded in culture dishes in a final volume of 5 ml. For Western blotting, 5×10^5 cells were seeded in six-well plates in a final volume of 2 ml/well. Finally, for confocal microscopy experiments, 5×10^4 cells were grown on polylysine slides placed in 24-well plates at a final volume of 1 ml/well.

In order to study METH-induced toxicity, PC12 cells were treated with different doses of METH (1 nM, 10 nM, 100 nM, 1 μM, and 10 μM) for 72 hours. In a second set of experiments, PC12 cells were treated with 1 μM or 10 μM of METH for different time exposures (12, 24, and 72 hours). A study from Melega et al. [50] reports data deriving from an i.v. intake of 1000 mg/day METH in humans, approximately corresponding to 10 mg/kg, which can produce neurotoxicity (i.e., loss of DA terminals and neurons) in mice. However, since the present study was designed to assess the ultrastructural effects of METH on specific subcellular organelles, apart from neurotoxicity, we chose METH doses from $1 \mu M$ to $10 \mu M$ based on the previous studies [6, 15, 37]. In our hands, at doses between 10 and $100 \mu M$ of METH in PC12 cell lines, only a few cells survive, and this is further exacerbated by METH doses above $100 \mu M$ [6, 43]. This is also due to intrinsic vulnerability of PC12 cells to DA-increasing agents, which explains such a discrepancy with DA neurons [49]. In fact, PC12 cells possess inherent features, which render these cells particularly sensitive to high doses of DA. These include (i) the presence of VMAT-1, which is less specific for the vesicular uptake of catecholamines when compared with its homolog VMAT-2 expressed in the brain, and (ii) low levels of the DAT, thus reduced cytosolic reuptake of DA. Thus, these cells have a limited ability to adapt the neurotransmitter synthesis and vesicle trafficking/release to the synaptic needs, which contrasts with the flexibility of DA neurons to respond appropriately to a releasing stimulus.

Further experiments were carried out to evaluate the effects produced on METH toxicity and APP components by the modulation of mTOR activity. In these experiments, cells were exposed to 100 nM rapamycin and 50 mM asparagine, alone or in combination with $10 \mu M$ METH, for 72 hours. When it was combined with METH, rapamycin was added 2 h before METH, while asparagine was administered 30 min before METH. The doses of asparagine and rapamycin were selected based on the previous papers [32, 47]. However, to validate these doses in these experimental conditions, the inhibition or activation of mTOR activity for each compound was tested by measuring the downstream product pS6.

METH and asparagine were dissolved directly in the culture medium. Dilutions of rapamycin were obtained by a stock solution (1 mM of rapamycin dissolved in the culture medium containing 10% DMSO).

2.2. Transmission Electron Microscopy.

PC12 cells were centrifuged at $1000g$ for 5 min. After removal of the supernatant, the pellet was rinsed in PBS before being fixed. The fixing procedure was carried out with a solution containing 2.0% paraformaldehyde and 0.1% glutaraldehyde in 0.1 M PBS (pH 7.4) for 90 min at 4°C. This aldehyde concentration minimally covers antigen epitopes, while fairly preserving tissue architecture. After removal of the fixing solution, specimens were postfixed in 1% OsO_4 for 1 h at 4°C; they were dehydrated in ethanol and finally embedded in epoxy resin.

For ultrastructural morphometry, grids containing nonserial ultrathin sections (40–50 nm thick) were examined at TEM, at a magnification of 8000x. Several grids were analyzed in order to count a total number of 50–100 cells for each experimental group. In particular, when counting cell death, 50 cells per group were sampled, while 50 cells per group were sampled to carry out ultrastructural morphometry and immunogold counts; when counting APP, 100 cells per group were used. Each count was repeated at least 3 times by three blind observers.

Plain TEM was implemented by a postembedding immunocytochemistry procedure for antibodies against LC3 and

TABLE 1: Sources and references for antibodies reported in the present study.

Antibodies	References
LC3 (Abcam)	[47, 51–54]
LC3 (Sigma)	[55–57]
Proteasome 20S (Abcam)	[47, 58–61]
Alpha-synuclein (BD Biosciences)	[62–66]
SQSTM1-p62 (Abcam)	[67–71]
Phospho-p70 S6 kinase (Thr421/Ser424) (Cell Signaling Technologies)	[72–76]

P20S, which were used as markers of ATG and UP pathways, respectively. Antibody specificity was assessed by a number of studies which were partially reported in Table 1 (extramural evidence), and they were routinely used for at least 10 years in our lab (intramural evidence) [51–76].

It is worth mentioning that LC3 and P20S antigens were chosen as markers of ATG vacuoles (LC3 alone) or APP vacuoles (LC3 combined with P20S) accordingly to the manuscript "Guidelines for the Use and Interpretation of Assays for Monitoring Autophagy (3rd Edition)" [48].

Sometimes, in order to validate the count for ATG vacuoles, beclin 1 was used instead of or in combination with LC3 for detecting early time points. No significant difference between LC3- and beclin 1-based counts was detected; thus, results fully express the amount of LC3. At the end of the plain TEM or immunocytochemistry procedure, ultrathin sections were stained with uranyl acetate and lead citrate, and they were finally examined using a JEOL JEM-100SX transmission electron microscope (JEOL, Tokyo, Japan).

2.2.1. Postembedding Immunocytochemistry.

Fixing and postfixing solutions and the use of epoxy resin were validated in our previous studies for immunogold-based ultrastructural morphometry [47]. In fact, a combination of aldehydes, OsO_4, and epoxy resin allows a minimal epitope covering, while preserving cell ultrastructure [47, 77, 78]. In particular, OsO_4 binds to cell membranes, thus enhancing the contrast of cytosolic compartments, and it prevents the formation of membrane's artifacts, which may mimic vacuoles. Moreover, epoxy resin is advantageous over acrylic resin in preserving cell morphology.

Postembedding procedure was carried out on ultrathin sections collected on nickel grids, which were incubated on droplets of aqueous sodium metaperiodate ($NaIO_4$), for 30 min, at room temperature in order to remove OsO_4. $NaIO_4$ is an oxidizing agent allowing a closer contact between antibodies and antigens by removing OsO_4 [77]. This step improves the visualization of immunogold particles specifically located within a sharp context of cell integrity, and it allows the counting of molecules within specific cell compartments. Then, grids were washed in PBS and incubated in a blocking solution containing 10% goat serum and 0.2% saponin for 20 min, at room temperature. Grids were then incubated with the primary antibody solution containing both rabbit anti-LC3 (Abcam, Cambridge, UK, diluted 1:50) and mouse anti-P20S (Abcam, Cambridge,

UK, diluted 1 : 50), with 0.2% saponin and 1% goat serum in a humidified chamber overnight, at 4°C. After washing in PBS, grids were incubated with the secondary antibodies conjugated with gold particles (10 nm mean diameter, for gold particle anti-rabbit; 20 nm mean diameter, for gold particle anti-mouse, BB International), diluted 1 : 30 in PBS containing 0.2% saponin and 1% goat serum for 1 h, at room temperature. Control sections were incubated with the secondary antibody only. After washing in PBS, grids were incubated on droplets of 1% glutaraldehyde for 3 min; additional extensive washing of grids on droplets of distilled water was carried out to remove extensive salt traces and prevent precipitation of uranyl acetate.

2.2.2. Ultrastructural Morphometry. In order to distinguish vacuoles (ATG from APP) and to count immunogold particles (ranging from 10 nm to 20 nm), observations were performed directly at TEM at a magnification of 8000x [79] since this represents the minimal magnification at which immunogold particles and all cell organelles can be concomitantly identified.

We started to count from a grid square corner in order to scan the whole cell pellet within that grid square, which was randomly identified. Assessments of vacuoles and measurement of immunogold particles were carried out according to Lenzi et al. [47].

Briefly, we counted the number of unstained vacuoles per cell as vacuoles with single, double, or multiple membranes possessing the same electron density of the surrounding cytoplasm or partly containing some electron dense structure. In each cell, we counted the total number of immunogold anti-LC3 and/or anti-P20S particles placed either in the cytoplasm or within vacuoles and we expressed the number of immunogold particles as the mean per cell. Finally, we counted the number of APPs per cell as a single, double, and multiple membrane vacuoles, in which immunogold particles of LC3 (10 nm) and P20S (20 nm) were colocalized.

2.3. Light Microscopy. For light microscopy, PC12 cells were harvested and centrifuged at 800 *g* for 5 min to obtain a pellet, which was further resuspended in 0.5 ml of the culture medium in order to obtain a dense cell suspension. This was layered on glass slide spinning at 15,000 *g* for 10 min by cytospin (Cytospin 4, Thermo Fisher).

2.3.1. Haematoxylin and Eosin Staining and Cell Count. Cells were fixed with 4% paraformaldehyde in PBS for 15 min and plunged in PBS and then in haematoxylin solution (Sigma) for 20 min. Haematoxylin staining was stopped by washing in distilled water and followed by plunging cells in the eosin solution (Sigma) for a few min. After repeated washing to remove the excess of dye, cells were dehydrated in increasing alcohol solutions, clarified in xylene, and finally covered with the DPX mounting medium (Sigma). Cell count was performed at light microscopy at 40x magnification. Briefly, for each experimental group, the number of stained cells detectable after each specific treatment was counted and expressed as a percentage of the control group. These values represent the means of six independent cell counts.

Moreover, we counted the number of giant cells occasionally observed after 10 *μ*M METH. We considered as giant cells those owning a diameter higher than 14–15 *μ*m. The amount of giant cells out of the total number of cells counted on the glass slide was expressed as a percentage, for each experimental group. The values represent the means of six independent cell counts.

2.3.2. Trypan Blue. For trypan blue staining, PC12 cells were seeded at a density of 1×10^4 cells/well and they were preincubated for 24 h. After METH treatments, PC12 cells were collected and centrifuged at 800 *g* for 5 min. The cell pellet was suspended in the culture medium, and 25 *μ*l of cell suspension was added to a solution of 1% trypan blue (62.5 *μ*l) and PBS (37.5 *μ*l). Cells were then incubated for 10 min, at room temperature. Soon after, 10 *μ*l aliquot of this solution was counted at light microscopy using a Bürker glass chamber. Viable and nonviable cells were counted, and cell death was expressed as percentage of trypan blue frankly positive cells out of the total cells. The values represent the means of three independent cell counts.

2.4. Confocal Microscopy. PC12 cells were washed in PBS and fixed with paraformaldehyde 4% for 5 min at room temperature. Antigen retrieval was carried out in 100 mM Tris-HCl, 5% urea at 95°C, for 10 min. After washing in PBS, cells were permeabilized in 0.2% Triton X-100, for 10 min. They were blocked in PBS containing 0.1% Tween-20, supplemented with 1% bovine serum albumin (BSA) and 23 mg/ml of glycine, for 30 min. Afterwards, cells were incubated overnight at 4°C in 1% BSA in PBS-T containing 1 : 50 anti-LC3 antibody (Abcam) and 1 : 30 anti-P20S (Abcam). Finally, cells were incubated for 1 h with fluorophore-conjugated secondary antibodies (1 : 200; goat anti-rabbit Alexa 488 and goat anti-mouse Alexa 594, Molecular Probes, Life Technologies) in 1% BSA in PBS-T at room temperature. Then, cells were washed in PBS, and they were mounted in ProLong Diamond Antifade Mountant (Molecular Probes, Life Technologies). The analysis was performed using a Leica TCSSP5 confocal laser scanning microscope (Leica Microsystems, Mannheim, Germany) using a sequential scanning procedure. Confocal images were collected every 400 nm intervals through the *z*-axis of each section by means of 63x oil lenses. Z-stacks of serial optical planes were analyzed using the Multicolor Package software (Leica Microsystems). Negative controls were carried out by omitting primary antibodies.

2.5. Coimmunoprecipitation Assay. PC12 cells were homogenized at 4°C in an ice-cold lysis buffer. One microliter of homogenates was used for protein determinations. 30 *μ*g of proteins from whole cell lysates was loaded to perform Western blotting before coimmunoprecipitation. *β*-Actin was used as a loading control for protein levels from the whole cell lysates, on which immunoprecipitation of LC3 was then performed.

Proteins (800 *μ*g) were incubated at 4°C overnight with primary rabbit anti-LC3 antibody (2 *μ*g for each sample; Sigma-Aldrich, Milan, Italy). The antibody/antigen complex was pulled out of the sample using protein A-Sepharose beads. This process isolated the protein of interest from the rest of the sample. Proteins were separated on sodium dodecyl sulphate-polyacrylamide gel (12%) and transferred on immuno-PVDF membrane (Bio-Rad, Milan, Italy) for 1 h. Filter was blocked for 1 h in Tween-20 Tris-buffered saline (TTBS) (100 mM Tris-HCl, 0.9% NaCl, 1% Tween 20, pH 7.4) containing 5% nonfat dry milk. Blot was incubated at 4°C overnight with mouse monoclonal primary antibody anti-P20S (1 : 100, Abcam), mouse monoclonal anti-alpha-synuclein (1 : 1000, BD Biosciences), and rabbit monoclonal anti-SQSTM1 (anti-p62, 1 : 1000, Abcam, Milan, Italy); it was washed 3 times with the TTBS buffer and then incubated for 1 h with secondary peroxidase-coupled antibody (anti-mouse, 1 : 7000; anti-rabbit, 1 : 7000; Calbiochem, Milan, Italy). Then, blot was stripped with a solution of distilled water and 3.5% acetic acid in the presence of 1% NaCl 5 M. Blot was kept in this solution for 20 min, and then, it was washed in TTBS (8 washes for 5 min). Finally, to verify the correct immunoprecipitation, blot was incubated with primary rabbit anti-LC3 antibody (1 : 6000, Sigma-Aldrich), for 1 h, at room temperature. Filter was washed 3 times with the TTBS buffer and then incubated for 1 h with secondary peroxidase-coupled antibody (anti-rabbit, 1 : 7000; Calbiochem, Milan, Italy). Immunostaining was revealed by enhanced chemiluminescence (GE Healthcare, Milan, Italy). The total amount of proteins measured through optical density was normalized for total β-actin, which was measured in whole cell lysates, since β-actin is not present in LC3 immunoprecipitates. Thus, readers should consider that such a normalization could not refer to the immunoprecipitated blotted proteins, but rather to the total amount of proteins in the very same cells used to carry out the immunoprecipitate.

2.6. Western Blotting. PC12 cells were lysed in a buffer (100 mM Tris-HCl, pH 7.5, 5 M NaCl, 0.5 m EDTA, 10% SDS, 1% NP40, IGEPAL), containing protease and phosphatase inhibitor, and centrifuged at 15,000 g for 20 min at 4°C. The supernatant was collected, and protein concentration was determined using a protein assay kit (Sigma). Samples containing 40 μg of total proteins were solubilized and electrophoresed on a 12% sodium dodecyl sulphate- (SDS-) polyacrylamide gel. Following electrophoresis, proteins were transferred to the nitrocellulose membrane (Bio-Rad Laboratories, MI, Italy). The membrane was immersed in a blocking solution (3% nonfat dried milk in 20 mM Tris and 137 mM NaCl at pH 7.6 containing 0.05% Tween-20) for 2 h on a plate shaker. Subsequently, the membrane was incubated with mouse anti-pS6 primary antibody (1 : 2000; Millipore, Burlington, MA, USA) overnight at 4°C on the plate shaker. Blot was probed with horseradish peroxidase-labeled secondary antibodies, and the bands were visualized with enhanced chemiluminescence reagents (Bio-Rad Laboratories). Image analysis was carried out by ChemiDoc System (Bio-Rad Laboratories).

2.7. Statistics. For ultrastructural morphometry data were given as an absolute number concerning the following measurements: (i) unstained vacuoles, (ii) LC3-positive vacuoles,

(iii) P20S-positive vacuoles, (iv) LC3 + P20S-positive vacuoles (APP), and (v) immunogold particles (including LC3 and P20S). Ratios were used to express (i) the number of LC3 immunogold particles within vacuoles out of the number of cytoplasmic LC3 immunogold particles and (ii) the number of P20S immunogold particles within vacuoles out of the number of cytoplasmic P20S immunogold particles. All data were reported as the means ± SEM per cell from 50 cells per group in all counts but the LC3 + P20S which was expressed as the means ± SEM from 100 cells per group.

Data on the amount of cell death were expressed as the percentage of the mean ± SEM dead cells out of the total cell number in each grid being analyzed (i.e., 5 total grids, each containing at least 10 cells, for a total of 50 cells for each experimental group).

For confocal microscopy, the amount of P20S + LC3 puncta was counted. Values were expressed as the mean number of puncta ± SEM per cell counted in each slide in two separate experiments (each one carried out in duplicate).

For Western blot optical density was expressed as the means ± SEM calculated in six separate experiments.

All statistical analyses were carried out by using one-way analysis of variance, ANOVA, followed by Sheffè's post hoc analysis. Null hypothesis (H0) was rejected for $p \leq 0.05$.

3. Results and Discussion

3.1. Dose and Time Dependencies of METH-Induced Unstained Vacuoles. Confirming previous data, METH administration for 72 h filled catecholamine cells with vacuoles, as reported in representative micrographs (Figure 1(a)) and counted in the graph of Figure 1(b). As measured in Figure 1(b), unstained vacuoles increase dose-dependently within a wide range of METH doses (from 1 nM up to 1 μM). At the dose of 1 μM, the number of METH-induced unstained vacuoles reached the peak. Whereas, for the highest dose of METH (10 μM), the number of unstained vacuoles dropped down to levels measured following low METH doses (1 nM and 10 nM). This suggests that at 10 μM METH dose, toxicity occludes the development of novel intracellular structures, even in spared cells. Therefore, the doses of METH 1 μM and 10 μM were chosen for the time dependence study. As reported in representative micrographs of Figure 1(c), a time-dependent increase of unstained vacuoles was produced by METH at the 1 μM dose from 12 h up to 72 h. These effects were evidenced by staining with arrows the unstained vacuoles in each experimental condition to relate representative pictures to counts reported in the graph in Figure 1(d). As expected, even the dose of 10 μM METH at 72 h time-dependently increases the number of unstained vacuoles (Figure 1(f)). This was evident in representative micrographs of Figure 1(e); we investigated the effects of such a METH dose at earlier time intervals (representative pictures of Figure 1(e)). These effects were evidenced by staining with arrows the unstained vacuoles at each time interval to relate representative pictures to counts reported in the graph in Figure 1(f). The number of unstained vacuoles is consistent with the time course and dose dependency of multilamellar

(a)

(b)

(c)

(d)

(e)

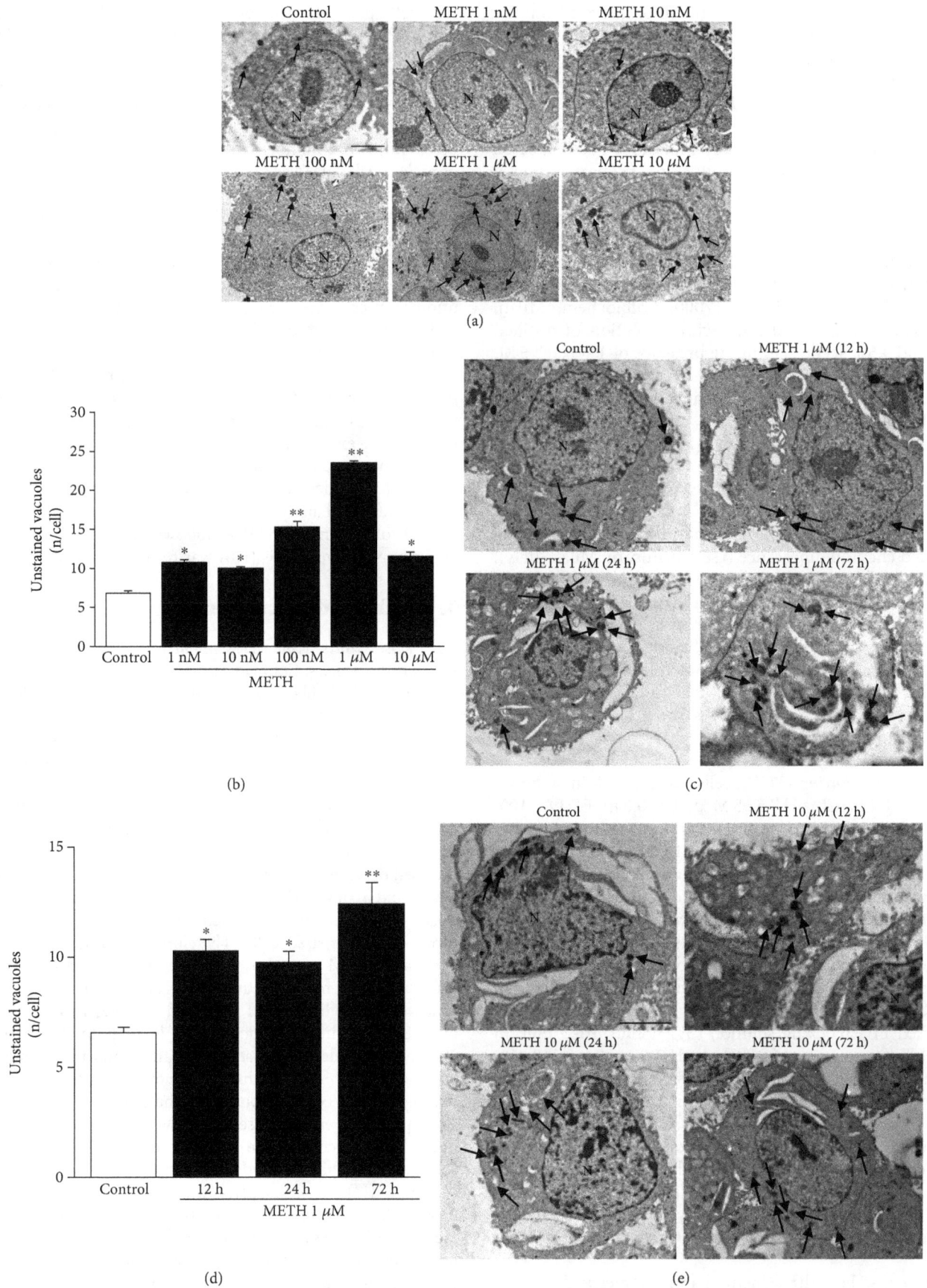

Figure 1: Continued.

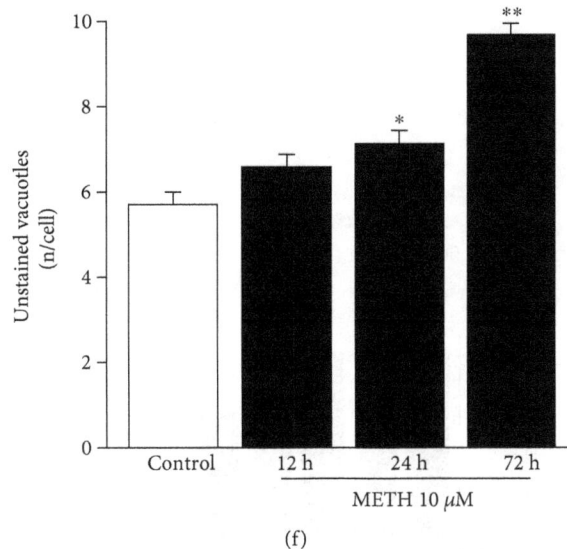

(f)

FIGURE 1: METH increases the amount of unstained vacuoles dose- and time-dependently. (a) Dose-dependent representative pictures of unstained vacuoles (arrows) of control and METH at 72 h treated cells at different doses. (b) Dose-dependent graph of unstained vacuoles per cell at 72 h. (c) Time-dependent representative pictures of unstained vacuoles (arrows) of control and 1 μM METH-treated cells. (d) Time-dependent graph of unstained vacuoles per cell of control and 1 μM METH-treated cells. (e) Time-dependent representative pictures of unstained vacuoles (arrows) of control and 10 μM METH-treated cells. (f) Time-dependent graph of unstained vacuoles per cell of control and 10 μM METH-treated cells. Values are given as the mean number of unstained vacuoles, which were counted in 50 cells per group. Error bars represent the standard error of the mean. $^*p \leq 0.05$ vs. control; $^{**}p \leq 0.05$ vs. other groups. N = nucleus. Scale bar = 1 μm.

bodies produced by METH, which we previously described under a different name (whorls) in this cell line [6].

3.2. Dose and Time Dependencies of METH-Induced Cell Death.

When assessing the effects produced by a 10 μM dose of METH, there was a dramatic increase (roughly by half) in the amount of cell loss compared with controls and occasionally, giant cells appeared, which were never observed in controls (representative H&E staining of Figures 2(a) and 2(b); graph of Figure 2(c)). The counts for surviving cells carried out at H&E staining revealed a dose- and time-dependent decrease in cell survival (graphs of Figures 2(d) and 2(e), respectively). This was dramatic at 72 h following 10 μM METH. These same results were reproduced by trypan blue-positive counts for dying cells, which confirmed a dose- and time-dependent increase in dying cells (graphs of Figures 2(f) and 2(g), respectively). A similar phenomenon (cell death in the same range of doses and times induced by METH administration) was detected at TEM (representative TEM micrographs of Figures 2(g) and 2(h), respectively). The count of dying cells (either necrotic or apoptotic) at TEM for METH and controls (Figures 2(h) and 2(i), respectively) was overlapping with that reported for trypan blue staining. Remarkably dying cells were higher than controls also following the dose of 1 μM (at 72 h, Figures 2(j) and 2(k)). The pronounced toxicity induced by 10 μM METH is likely to impair cell metabolism even in spared cells, which when analyzed at 72 h own much less vacuoles compared with other doses.

3.3. METH Alters Dose and Time Dependency of the Amount and Placement of LC3 Particles.

In order to identify ATG and UP components within METH-treated cells, we carried out ultrastructural morphometry by using 10 nm immunogold particles to reveal LC3, while 20 nm immunogold particles were used to stain P20S. Following METH administration, an increase in LC3-stained vacuoles was detected starting at the dose of 100 nM METH, while no increase compared with controls was counted in a lower range of doses (between 1 nM and 10 nM, Figure 3(a)). This was quite unexpected since the count of unstained vacuoles provided in Figure 1(b) indicates a significant increase (almost two-fold) compared with controls even at the dose of 1 nM METH. This is a key point, since unstained vacuoles are considered to correspond to pure ATG vacuoles. Thus, one would expect an overlapping between unstained and LC3-positive vacuoles. Such a discrepancy leaves the issue open on which the nature of METH-induced unstained vacuoles might be. In fact, these vacuoles were induced by METH administration since they increased two-fold compared with controls at the dose of 1 nM and 10 nM METH.

A lack of LC3 staining in these vacuoles for low METH doses suggests that these may not correspond to authentic ATG vacuoles, although they increase two-fold with respect to controls. Although the nature of these unstained vacuoles remains to be defined, the possibility exists that LC3 particles moving within ATG vacuoles remain undetected for these low METH doses. However, as shown in the graph of Figure 3(b), total LC3 particles in the cell for 1 nM and 10 nM METH do not increase either. This indicates a lack of ATG induction for low METH doses. Another possibility

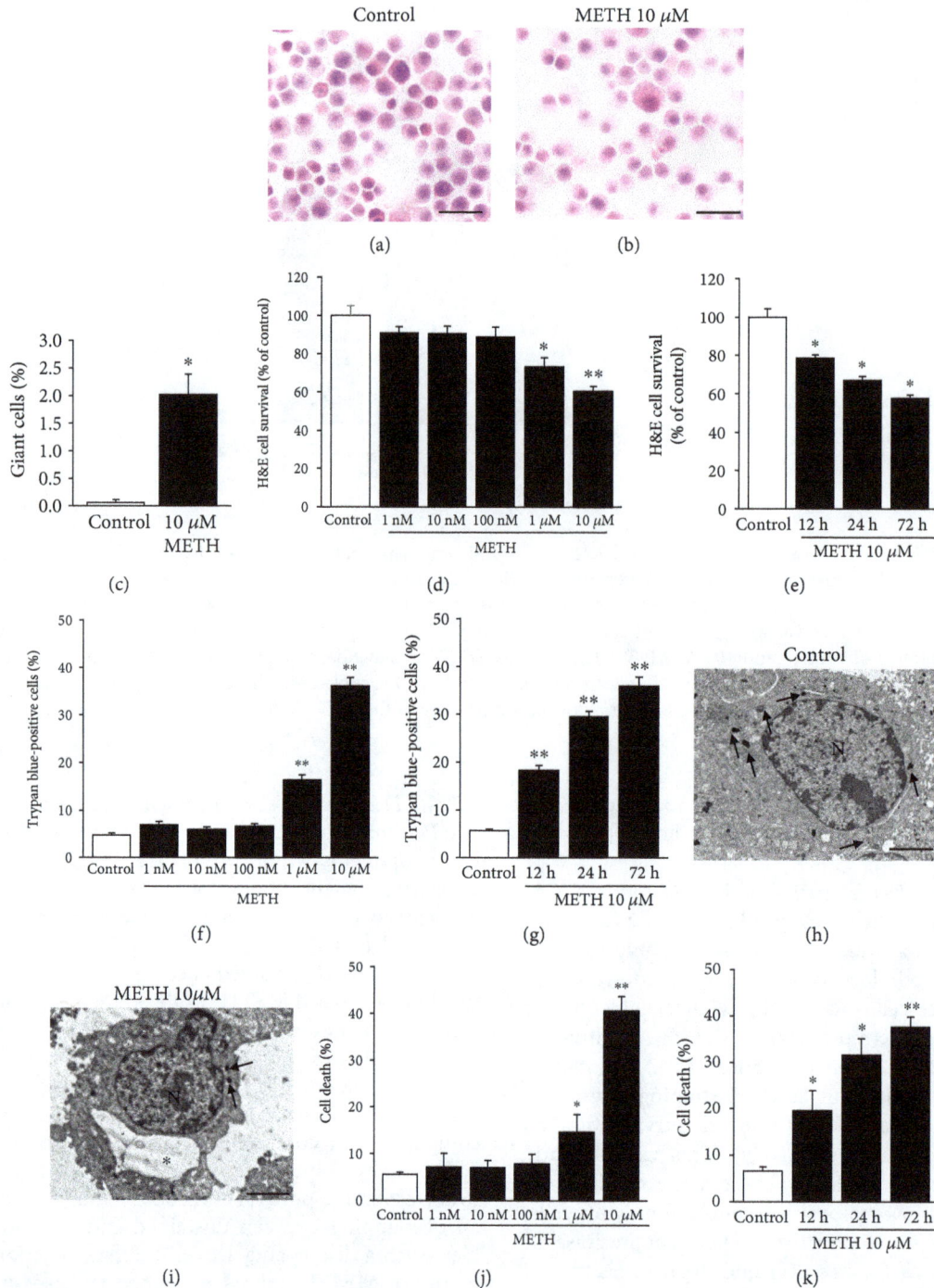

FIGURE 2: METH induces cell death time- and dose-dependently with a maximal effect at the 1 μM and 10 μM doses. (a) Representative H&E-stained picture from controls. (b) Representative H&E-stained picture following 10 μM METH at 72 h. (c) Graph reporting the percentage of giant cells counted in H&E-stained total cells from controls and METH at 72 h. (d) Dose-dependent graph of H&E-stained cells from control and METH at 72 h. (e) Time-dependent graph of H&E-stained cells from control and 10 μM METH-treated cells. (f) Dose-dependent graph of trypan blue-stained cells from control and METH at 72 h. (g) Time-dependent graph of trypan blue-stained cells from control and 10 μM METH-treated cells. (h) Representative micrograph from a control cell. (h) Representative micrograph from a control cell. (i) Representative micrograph from a METH cell at 72 h. (j) Dose-dependent graph of cell death from control and METH at 72 h. (m) Time-dependent graph of cell death from control and 10 μM METH-treated cells. For the graphs in (c)–(g), values are given as the percentage of cell counted in two triplicates ($n = 6$). For the graphs in (j) and (k), values are given as the percentage of cell counted on 5 grids. Error bars represent the standard error of the mean. $^{*}p \leq 0.05$ vs. control, $^{**}p \leq 0.05$ vs. other groups. Arrows point to vacuoles; asterisk (*) indicates a large vacuole. N = nucleus. Scale bar = 23.4 μm (a, b) and 2 μm (h, i).

(a)

(b)

(c)

(d)

(e)

(f)

(g)

(h)

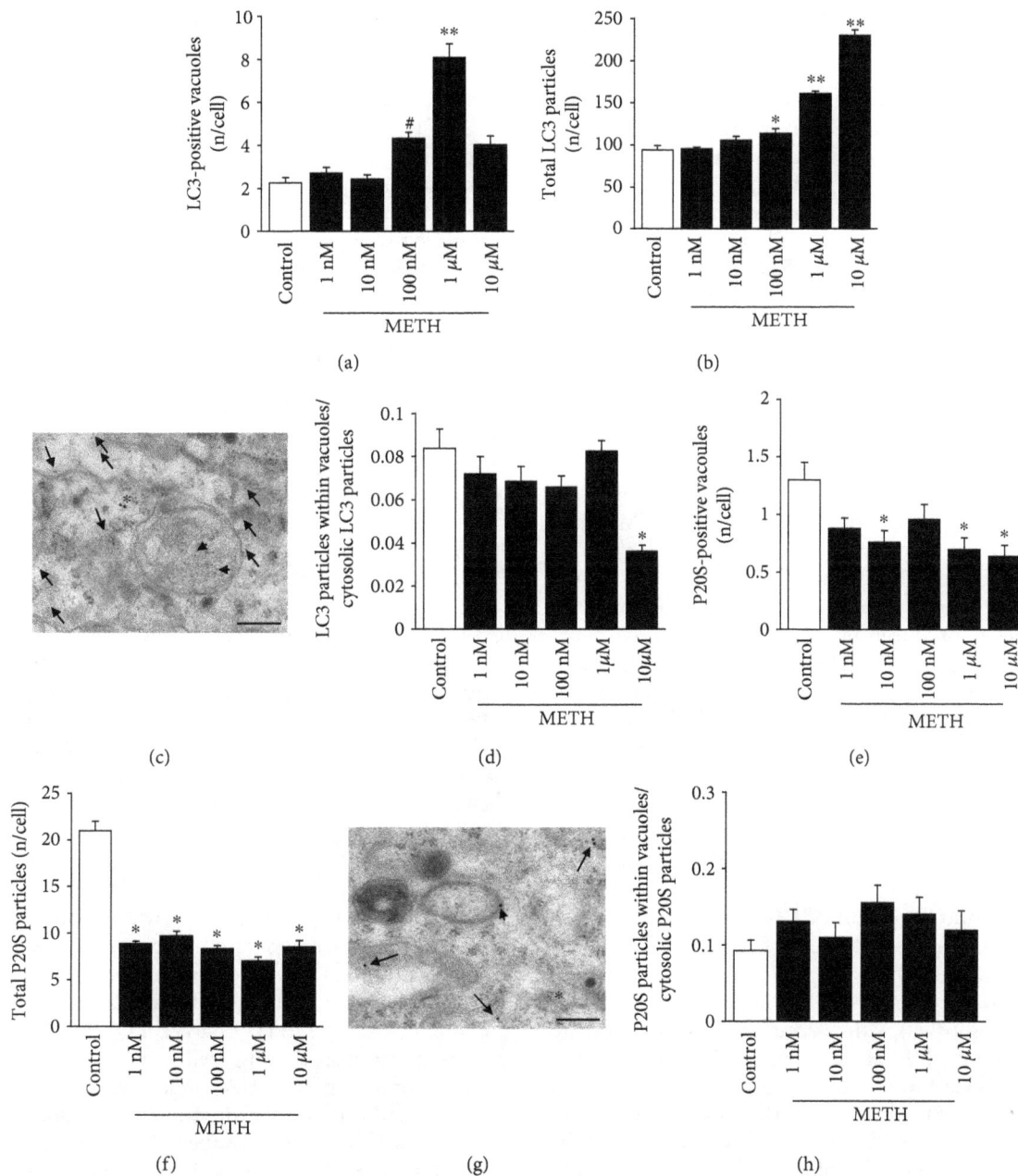

FIGURE 3: METH alters the amount and placement of LC3 and P20S particles dose-dependently, with P20S being more sensitive than LC3. (a) Dose-dependent graph of the number of LC3-positive vacuoles per cell from controls and METH at 72 h. (b) Dose-dependent graph of total LC3 particles per cell from controls and METH at 72 h. (c) Representative micrograph of LC3-positive vacuole from 10 μM METH at 72 h. (d) Dose-dependent graph of the ratio between the numbers of LC3 particles within vacuoles with respect to cytosolic LC3 particles from controls and METH at 72 h. (e) Dose-dependent graph of the number of P20S-positive vacuoles per cell from controls and METH at 72 h. (f) Dose-dependent graph of total P20S particles per cell from controls and METH at 72 h. (g) Representative micrograph of P20S-positive vacuoles from 10 μM METH at 72 h. (h) Dose-dependent graph of the ratio between the numbers of P20S particles within vacuoles with respect to cytosolic P20S particles from controls and METH at 72 h. Values are given as the mean number of LC3 or P20S particles and vacuoles counted in 50 cells per group. Error bars represent the standard error of the mean. $^*p \leq 0.05$ vs. control; $^{**}p \leq 0.05$ vs. other groups; $^\#p \leq 0.05$ vs. control and 1 nM and 10 nM METH. Arrows point to free cytosolic LC3 (10 nm) or P20S (20 nm); arrowheads point to LC3 (10 nm) or P20S (20 nm) within vacuoles; asterisk (*) indicates P20S in the cytosol (c) and LC3 in the cytosol (g). Scale bar = 200 nm.

deals with the dynamics of ATG vacuoles, which could mature before LC3 is increased. This hypothesis remains unlikely, since other markers, such as beclin 1, which stains ATG vacuoles earlier than LC3, do not provide any staining either. Moreover, LC3 staining is a gold standard to define

autophagosomes, and 72 h should be enough to complete the process. Instead, even at this time interval for low (1 nM and 10 nM) METH doses, LC3 particles do not increase in any cell compartments including the cytosol. This suggests that 1 nM and 10 nM METH do not really increase

ATG. Therefore, unstained vacuoles, which minimally occur in control cells and selectively increase following very low METH doses, are likely to belong to other pathways (such as the exosomal compartment). This hypothesis is currently under investigation in the lab. Vacuolar compartments other than ATG may be recruited for low METH doses. It is likely that DA turnover promoted by METH increases vesicle recycling, which may account for these unstained vacuoles. On the other hand, the lowest effects of METH on membrane trafficking may affect other compartments such as retromers or exosomes, which are more bound to cell release than ATG activation.

The increase in vacuoles measured for doses above 10 nM corresponds to LC3-positive (ATG) vacuoles. Data on the amount of LC3-positive vacuoles (shown in representative Figure 3(c)) parallels data on LC3 particles reported in the graph of Figure 3(b). In fact, they increase significantly only at the dose of 100 nM, while they do not differ from controls at low METH doses (1 nM and 10 nM METH). Thus, METH increases LC3 particles (Figure 3(b)) and LC3-positive vacuoles (Figure 3(a)) only at doses higher than 10 nM, although no compartmentalization of LC3 within vacuoles is produced by any dose of METH (graph of Figure 3(d)). In contrast, the trend indicates a dispersion rather than a polarization of LC3 particles from cell vacuoles towards the cytosol. This is indicated by the finding that the ratio of vacuolar vs. cytosolic LC3 particles following METH decreases dose-dependently (Figure 3(d)), which indicates a METH-induced loss of LC3 compartmentalization. Such an uncoupling between LC3 and ATG vacuoles is a novel finding in METH toxicity. In fact, so far, METH was thought to impair ATG machinery by engulfing ATG vacuoles, which become stagnant and filled with LC3. The present data show that, under METH, ATG vacuoles are impaired already in their maturation. In fact, for low METH doses, LC3 is not increased, while for higher METH doses, LC3 increases more in the cytosol than within vacuoles. It looks like that in these conditions (METH doses up to 1 μM), the drive which polarizes LC3 towards the ATG machinery is weakened. At 10 μM METH, there is a further drop in the ratio between vacuolar and cytosolic LC3 particles, which is likely to be due to a concomitant loss of cell ability to build organelles for toxic METH doses. This latter finding is confirmed by the fact that 10 μM METH strongly increases free LC3 particles compared with the dose of 1 μM, but the number of LC3-positive ATG vacuoles at 10 μM is roughly a half of that counted at 1 μM.

These observations, despite being unexpected, provide also novel methodological insights into ATG. In fact, when using confocal microscopy following high METH doses, there is a strong increase in LC3 immunofluorescence, which is routinely interpreted as produced by stagnant vacuoles. However, ultrastructural morphometry demonstrates that an increase in LC3 immunostaining is indeed driven by free cytosolic noncompartmentalized LC3 rather than by vacuolar LC3.

We may summarize these latter data by stating that, under METH administration, there is a loss of compartmentalization of LC3 particles within vacuoles, despite an increased amount of both LC3 particles and vacuoles per se, which represents a novel insight in ATG and METH toxicity.

This leads to reconsider the significance of densely fluorescent LC3 spots detected at confocal microscopy following METH [16, 80]. The stoichiometric counts at TEM demonstrate that a greater contribution is provided by free cytosolic LC3. This is representatively evidenced in micrograph of Figure 3(c), and it is remarked by the ratio between compartmentalized LC3 particles in ATG vacuoles and free cytosolic LC3 particles (graph of Figure 3(d)). This demonstrates a lack of METH-induced LC3 compartmentalization with a trend towards "METH-induced LC3 dispersion." This is frankly evident for a neurotoxic dose of METH (10 μM) where a loss of fine subcellular compartments take place. As discussed for Figure 1(b), this is likely to reflect a degeneration of the subcellular trim of spared cells, which organize protein trafficking, where the ability to create various cell compartments is reduced.

3.4. METH Alters the Amount and Placement of P20S Particles. When counting P20S-positive vacuoles, these were consistently decreased compared with controls for all METH doses (Figures 3(e) and 3(g)). These findings were reproduced when counting P20S immunogold particles, which were markedly decreased following all METH doses (ranging between 1 nM and 10 μM, Figure 3(f)). Remarkably, this was replicated even for the highest dose of 10 μM METH, which was shown to suppress compartmentalization of LC3 within vacuoles (Figure 3(d)). It is likely that such a discrepancy is related to a different sensitivity of P20S compared with LC3 to the effects of METH. Again, no polarization of P20S towards vacuoles was induced by METH, which left the ratio unmodified between P20S particles within vacuoles and cytosolic P20S particles compared with controls (Figure 3(h)), although the trend was different compared with LC3.

It is surprising that the effects induced by METH on the number of the ATG marker LC3 follow a different dose-response curve compared with the effects induced on the number of the UP marker P20S. In fact, in the range of 1 nM to 10 nM doses, no alterations were produced by METH in the number of LC3 immunogold particles (Figure 3(b)), while at the dose of 1 nM of METH, the reduction of P20S immunogold particles was already maximal (roughly, a half of controls, Figure 3(f)). This suggests that the biochemical pathways involved (regulating either ATG or UP) possess a different dose-response curve being the UP maximally affected already at the lowest dose of METH. Thus, the P20S protein component is markedly sensitive to doses of METH, which are likely to be in the picomolar range.

As previously discussed, the lowest dose of METH (1 nM) doubled the number of unstained vacuoles without affecting neither LC3 particles nor LC3 vacuoles. In contrast, this very same dose reduced roughly to a half both P20S particles and P20S-positive vacuoles. It is worth noting that this METH dose is sufficient to double the DA release in PC12 cells [6]. Thus, it is likely that an increased amount of free DA may already impair the P20S proteasome. This is consistent with our previous study showing that, at the dose of 1 nM of

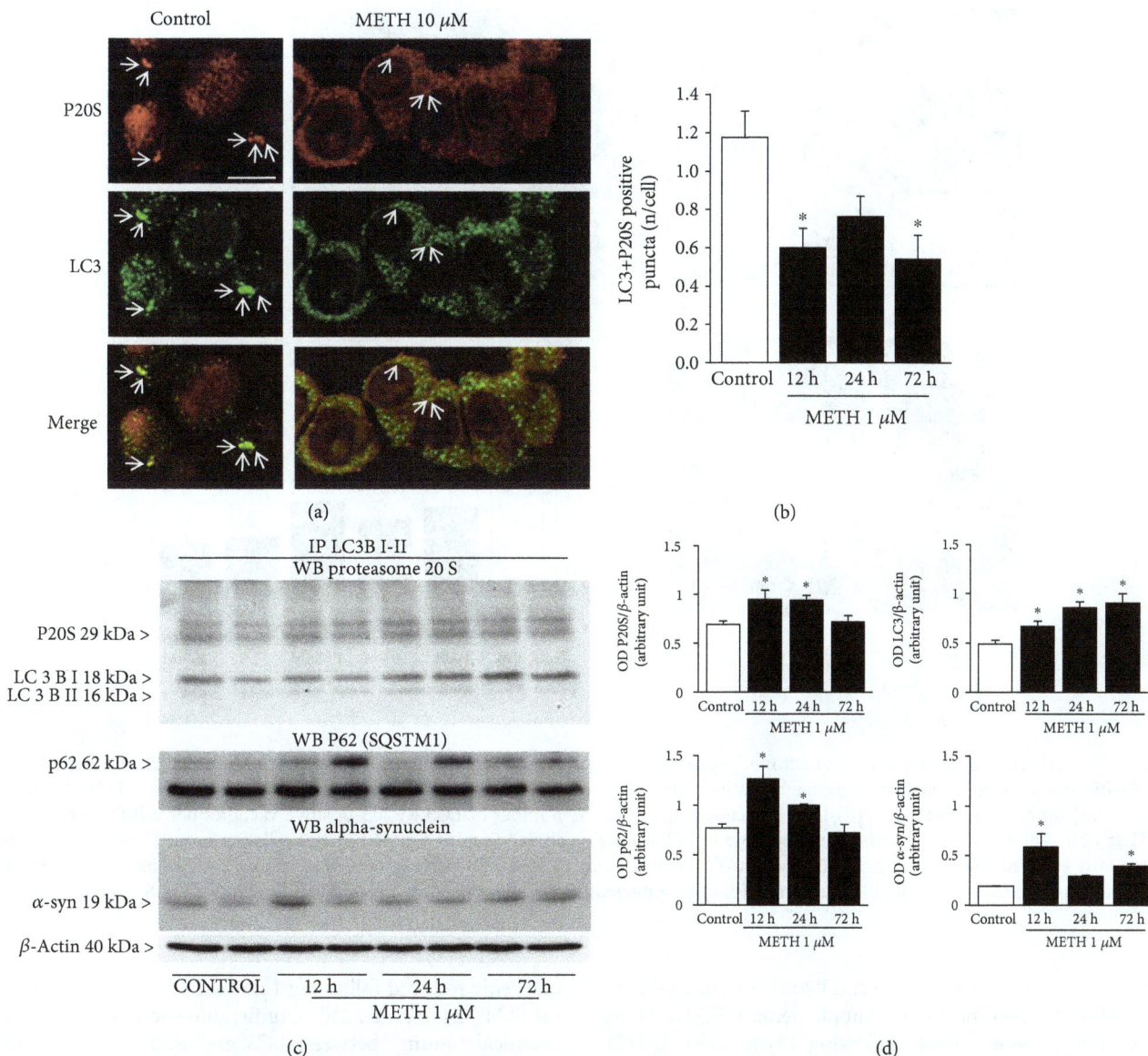

FIGURE 4: METH reduces the occurrence of the autophagoproteasome (APP) which hosts LC3, P20S, p62, and alpha-synuclein. (a) Representative immunofluorescence from controls and METH at 72 h. (b) Time-dependent graph of the number of LC3 + P20S-positive puncta per cell from control and METH at 1 μM. (c) P20S, p62, and alpha-synuclein Western blotting on LC3BI-II immunoprecipitates. (d) Densitometric analysis. Values are given as the optical density detected in four separate replicates ($n = 4$). Values are given as the mean number of LC3 + P20S puncta counted in 4 slides. Error bars represent the standard error of the mean. *$p \leq 0.05$ vs. control. Arrows point to P20S (red fluorescence) or LC3 (green fluorescence) or merge P20S and LC3 (orange fluorescence). Scale bar = 6.6 μm.

METH, P20S is already suppressed [43]. While this corresponds to a two-fold decrease in P20S-positive vacuoles (Figure 3(e)), the number of unstained METH-induced vacuoles increases by 2-fold ([6, 43]; present study in Figure 1(b)). Remarkably, UP inhibition enhances neurotransmitter release [81, 82]; in fact, proteasome inhibitors produce striatal DA release [83]. This is due to an effect of proteasome activity in the recycling of short-lived proteins from and towards the plasma membrane including DA receptors [84], which is compatible with the retromer hypothesis for unstained vacuoles expressed above [85]. It is demonstrated that increased DA stimulation disassembles

the proteasome structure, and it is related to sensitization [84]. Thus, a vicious circle may establish in which METH-induced DA release alters the proteasome structure, which in turn enhances DA release. This issue opens novel avenues to study the role of protein clearing systems in determining METH-induced sensitization. Thus, the increase in DA release occurring after 1 nM METH may be due to altered proteasome levels shown in this study. This is in line with imaging of P20S following METH compared with controls at confocal microscopy. In METH-treated cells, perimembranous rings of fluorescence appear instead of the diffuse fluorescent P20S staining occurring in controls (Figure 4(a)).

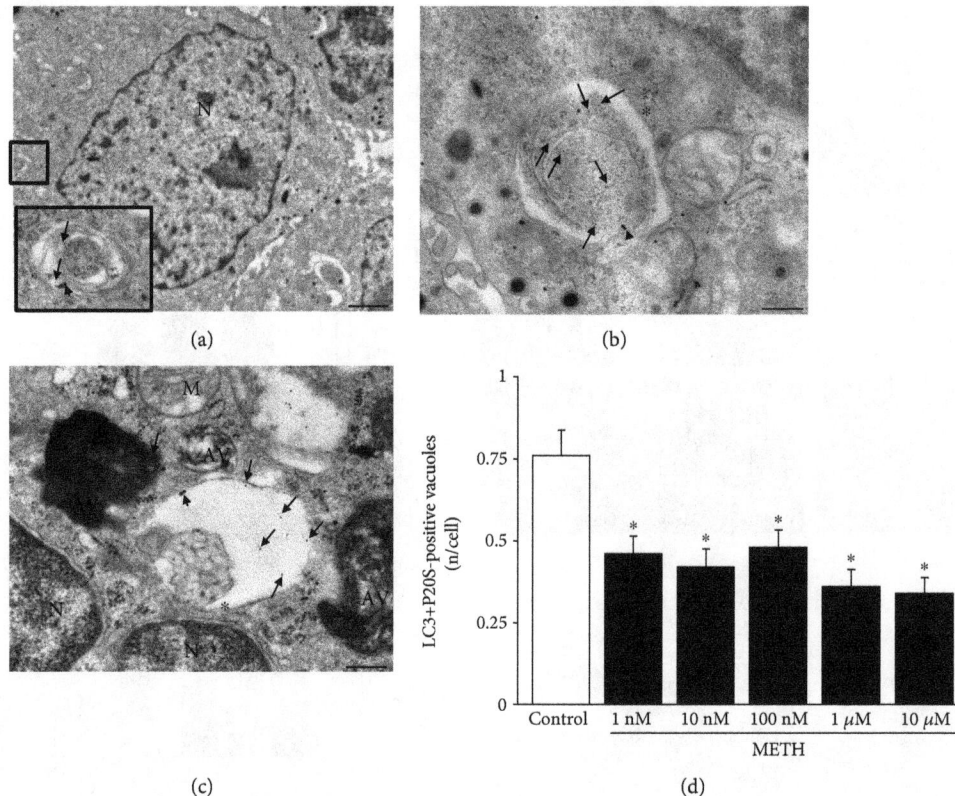

FIGURE 5: METH reduces the occurrence of autophagoproteasomes (APPs) dose-dependently. (a) Representative picture of a PC12 cell (low magnification) and an APP vacuole (high magnification). (b, c) Representative pictures of APP vacuoles stained for both LC3 (10 nm) and P20S (20 nm) immunogold particles. (d) Dose-dependent graph of the number of LC3 + P20S-positive vacuoles per cell from control and METH at 72 h. Values are given as the mean number of LC3 + P20S-positive vacuoles counted in 100 cells per group. Error bars represent the standard error of the mean. $^*p \leq 0.05$ vs. control. Arrows point to free LC3 particles (10 nm); arrowheads point to P20S particles (20 nm); asterisk (*) indicates a double membrane (b, c). N = nucleus; AV = autophagic vacuoles; M = mitochondrion. Scale bar = 220 nm.

The discrepancy between LC3 and P20S immunogold particles extends to the time course (Supplementary Figure 1). In fact, for longer time intervals following 10 μM METH, LC3 particles increase progressively (Supplementary Figure 1a), along with LC3-positive vacuoles (Supplementary Figure 1b) with a decreasing ratio between LC3 in vacuoles and LC3 in cytosol, which is time-dependent (Supplementary Figure 1c). P20S particles and vacuoles decrease slightly (Supplementary Figure 1d and Figure 1(e), respectively). The ratio between P20S in vacuoles and P20S in cytosol was similar for all time intervals (Supplementary Figure 1f). This suggests that a loss of compartmentalization for P20S is maximal already for the lowest dose of METH.

3.5. METH and Autophagoproteasome (APP).
In order to document the occurrence of APP in PC12 cells and its modulation at various doses and time intervals following METH, we used confocal microscopy to document the merging between P20S and LC3 particles. As shown in representative Figure 4(a), the punctum staining for P20S and LC3 was fairly merging in baseline conditions, while only some merging could be detected also following the highest dose of METH. When we counted the amount of merging puncta detected at confocal microscopy (Figure 4(b)), these were

markedly reduced following 1 μM METH at each time interval (12 h, 24 h, and 72 h). Confirming the hypothesis that a chemical binding between LC3 and P20S within vacuoles exists, we carried out Western blotting on LC3BI-II immunoprecipitates from whole cell lysates. In these experimental conditions, P20S was detected along with p62 (Figures 4(c) and 4(d)). The occurrence of p62 is the key since, as recently shown by Cohen-Kaplan et al. [86], p62 is pivotal in shuttling proteasome subunits within LC3-positive autophagosomes. In line with the key role played by both ATG and proteasome to metabolize alpha-synuclein [87, 88], we checked whether these merging organelles contain alpha-synuclein. In fact, alpha-synuclein is detected here within immunoprecipitates (Figures 4(c) and 4(d)). Incidentally, these findings indicate why, in biochemical studies, the metabolism of alpha-synuclein was attributed to ATG, UP, or both, depending on the study [89–91]. The present research paper demonstrates at the morphological level the occurrence of a single organelle hosting both UP and ATG components, which recruits alpha-synuclein (Figure 4(c)). When analyzed at ultrastructural morphometry, these merging units between P20S and LC3 appear as vacuoles owning different shapes and structures corresponding to autophagoproteasomes (APPs, Figures 4(a), 5(b), and 5(c)). It is remarkable that,

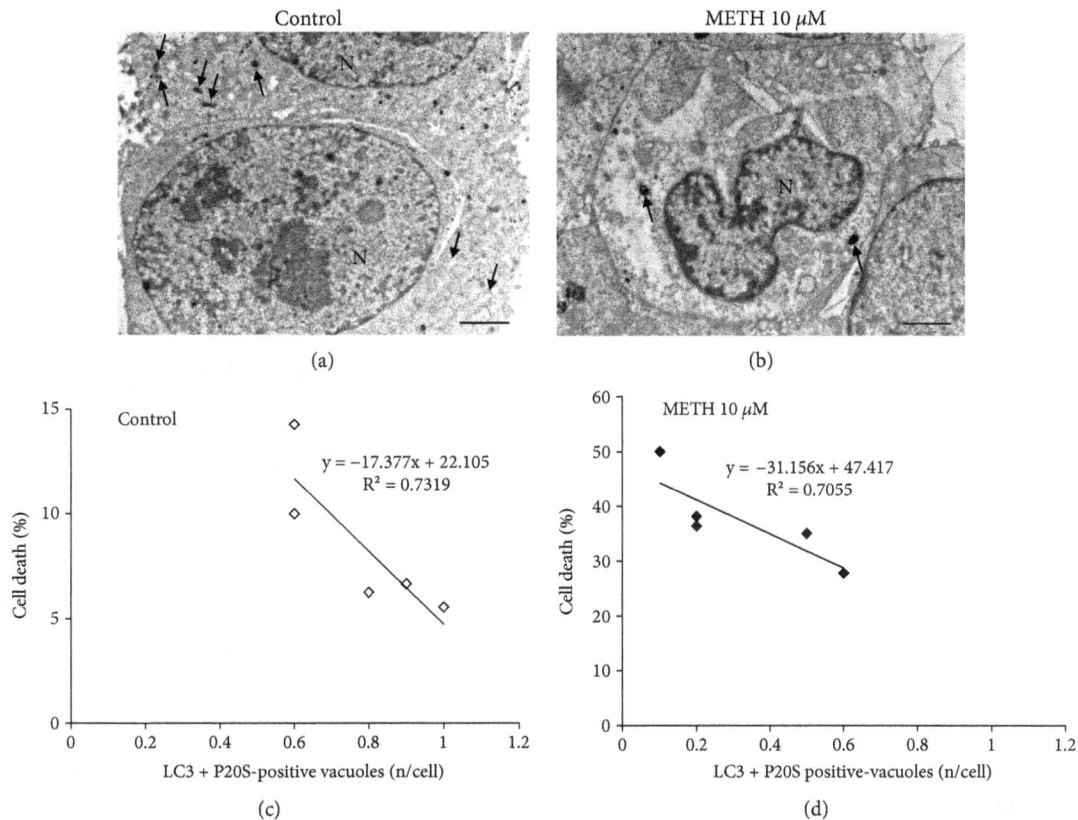

(a)

(b)

(c)

(d)

FIGURE 6: Inverse correlation between the occurrence of APP and METH-induced toxicity. (a) Representative micrograph from a control cell. (b) Representative micrograph from a cell following METH at 72 h. (c) Linear regression between the percentage of cell death and the number of LC3 + P20S-positive vacuoles in control. (d) Linear regression between the percentage of cell death and the number of LC3 + P20S-positive vacuoles following METH at 72 h. The puncta reported in the graphs ((c) white square and (d) black square) correspond to the number of grid ($n = 5$). Arrows point to vacuoles. N = nucleus. Scale bar = 1 μm.

according to confocal microscopy, under METH administration, a marked suppression was counted for APP for each dose of METH ranging between 1 nM and 10 μM as shown in the graph of Figure 5(d). Similarly, just like it was described for the time course detected at confocal microscopy, even at TEM, APP was similarly depressed by METH at 12, 24, and 72 h (Supplementary Figure 2). The number of APP in controls (representative Figure 6(a)) and following METH (Figure 6(b)) was plotted for a regression analysis between the amount of APPs and the number of dead cells in controls (graph of Figure 6(c)) and following METH (graph of Figure 6(d)). A negative correlation was detected between cell death and the number of APPs with a slope, which was consistent in control conditions and following METH at 10 μM. In fact, in both experimental conditions, cell death was lesser and lesser when APPs were more and more expressed. In controls, dead cells exceeded 10% in those samples owning only a few APPs/cell (roughly 0.6), while cell death was occluded down to 5% when APPs increased two-fold (graph of Figure 6(c)). As expected, the percentage of cell death reached almost 50% following the 10 μM dose of METH, when only a few APPs were produced (roughly 0.1 per cell); in contrast, cell death was toned down to 30% in those samples in which the amount of APPs was six-fold higher (roughly 0.6 per cell, graph of Figure 6(d)).

3.6. The Effects of mTOR Modulation on P20S, LC3, and Autophagoproteasome Related with METH Neurotoxicity. As previously published, mTOR activity finely tunes APP [47]. Therefore, in order to test in the present experiments the effects of specific doses of compounds, which are known to act either as mTOR inhibitors or activators, we measured the amount of the downstream product of mTOR activity (pS6). Asparagine is a well-known mTORC1 activator [92] while rapamycin is the gold standard mTORC1 inhibitor [93, 94]. The doses of these compounds were tested as reported in Figure 7. Asparagine at the dose of 50 mM activates mTOR while rapamycin at the dose of 100 nM inhibits mTOR as calculated by the amount of Western blotted pS6. Therefore, owning the right compounds at appropriated doses, we tested the effects of these compounds on cell death and amount of APPs. As shown in representative micrographs of Figure 8, we observed a variety of effects, which are in line with the key role of mTOR in METH toxicity and APP stimulation [80, 94, 95]. In fact, the dose of 10 μM METH produces roughly 35% cell death, which was totally prevented by rapamycin (100 nM). Remarkably, rapamycin alone further reduced cell death significantly below levels found in control cells. This witnesses for the presence of a baseline inherent aberrancy of mTOR regulation in this cell line, which is reminiscent of neurodegeneration [49].

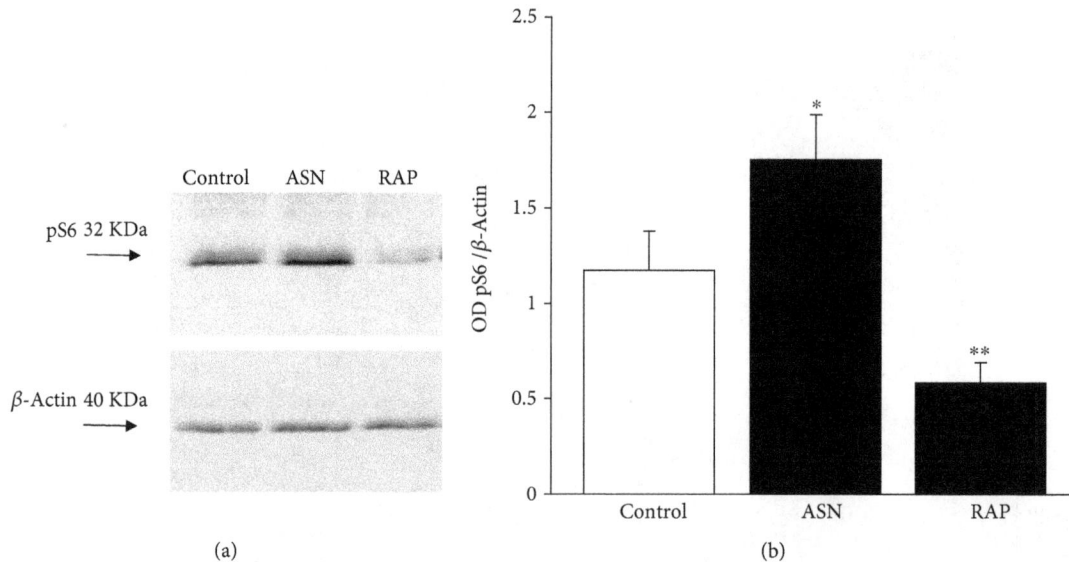

(a)   (b)

FIGURE 7: Modulation of pS6 levels underlie mTOR inhibition and activation by rapamycin and asparagine, respectively. (a) Representative SDS-PAGE immunoblotting of pS6 protein. (d) Densitometric analysis. Values are given as the optical density detected in six separate replicates ($n = 6$). Error bars represent the standard error of the mean. $^{*}p \leq 0.05$ vs. control; $^{**}p \leq 0.05$ vs. control and METH. ASN = asparagine; RAP = rapamycin.

Incidentally, this is the first report showing that the gold standard inhibitor of mTOR rapamycin prevents METH toxicity. This key finding provided here as side observation is in need of a dedicated experimental project. So far, only taurine and melatonin were shown to slightly prevent METH toxicity with an indirect evidence of mTOR-mediated mechanisms [94, 96], although this was interpreted using a multifaceted hypothesis. Remarkably, recent evidence, despite not addressing directly METH neurotoxicity, demonstrated that METH-induced behavioral sensitization associates with mTOR overexpression, while rapamycin reverts such an effect [97]. Again, the stimulation of DA D1 receptors, which are key in both METH-induced toxicity and behavioral sensitization [9, 98], directly promotes mTOR activation while inhibiting autophagy [99].

The present study directly relates neuroprotection with mTOR inhibition, while showing that METH impairs autophagy. This was consolidated by the deleterious effects of asparagine. In fact, in the graph of Figure 8(b), we found that asparagine alone was slightly increasing the natural cell death occurring in control cells but it did not really increase much the amount of METH-induced cell death. When all the three compounds were coadministered, the protective effects of rapamycin prevailed, with a robust suppression of cell death occurring following METH + asparagine (graph of Figure 8). These data concerning cell death were almost mirrored by each treatment in the count of APPs. In detail, METH suppressed APPs while rapamycin increased their number almost two-fold of controls. Asparagine, as expected, depressed APPs similarly to METH, while the combination METH + asparagine produced the lowest number of APPs (3-fold less than controls). It is remarkable that rapamycin rescued the loss of APPs induced following either asparagine alone or asparagine + METH

(Figure 8(c)). This strengthens the significance of the present data concerning the role of mTOR in tuning METH toxicity and APPs in a reciprocal pattern.

Here, we wish to emphasize the protective effects of mTOR inhibition on natural cell death which occurs in the PC12 cell line. In fact, these cells possess an inherent aberrancy, which is useful in understanding neuronal degeneration [49]. This is partly due to an aberrancy in DA compartmentalization and vesicle polarization, where in baseline conditions most neurotransmitter is docking to the cell membrane, making this cell line highly prone to produce massive amount of self-oxidized DA metabolites [49]. It is remarkable that upgrading APPs through mTOR inhibition erases such an inborn trend to degenerate. Since UP inhibition enhances DA release, which is related to METH toxicity, it is expected that mTOR activation, by inhibiting UP activity and compartmentalization, enhances METH-induced cell death. The present research seems to uncover the molecular determinants of inherent vulnerability of the DA-PC12 cell line, by targeting specifically mTORC1 complex dysregulation.

3.7. The Effects of mTOR Modulation on Unstained Vacuoles.
When these experimental conditions were applied to unstained vacuoles (representative picture of Supplementary Figure 3), data obtained were quite similar to APPs, though with some exceptions. In fact, METH increases the number of unstained vacuoles, which were further increased by rapamycin alone, way more compared with LC3-positive vacuoles (roughly 20 per cell and roughly 8 per cell, respectively). This adds further information about the previous question concerning the nature of these unstained vacuoles, which turn out to be mTOR-dependent. Unexpectedly, combined administration of METH and rapamycin instead of further increasing the number of

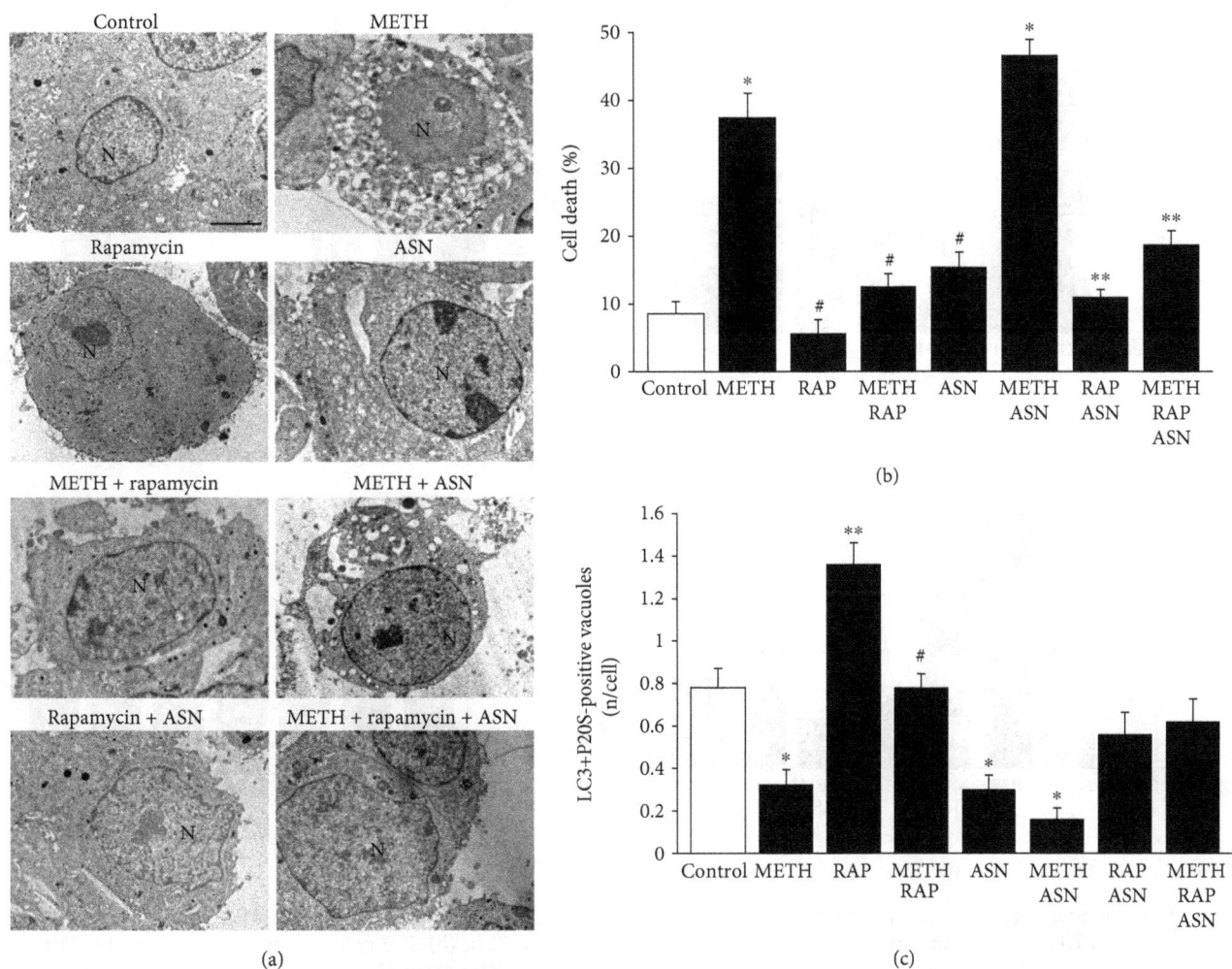

(a)

(b)

(c)

FIGURE 8: mTOR inhibition prevents cell death and rescues the amount of APPs induced by METH and the mTOR activator asparagine. (a) Representative micrographs of control and following METH 10 μM, rapamycin 100 nM, and asparagine 50 mM, at 72 h. (b) Graph of the percentage of cell death in control and following METH 10 μM, rapamycin 100 nM, and asparagine 50 mM, at 72 h. (c) Graph of the number of LC3 + P20S-positive vacuoles in control and following METH 10 μM, rapamycin 100 nM, and asparagine 50 mM, at 72 h. For the graph in (b), values are given as the percentage of cell counted on 5 grids. For the graph in (c), values are given as the mean number of LC3 + P20S-positive vacuoles counted in 100 cells per group. Error bars represent the standard error of the mean. $^*p \leq 0.05$ vs. control; $^{**}p \leq 0.05$ vs. control and METH; $^\#p \leq 0.05$ vs. METH. N = nucleus; ASN = asparagine; RAP = rapamycin. Scale bar = 0.5 μm.

unstained vacuoles compared with rapamycin alone produces a decrease in these vacuoles (which remain higher than controls). It is likely that, in the presence of rapamycin, there is no longer an oxidative stress, which produces an altered vesicle trafficking. In fact, mTOR inhibition stimulates both the activity and the amount of the proteasome subunit, which suppresses DA release. Thus, according to the hypothesis that unstained vacuoles are due to DA release and proteasome dysfunction mutually enhancing each other, it is expected that rapamycin occludes this component. Thus, combined METH and rapamycin administration produces a number of unstained vacuoles which is still higher than controls but lower than rapamycin alone. Asparagine alone or in combination with METH decreased unstained vacuoles, which were brought up to control the levels by adding rapamycin (Supplementary Figure 3).

These data suggest that the mechanisms by which unstained vacuoles are increased are different following rapamycin compared with METH administration, since double treatment occludes this effect instead of enhancing it. This is consistent with the opposite effects on cell death, which is induced by METH and rescued by rapamycin. In contrast, APP vacuoles despite being decreased by METH were increased by rapamycin, which witnesses for a different regulation of unstained compared with APP vacuoles.

3.8. The Effects of mTOR Modulation on LC3. Following mTOR inhibition by rapamycin, LC3 particles were never depressed below control values, even when METH and asparagine were combined. In these experimental conditions, compartmentalization of LC3 particles within vacuoles was dramatically enhanced by rapamycin. This mechanism was

(a)

(b)

(c)

(d)

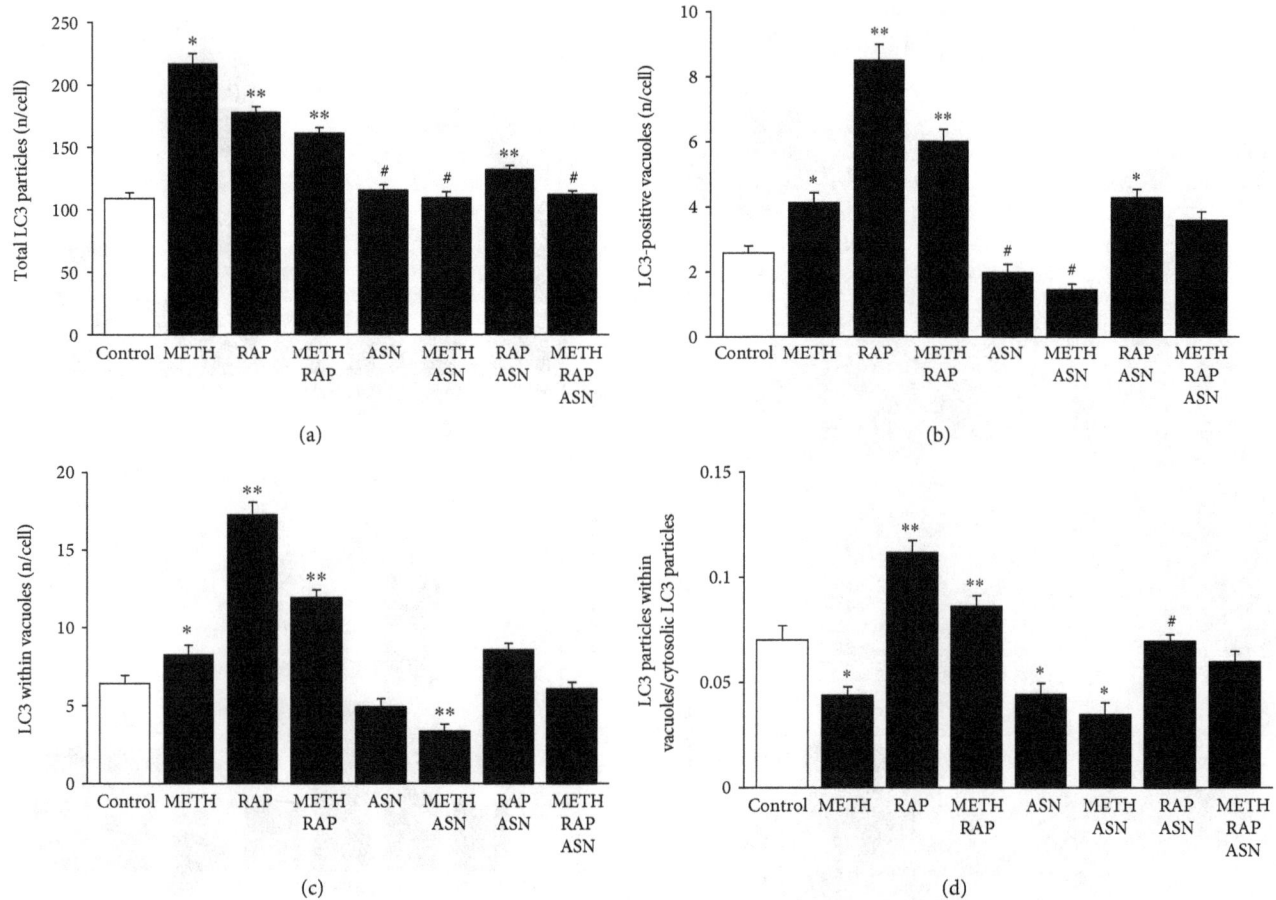

FIGURE 9: mTOR modulates the number and placement of LC3 particles. (a) The graph shows the number of total LC3 particles per cell in control, following METH 10 μM, rapamycin 100 nM, and asparagine 50 mM, at 72 h. (b) The graph shows the number of LC3-positive vacuoles per cell in control, following METH 10 μM, rapamycin 100 nM, and asparagine 50 mM, at 72 h. (c) The graph shows the number of LC3-positive vacuoles in control and following METH 10 μM, rapamycin 100 nM, and asparagine 50 mM, at 72 h. (d) The graph shows the ratio between the number of LC3 particles within vacuoles and cytosolic LC3 particles. Values are given as the mean number of LC3 particles and vacuoles counted in 50 cells per group. Error bars represent the standard error of the mean. $^{*}p \leq 0.05$ vs. control; $^{**}p \leq 0.05$ vs. control and METH; $^{\#}p \leq 0.05$ vs. METH.

independent from the one produced by METH; in fact, despite METH 10 μM was more effective than rapamycin 100 nM to increase total LC3 particles in the cell, rapamycin alone was much more powerful than METH alone in increasing LC3 within vacuoles (Figure 9(a)). Again, when rapamycin was combined with METH, a decrease of vacuolar LC3 was detected compared with rapamycin alone (Figure 9(b)). This indicates a strong compartmentalizing effect of rapamycin, which sharply contrasts with METH-induced LC3 dispersion (the generalized and nonspecific increase of LC3 promoted by METH, Figure 9(a)). The mTOR activator asparagine alone or in combination with METH further dispersed LC3 particles, since it decreased the placement of LC3 within vacuoles. This witnesses for a strong modulation by mTOR of LC3 compartmentalization (Figure 9(c)). This was further evidenced by counting the number of LC3 particles in the vacuoles versus LC3 particles within the cytosol (Figure 9(d)). In this case, METH decreases the ratio compared with controls, while rapamycin was increasing two-fold the ratio compared with controls and reverted

the effects of METH. Asparagine alone was similar to METH and further suppressed the ratio when it was combined with METH.

3.9. The Effects of mTOR Modulation on P20S. The effects of mTOR inhibition were sharply contrasting with the effects of METH concerning the amount and placement of P20S particles. In fact, while METH depressed, rapamycin increased total P20S (Figure 10(a)). Moreover, rapamycin reverted the suppression induced by METH, while the effect of asparagine alone was less effective compared with METH. Combined administration of asparagine and METH did not alter the effects produced by METH alone. The effects of asparagine were antagonized by rapamycin. This was replicated by the number of P20S in the vacuoles (Figures 10(b) and 10(c)). When counting P20S-positive vacuoles or P20S in the vacuoles (Figures 10(b) and 10(c), respectively), although the general trend was similar to what is described in Figure 10(a), there was a remarkable difference concerning asparagine. In fact, the polarization of P20S within vacuoles was dramatically suppressed

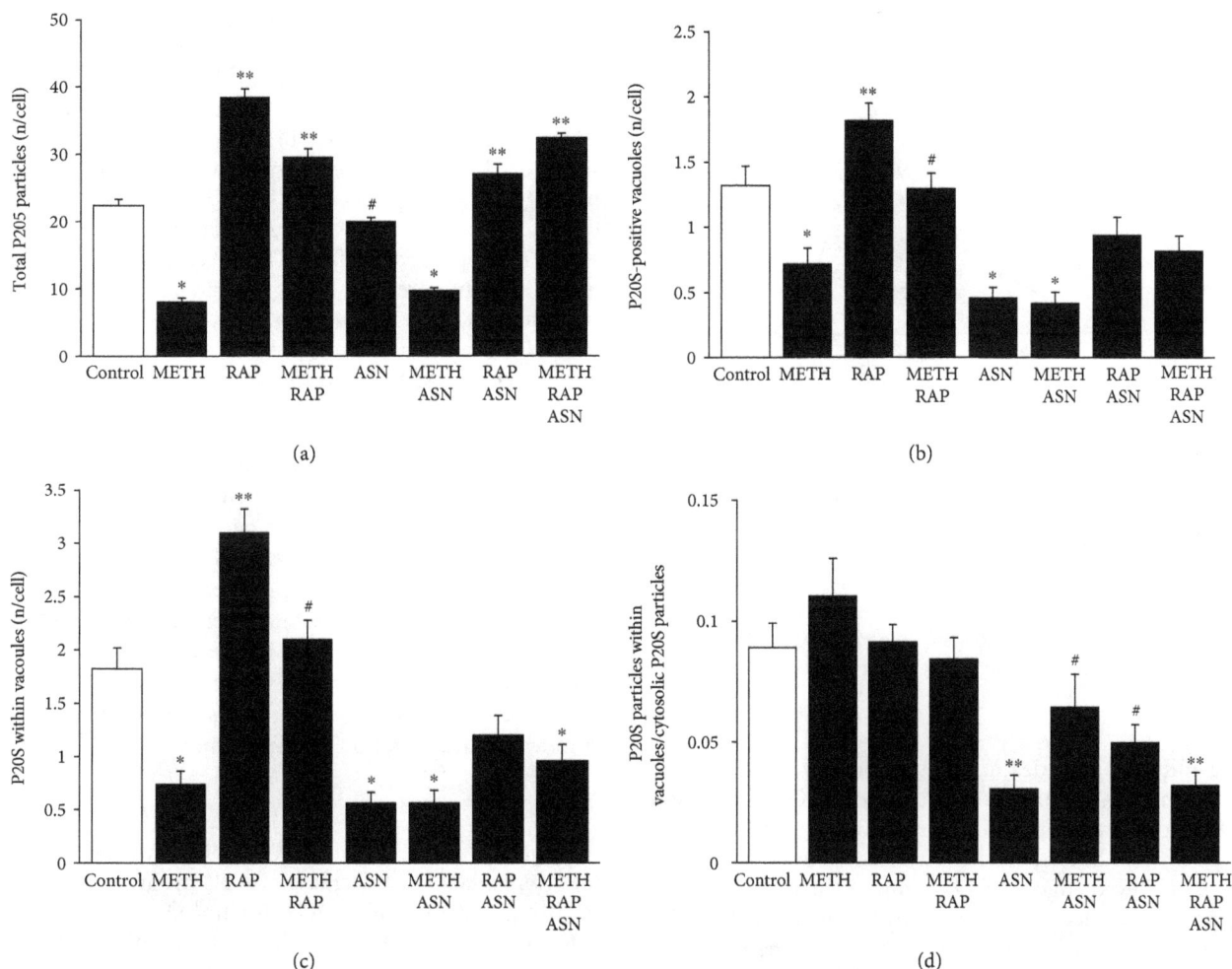

(a)

(b)

(c)

(d)

FIGURE 10: mTOR modulates the number and placement of P20S particles. (a) The graph shows the number of total P20S particles per cell in control, following METH 10 μM, rapamycin 100 nM, and asparagine 50 mM, at 72 h. (b) The graph shows the number of P20S-positive vacuoles per cell in control, following METH 10 μM, rapamycin 100 nM, and asparagine 50 mM, at 72 h. (c) The graph shows the number of P20S-positive vacuoles in control and following METH 10 μM, rapamycin 100 nM, and asparagine 50 mM, at 72 h. (d) The graph shows the ratio between the number of P20S particles within vacuoles and cytosolic P20S particles. Values are given as the mean number of P20S particles and vacuoles counted in 50 cells per group. Error bars represent the standard error of the mean. $^{*}p \leq 0.05$ vs. control; ** $p \leq 0.05$ vs. control and METH; $^{\#}p \leq 0.05$ vs. METH. ASN = asparagine; RAP = rapamycin.

by this mTOR activator even when compared with METH. Moreover, the effects of asparagine on the dispersion of P20S was so powerful that even rapamycin was not able to prevent it (Figure 10(d)).

3.10. Correlation between Autophagoproteasomes and Cell Death. The effects of all these treatments on the amount of APPs versus the occurrence of cell death were plotted in the graph of Figure 11, which remarks for various mTOR modulators and a powerful negative correlation between the number of APPs and the number of dead cells.

In conclusions, the negative correlation which was described for APP and cell death in controls and following a 10 μM dose of METH (Figure 6) was strengthened by the analysis carried out with mTOR modulators (Figure 8). This final plotting shows, at one glance, how mTOR inhibition is key for producing the merging between proteasome and

autophagy to build autophagoproteasome, while it is compatible with a strong neuroprotective role exerted by such a merging organelle.

4. Concluding Remarks

METH administration is known to increase the number of ATG vacuoles within catecholamine-containing cells. This was originally published by Cubells et al. [22], and at first, it was suggested to produce ATG-mediated cell damage [22].

Nonetheless, in 2008, we demonstrated that the inhibition of ATG in METH-treated catecholamine cells instead of producing neuroprotection worsened METH neurotoxicity indicating a compensatory neuroprotection for ATG induction during METH toxicity, as confirmed by several studies [16, 37, 80, 100–102].

In line with this, in the present manuscript, we demonstrate that rapamycin administration fully rescues

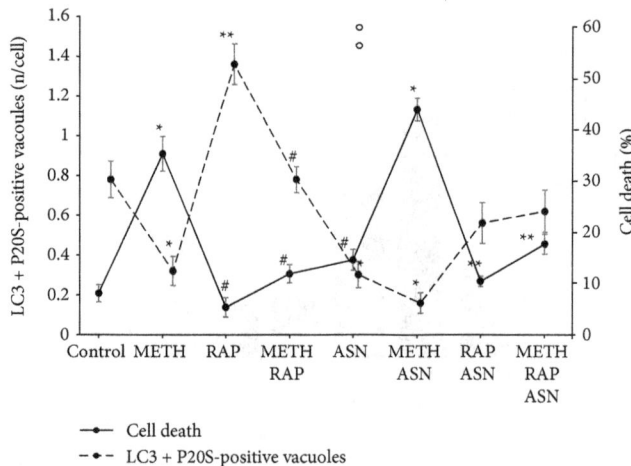

FIGURE 11: Inverse correlation between cell death and amount of APPs following mTOR modulation. The dashed line shows the amount of APPs while the continuous line shows the percentage of cell death. For each treatment, the values of the two lines produce a mirror image, which indicates a negative correlation. $^*p \leq 0.05$ vs. control; $^{**}p \leq 0.05$ vs. control and METH; $^{\#}p \leq 0.05$ vs. METH. ASN = asparagine; RAP = rapamycin.

METH-induced cell death. In the present paper, apart from strengthening the concept that mTOR inhibition and ATG protect against METH toxicity, we further detail the significance of specific ATG-related structures.

It is believed that METH-induced increase in LC3 immunofluorescence is produced by an increase in LC3-positive stagnant ATG vacuoles with an impairment of the autophagy flux [37]. However, in the present study, we demonstrate that, under METH administration, there is a loss of compartmentalization of LC3 particles within vacuoles. In fact, LC3 particles increase more in the cytosol than within vacuoles, which represents a novel insight in ATG and METH toxicity.

This leads to reconsider the significance of densely fluorescent LC3 spots detected at confocal microscopy following METH, since the greatest contribution is provided by free cytosolic LC3.

In these experimental conditions, the effects of rapamycin are demonstrated to be neuroprotective against cell death while reinstating vacuolar compartmentalization of both LC3 and P20S.

It is likely that a concomitant acceleration of activity within stagnant ATG vacuoles may concur to provide neuroprotection. In fact, asparagine, which also impairs the merge between autophagosomes and lysosomes, produces a dramatic effect.

In these experimental conditions, the occurrence of ATG vacuoles is further dissected for the concomitant presence of the P20S proteasome component. It is now well established that these LC3 + P20S vacuoles contain both ATG and proteasome markers and are named "autophagoproteasomes" (APPs) [48].

In the present study, we demonstrate that LC3 + P20S-positive vacuoles (APP) represents a clearing compartment

which behaves distinctly and sometimes opposite to classic ATG (LC3-positive) compartment. This specific compartment correlates with cell survival. In line with this, alpha-synuclein, which is known to buffer oxidative species [103, 104], is involved in METH toxicity, since in alpha-synuclein knockout mice, a potentiation of METH-induced nigrostriatal damage occurs [105]. The coimmunoprecipitation of alpha-synuclein within APPs found here corroborates such a neuroprotective effect. This novel organelle may counteract also impaired mitophagy during METH administration. In fact, few key steps in mitochondrial removal are carried out by proteasome components acting during early autophagosome formation [39, 106, 107].

As a proof of principle, we cannot be satisfied yet, since one might argue that a defect in ATG progression may lead ATG vacuoles not to be able to take up the proteasome component due to a failure in the p62-driven uptake of ubiquitinated proteasomes. When such an alternative explanation is consistent, then an increased amount of P20S should be measured in the cytosol. However, the number of P20S in the cytosol was decreased by METH administration, and it was further suppressed by the concomitant administration of asparagine.

Again, if the decreased amount of UP within ATG vacuoles were related to a decrease of ATG progression (impaired shuttling of P20S within ATG vacuoles), the ratio between cytosolic vs. vacuolar P20S should be modified by METH, while this ratio stays steady.

Authors' Contributions

Gloria Lazzeri and Francesca Biagioni equally contributed to the present manuscript.

Acknowledgments

We are grateful to Dr. Marina Flaibani for the precious technical support. This work was supported by Ricerca Corrente 2018 (Ministero della Salute).

Supplementary Materials

Supplementary Figures 1, 2, and 3: further evidence about various METH-induced ultrastructural alterations. In all these graphs, the dose of METH was kept constant 10 μM. Supplementary Figure 1: the time dependency of METH-induced variations in LC3 and P20S particles (12 h, 24 h, and 72 h). Counts refer to whole cytosol or selectively within vacuoles. Moreover, the ratio between compartmentalized particles within vacuoles and total cytosolic particles at these time intervals is reported. Supplementary Figure 2: the time dependency of METH-induced suppression of APPs, which concerns selectively with the number of LC3 + P20S-positive vacuoles (autophagoproteasomes) in the whole cytosol. Supplementary Figure 3: the number of unstained vacuoles in the whole cytosol following various single and combined treatments with mTOR modulators. *(Supplementary Materials)*

References

[1] N. D. Volkow, L. Chang, G. J. Wang et al., "Association of dopamine transporter reduction with psychomotor impairment in methamphetamine abusers," *American Journal of Psychiatry*, vol. 158, no. 3, pp. 377–382, 2001.

[2] D. E. Rusyniak, "Neurologic manifestations of chronic methamphetamine abuse," *Neurologic Clinics*, vol. 29, no. 3, pp. 641–655, 2011.

[3] G. C. Wagner, G. A. Ricaurte, L. S. Seiden, C. R. Schuster, R. J. Miller, and J. Westley, "Long-lasting depletions of striatal dopamine and loss of dopamine uptake sites following repeated administration of methamphetamine," *Brain Research*, vol. 181, no. 1, pp. 151–160, 1980.

[4] G. A. Ricaurte, R. W. Guillery, and L. S. Seiden, "Dopamine nerve terminal degeneration produced by high doses of methylamphetamine in the rat brain," *Brain Research*, vol. 235, no. 1, pp. 93–103, 1982.

[5] J. M. Wilson, K. S. Kalasinsky, A. I. Levey et al., "Striatal dopamine nerve terminal markers in human, chronic methamphetamine users," *Nature Medicine*, vol. 2, no. 6, pp. 699–703, 1996.

[6] F. Fornai, P. Lenzi, M. Gesi et al., "Methamphetamine produces neuronal inclusions in the nigrostriatal system and in PC12 cells," *Journal of Neurochemistry*, vol. 88, no. 1, pp. 114–123, 2004.

[7] B. Liu and D. E. Dluzen, "Effect of estrogen upon methamphetamine-induced neurotoxicity within the impaired nigrostriatal dopaminergic system," *Synapse*, vol. 60, no. 5, pp. 354–361, 2006.

[8] S. Ares-Santos, N. Granado, I. Espadas, R. Martinez-Murillo, and R. Moratalla, "Methamphetamine causes degeneration of dopamine cell bodies and terminals of the nigrostriatal pathway evidenced by silver staining," *Neuropsychopharmacology*, vol. 39, no. 5, pp. 1066–1080, 2014.

[9] S. Ares-Santos, N. Granado, I. Oliva et al., "Dopamine D(1) receptor deletion strongly reduces neurotoxic effects of methamphetamine," *Neurobiology of Disease*, vol. 45, no. 2, pp. 810–820, 2012.

[10] N. Granado, S. Ares-Santos, E. O'Shea, C. Vicario-Abejón, M. I. Colado, and R. Moratalla, "Selective vulnerability in striosomes and in the nigrostriatal dopaminergic pathway after methamphetamine administration: early loss of TH in striosomes after methamphetamine," *Neurotoxicity Research*, vol. 18, no. 1, pp. 48–58, 2010.

[11] N. Granado, S. Ares-Santos, and R. Moratalla, "D1 but not D4 dopamine receptors are critical for MDMA-induced neurotoxicity in mice," *Neurotoxicity Research*, vol. 25, no. 1, pp. 100–109, 2014.

[12] N. Granado, S. Ares-Santos, Y. Tizabi, and R. Moratalla, "Striatal reinnervation process after acute methamphetamine-induced dopaminergic degeneration in mice," *Neurotoxicity Research*, vol. 34, no. 3, pp. 627–639, 2018.

[13] F. Fornai, P. Lenzi, M. Gesi et al., "Similarities between methamphetamine toxicity and proteasome inhibition," *Annals of the New York Academy of Sciences*, vol. 1025, no. 1, pp. 162–170, 2004.

[14] F. Fornai, G. Lazzeri, A. Bandettini Di Poggio et al., "Convergent roles of α-synuclein, DA metabolism, and the ubiquitin-proteasome system in nigrostriatal toxicity," *Annals of the New York Academy of Sciences*, vol. 1074, no. 1, pp. 84–89, 2006.

[15] G. Lazzeri, P. Lenzi, C. L. Busceti et al., "Mechanisms involved in the formation of dopamine-induced intracellular bodies within striatal neurons," *Journal of Neurochemistry*, vol. 101, no. 5, pp. 1414–1427, 2007.

[16] M. Lin, P. Chandramani-Shivalingappa, H. Jin et al., "Methamphetamine-induced neurotoxicity linked to ubiquitin-proteasome system dysfunction and autophagy-related changes that can be modulated by protein kinase C delta in dopaminergic neuronal cells," *Neuroscience*, vol. 210, pp. 308–332, 2012.

[17] L. Quan, T. Ishikawa, T. Michiue et al., "Ubiquitin-immunoreactive structures in the midbrain of methamphetamine abusers," *Legal Medicine*, vol. 7, no. 3, pp. 144–150, 2005.

[18] P. K. Sonsalla, J. W. Gibb, and G. R. Hanson, "Roles of D1 and D2 dopamine receptor subtypes in mediating the methamphetamine-induced changes in monoamine systems," *Journal of Pharmacology and Experimental Therapeutics*, vol. 238, no. 3, pp. 932–937, 1986.

[19] J. W. Gibb, M. Johnson, and G. R. Hanson, "Neurochemical basis of neurotoxicity," *Neurotoxicology*, vol. 11, no. 2, pp. 317–321, 1990.

[20] D. Sulzer and S. Rayport, "Amphetamine and other psychostimulants reduce pH gradients in midbrain dopaminergic neurons and chromaffin granules: a mechanism of action," *Neuron*, vol. 5, no. 6, pp. 797–808, 1990.

[21] D. Sulzer, E. Pothos, H. M. Sung, N. T. Maidment, B. G. Hoebel, and S. Rayport, "Weak base model of amphetamine action," *Annals of the New York Academy of Sciences*, vol. 654, no. 1, pp. 525–528, 1992.

[22] J. F. Cubells, S. Rayport, G. Rajendran, and D. Sulzer, "Methamphetamine neurotoxicity involves vacuolation of endocytic organelles and dopamine-dependent intracellular oxidative stress," *Journal of Neuroscience*, vol. 14, no. 4, pp. 2260–2271, 1994.

[23] O. Suzuki, H. Hattori, M. Asano, M. Oya, and Y. Katsumata, "Inhibition of monoamine oxidase by *d*-methamphetamine," *Biochemical Pharmacolgy*, vol. 29, no. 14, pp. 2071–2073, 1980.

[24] F. Fornai, K. Chen, F. S. Giorgi, M. Gesi, M. G. Alessandri, and J. C. Shih, "Striatal dopamine metabolism in monoamine oxidase B-deficient mice: a brain dialysis study," *Journal of Neurochemistry*, vol. 73, no. 6, pp. 2434–2440, 1999.

[25] C. J. Schmidt and J. W. Gibb, "Role of the dopamine uptake carrier in the neurochemical response to methamphetamine: effects of amfonelic acid," *European Journal of Pharmacology*, vol. 109, no. 1, pp. 73–80, 1985.

[26] R. Moratalla, A. Khairnar, N. Simola et al., "Amphetamine-related drugs neurotoxicity in humans and in experimental animals: main mechanisms," *Progress in Neurobiology*, vol. 155, pp. 149–170, 2017.

[27] J. L. Cadet, S. Ali, and C. Epstein, "Involvement of oxygen-based radicals in methamphetamine-induced neurotoxicity:

evidence from the use of CuZnSOD transgenic mice," *Annals of the New York Academy of Sciences*, vol. 738, no. 1, pp. 388–391, 2006.

[28] J. P. Spencer, M. Whiteman, P. Jenner, and B. Halliwell, "5-s-Cysteinyl-conjugates of catecholamines induce cell damage, extensive DNA base modification and increases in caspase-3 activity in neurons," *Journal of Neurochemistry*, vol. 81, no. 1, pp. 122–129, 2002.

[29] N. Granado, I. Lastres-Becker, S. Ares-Santos et al., "Nrf2 deficiency potentiates methamphetamine-induced dopaminergic axonal damage and gliosis in the striatum," *Glia*, vol. 59, no. 12, pp. 1850–1863, 2011.

[30] L. Mendieta, N. Granado, J. Aguilera, Y. Tizabi, and R. Moratalla, "Fragment C domain of tetanus toxin mitigates methamphetamine neurotoxicity and its motor consequences in mice," *International Journal of Neuropsychopharmacology*, vol. 19, no. 8, article pyw021, 2016.

[31] M. J. LaVoie and T. G. Hastings, "Dopamine quinone formation and protein modification associated with the striatal neurotoxicity of methamphetamine: evidence against a role for extracellular dopamine," *The Journal of Neuroscience*, vol. 19, no. 4, pp. 1484–1491, 1999.

[32] F. Fornai, P. Longone, M. Ferrucci et al., "Autophagy and amyotrophic lateral sclerosis: the multiple roles of lithium," *Autophagy*, vol. 4, no. 4, pp. 527–530, 2008.

[33] M. Ferrucci, L. Ryskalin, F. Biagioni et al., "Methamphetamine increases prion protein and induces dopamine-dependent expression of protease resistant PrPsc," *Archives Italiennes de Biologie*, vol. 155, no. 1-2, pp. 81–97, 2017.

[34] A. Moszczynska and B. K. Yamamoto, "Methamphetamine oxidatively damages parkin and decreases the activity of 26S proteasome in vivo," *Journal of Neurochemistry*, vol. 116, no. 6, pp. 1005–1017, 2011.

[35] J. M. Brown, M. S. Quinton, and B. K. Yamamoto, "Methamphetamine-induced inhibition of mitochondrial complex II: roles of glutamate and peroxynitrite," *Journal of Neurochemistry*, vol. 95, no. 2, pp. 429–436, 2005.

[36] D. J. Barbosa, J. P. Capela, R. Feio-Azevedo, A. Teixeira-Gomes, M. L. Bastos, and F. Carvalho, "Mitochondria: key players in the neurotoxic effects of amphetamines," *Archives of Toxicology*, vol. 89, no. 10, pp. 1695–1725, 2015.

[37] R. Castino, G. Lazzeri, P. Lenzi et al., "Suppression of autophagy precipitates neuronal cell death following low doses of methamphetamine," *Journal of Neurochemistry*, vol. 106, no. 3, pp. 1426–1439, 2008.

[38] G. Beauvais, K. Atwell, S. Jayanthi, B. Ladenheim, and J. L. Cadet, "Involvement of dopamine receptors in binge methamphetamine-induced activation of endoplasmic reticulum and mitochondrial stress pathways," *PLoS One*, vol. 6, no. 12, article e28946, 2011.

[39] P. Lenzi, R. Marongiu, A. Falleni et al., "A subcellular analysis of genetic modulation of PINK1 on mitochondrial alterations, autophagy and cell death," *Archives Italiennes de Biologie*, vol. 150, no. 2-3, pp. 194–217, 2012.

[40] B. K. Yamamoto and W. Zhu, "The effects of methamphetamine on the production of free radicals and oxidative stress," *The Journal of Pharmacology and Experimental Therapy*, vol. 287, no. 1, pp. 107–114, 1998.

[41] P. S. Fitzmaurice, J. Tong, M. Yazdanpanah, P. P. Liu, K. S. Kalasinsky, and S. J. Kish, "Levels of 4-hydroxynonenal and malondialdehyde are increased in brain of human chronic users of methamphetamine," *The Journal of Pharmacology and Experimental Therapy*, vol. 319, no. 2, pp. 703–709, 2006.

[42] F. Fornai, P. Lenzi, M. Gesi et al., "Fine structure and biochemical mechanisms underlying nigrostriatal inclusions and cell death after proteasome inhibition," *Journal of Neuroscience*, vol. 23, no. 26, pp. 8955–8966, 2003.

[43] G. Lazzeri, P. Lenzi, M. Gesi et al., "In PC12 cells neurotoxicity induced by methamphetamine is related to proteasome inhibition," *Annals of the New York Academy of Sciences*, vol. 1074, no. 1, pp. 174–177, 2006.

[44] K. E. Larsen, E. A. Fon, T. G. Hastings, R. H. Edwards, and D. Sulzer, "Methamphetamine-induced degeneration of dopaminergic neurons involves autophagy and upregulation of dopamine synthesis," *Journal of Neurochemistry*, vol. 22, no. 20, pp. 8951–8960, 2002.

[45] D. Weinshenker, M. Ferrucci, C. L. Busceti et al., "Genetic or pharmacological blockade of noradrenaline synthesis enhances the neurochemical, behavioral, and neurotoxic effects of methamphetamine," *Journal of Neurochemistry*, vol. 105, no. 2, pp. 471–483, 2008.

[46] X. L. Xie, J. T. He, Z. T. Wang et al., "Lactulose attenuates METH-induced neurotoxicity by alleviating the impaired autophagy, stabilizing the perturbed antioxidant system and suppressing apoptosis in rat striatum," *Toxicology Letters*, vol. 289, pp. 107–113, 2018.

[47] P. Lenzi, G. Lazzeri, F. Biagioni et al., "The autophagoproteasome a novel cell clearing organelle in baseline and stimulated conditions," *Frontiers in Neuroanatomy*, vol. 10, p. 78, 2016.

[48] D. J. Klionsky, K. Abdelmohsen, A. Abe et al., "Guidelines for the use and interpretation of assays for monitoring autophagy (3rd edition)," *Autophagy*, vol. 12, no. 1, pp. 1–222, 2016.

[49] F. Fornai, P. Lenzi, G. Lazzeri et al., "Fine ultrastructure and biochemistry of PC12 cells: a comparative approach to understand neurotoxicity," *Brain Research*, vol. 1129, no. 1, pp. 174–190, 2007.

[50] W. P. Melega, A. K. Cho, D. Harvey, and G. Laćan, "Methamphetamine blood concentrations in human abusers: application to pharmacokinetic modelling," *Synapse*, vol. 61, no. 4, pp. 216–220, 2007.

[51] Z. Wang, X. Shi, Y. Li et al., "Blocking autophagy enhanced cytotoxicity induced by recombinant human arginase in triple-negative breast cancer cells," *Cell Death & Disease*, vol. 5, no. 12, article e1563, 2014.

[52] Y. Chen, L. Hong, Y. Zeng, Y. Shen, and Q. Zeng, "Power frequency magnetic fields induced reactive oxygen species-related autophagy in mouse embryonic fibroblasts," *The International Journal of Biochemistry & Cell Biology*, vol. 57, pp. 108–114, 2014.

[53] A. Pla, M. Pascual, J. Renau-Piqueras, and C. Guerri, "TLR4 mediates the impairment of ubiquitin-proteasome and autophagy-lysosome pathways induced by ethanol treatment in brain," *Cell Death & Disease*, vol. 5, no. 2, article e1066, 2014.

[54] K. Porter, J. Nallathambi, Y. Lin, and P. B. Liton, "Lysosomal basification and decreased autophagic flux in oxidatively stressed trabecular meshwork cells: implications for glaucoma pathogenesis," *Autophagy*, vol. 9, no. 4, pp. 581–594, 2013.

[55] D. J. Klionsky and S. D. Emr, "Autophagy as a regulated pathway of cellular degradation," *Science*, vol. 290, no. 5497, pp. 1717–1721, 2000.

[56] A. Kuma, M. Hatano, M. Matsui et al., "The role of autophagy during the early neonatal starvation period," *Nature*, vol. 432, no. 7020, pp. 1032–1036, 2004.

[57] D. J. Klionsky, J. M. Cregg, W. A. Dunn Jr. et al., "A unified nomenclature for yeast autophagy-related genes," *Developmental Cell*, vol. 5, no. 4, pp. 539–545, 2003.

[58] G. J. Stout, E. C. Stigter, P. B. Essers et al., "Insulin/IGF-1-mediated longevity is marked by reduced protein metabolism," *Molecular Systems Biology*, vo., vol. 9, no. 1, p. 679, 2013.

[59] D. Vilchez, I. Morantte, Z. Liu et al., "RPN-6 determines *C. elegans* longevity under proteotoxic stress conditions," *Nature*, vol. 489, no. 7415, pp. 263–268, 2012.

[60] K. B. Hendil, P. Kristensen, and W. Uerkvitz, "Human proteasomes analysed with monoclonal antibodies," *Biochemical Journal*, vol. 305, no. 1, pp. 245–252, 1995.

[61] M. Kovarik, T. Muthny, L. Sispera, and M. Holecek, "Effects of β-hydroxy-β-methylbutyrate treatment in different types of skeletal muscle of intact and septic rats," *Journal of Physiology and Biochemistry*, vol. 66, no. 4, pp. 311–319, 2010.

[62] E. Jo, J. McLaurin, C. M. Yip, P. St. George-Hyslop, and P. E. Fraser, "α-Synuclein membrane interactions and lipid specificity," *Journal of Biological Chemistry*, vol. 275, no. 44, pp. 34328–34334, 2000.

[63] Y. Liu, L. Fallon, H. A. Lashuel, Z. Liu, and P. T. Lansbury Jr, "The UCH-L1 gene encodes two opposing enzymatic activities that affect alpha-synuclein degradation and Parkinson's disease susceptibility," *Cell*, vol. 111, no. 2, pp. 209–218, 2002.

[64] L. Maroteaux, J. T. Campanelli, and R. H. Scheller, "Synuclein: a neuron-specific protein localized to the nucleus and presynaptic nerve terminal," *Journal of Neuroscience*, vol. 8, no. 8, pp. 2804–2815, 1988.

[65] N. Ostrerova-Golts, L. Petrucelli, J. Hardy, J. M. Lee, M. Farer, and B. Wolozin, "The A53T alpha-synuclein mutation increases iron-dependent aggregation and toxicity," *Journal of Neuroscience*, vol. 20, no. 16, pp. 6048–6054, 2000.

[66] H. van der Putten, K. H. Wiederhold, A. Probst et al., "Neuropathology in mice expressing human alpha-synuclein," *Journal of Neuroscience*, vol. 20, no. 16, pp. 6021–6029, 2000.

[67] F. Bartolome, M. de la Cueva, C. Pascual et al., "Amyloid β-induced impairments on mitochondrial dynamics, hippocampal neurogenesis, and memory are restored by phosphodiesterase 7 inhibition," *Alzheimer's Research and Therapy*, vol. 10, no. 1, p. 24, 2018.

[68] R. Flores-Costa, J. Alcaraz-Quiles, E. Titos et al., "The soluble guanylate cyclase stimulator IW-1973 prevents inflammation and fibrosis in experimental non-alcoholic steatohepatitis," *British Journal of Pharmacology*, vol. 175, no. 6, pp. 953–967, 2018.

[69] P. Wang, L. Jiang, N. Zhou et al., "Resveratrol ameliorates autophagic flux to promote functional recovery in rats after spinal cord injury," *Oncotarget*, vol. 9, no. 9, pp. 8427–8440, 2018.

[70] D. Sun, W. Wang, X. Wang et al., "bFGF plays a neuroprotective role by suppressing excessive autophagy and apoptosis after transient global cerebral ischemia in rats," *Cell Death & Disease*, vol. 9, no. 2, p. 172, 2018.

[71] A. Du, S. Huang, X. Zhao et al., "Suppression of CHRN endocytosis by carbonic anhydrase CAR3 in the pathogenesis of myasthenia gravis," *Autophagy*, vol. 13, no. 11, pp. 1981–1994, 2017.

[72] N. Pullen and G. Thomas, "The modular phosphorylation and activation of p70s6k," *FEBS Letters*, vol. 410, no. 1, pp. 78–82, 1997.

[73] D. R. Alessi, M. T. Kozlowski, Q. P. Weng, N. Morrice, and J. Avruch, "3-Phosphoinositide-dependent protein kinase 1 (PDK1) phosphorylates and activates the p70 S6 kinase in vivo and in vitro," *Current Biology*, vol. 8, no. 2, pp. 69–81, 1998.

[74] R. D. Polakiewicz, S. M. Schieferl, A. C. Gingras, N. Sonenberg, and M. J. Comb, "μ-Opioid receptor activates signaling pathways implicated in cell survival and translational control," *Journal of Biological Chemistry*, vol. 273, no. 36, pp. 23534–23541, 1998.

[75] D. C. Finger, S. Salama, C. Tsou, E. Harlow, and J. Blenis, "Mammalian cell size is controlled by mTOR and its downstream targets S6K1 and 4EBP1/eIF4E," *Genes & Development*, vol. 16, no. 12, pp. 1472–1487, 2002.

[76] M. Saitoh, N. Pullen, P. Brennan, D. Cantrell, P. B. Dennis, and G. Thomas, "Regulation of an activated S6 kinase 1 variant reveals a novel mammalian target of rapamycin phosphorylation site," *Journal of Biological Chemistry*, vol. 277, no. 22, pp. 20104–20112, 2002.

[77] M. Bendayan and M. Zollinger, "Ultrastructural localization of antigenic sites on osmium-fixed tissues applying the protein A-gold technique," *The Journal of Histochemistry & Cytochemistry*, vol. 31, no. 1, pp. 101–109, 1983.

[78] D. D'Alessandro, L. Mattii, S. Moscato et al., "Immunohistochemical demonstration of the small GTPase RhoAA on epoxy-resin embedded sections," *Micron*, vol. 35, no. 4, pp. 287–296, 2004.

[79] J. M. Lucocq, A. Habermann, S. Watt, J. M. Backer, T. M. Mayhew, and G. Griffiths, "A rapid method for assessing the distribution of gold labeling on thin sections," *Journal of Histochemistry & Cytochemistry*, vol. 52, no. 8, pp. 991–1000, 2004.

[80] J. Ma, J. Wan, J. Meng, S. Banerjee, S. Ramakrishnan, and S. Roy, "Methamphetamine induces autophagy as a pro-survival response against apoptotic endothelial cell death through the Kappa opioid receptor," *Cell Death & Disease*, vol. 5, no. 3, article e1099, 2014.

[81] G. V. Rinetti and F. E. Schweizer, "Ubiquitination acutely regulates presynaptic neurotransmitter release in mammalian neurons," *Journal of Neuroscience*, vol. 30, no. 9, pp. 3157–3166, 2010.

[82] C. Wentzel, I. Delvendahl, S. Sydlik, O. Georgiev, and M. Müller, "Dysbindin links presynaptic proteasome function to homeostatic recruitment of low release probability vesicles," *Nature Communications*, vol. 9, no. 1, p. 267, 2018.

[83] J. Konieczny, T. Lenda, and A. Czarnecka, "Early increase in dopamine release in the ipsilateral striatum after unilateral intranigral administration of lactacystin produces spontaneous contralateral rotations in rats," *Neuroscience*, vol. 324, pp. 92–106, 2016.

[84] P. Barroso-Chinea, M. L. Thiolat, S. Bido et al., "D1 dopamine receptor stimulation impairs striatal proteasome activity in parkinsonism through 26S proteasome disassembly," *Neurobiology of Disease*, vol. 78, pp. 77–87, 2015.

[85] N. Ueda, T. Tomita, K. Yanagisawa, and N. Kimura, "Retromer and Rab2-dependent trafficking mediate PS1 degradation by proteasomes in endocytic disturbance," *Journal of Neurochemistry*, vol. 137, no. 4, pp. 647–658, 2016.

[86] V. Cohen-Kaplan, A. Ciechanover, and I. Livneh, "p62 at the crossroad of the ubiquitin-proteasome system and autophagy," *Oncotarget*, vol. 7, no. 51, pp. 83833-83834, 2016.

[87] S. Engelender, "α-Synuclein fate: proteasome or autophagy?," *Autophagy*, vol. 8, no. 3, pp. 418–420, 2012.

[88] M. Xilouri, O. R. Brekk, and L. Stefanis, "α-Synuclein and protein degradation systems: a reciprocal relationship," *Molecular Neurobiology*, vol. 47, no. 2, pp. 537–551, 2013.

[89] J. L. Webb, B. Ravikumar, J. Atkins, J. N. Skepper, and D. C. Rubinsztein, "Alpha-synuclein is degraded by both autophagy and the proteasome," *Journal of Biological Chemistry*, vol. 278, no. 27, pp. 25009–25013, 2003.

[90] M. Ferrucci, L. Pasquali, S. Ruggieri, A. Paparelli, and F. Fornai, "Alpha-synuclein and autophagy as common steps in neurodegeneration," *Parkinsonism & Related Disorders*, vol. 14, Supplement 2, pp. S180–S184, 2008.

[91] F. Yang, Y. P. Yang, C. J. Mao et al., "Crosstalk between the proteasome system and autophagy in the clearance of α-synuclein," *Acta Pharmacologica Sinica*, vol. 34, no. 5, pp. 674–680, 2013.

[92] A. S. Krall, S. Xu, T. G. Graeber, D. Braas, and H. R. Christofk, "Asparagine promotes cancer cell proliferation through use as an amino acid exchange factor," *Nature Communications*, vol. 7, article 11457, 2016.

[93] R. Loewith, E. Jacinto, S. Wullschleger et al., "Two TOR complexes, only one of which is rapamycin sensitive, have distinct roles in cell growth control," *Molecular Cell*, vol. 10, no. 3, article 10.1016/s1097-2765(02)00636-6, pp. 457–468, 2002.

[94] Y. Li, Z. Hu, B. Chen et al., "Taurine attenuates methamphetamine-induced autophagy and apoptosis in PC12 cells through mTOR signaling pathway," *Toxicology Letters*, vol. 215, no. 1, pp. 1–7, 2012.

[95] J. Wu, D. Zhu, J. Zhang, G. Li, Z. Liu, and J. Sun, "Lithium protects against methamphetamine-induced neurotoxicity in PC12 cells via Akt/GSK3β/mTOR pathway," *Biochemical and Biophysical Research Communication*, vol. 465, no. 3, pp. 368–373, 2015.

[96] P. Kongsuphol, S. Mukda, C. Nopparat, A. Villarroel, and P. Govitrapong, "Melatonin attenuates methamphetamine-induced deactivation of the mammalian target of rapamycin signaling to induce autophagy in SK-N-SH cells," *Journal of Pineal Research*, vol. 46, no. 2, pp. 199–206, 2008.

[97] S. H. Huang, W. R. Wu, L. M. Lee, P. R. Huang, and J. C. Chen, "mTOR signaling in the nucleus accumbens mediates behavioral sensitization to methamphetamine," *Progress in Neuro-Psychopharmacology & Biological Psychiatry*, vol. 86, pp. 331–339, 2018.

[98] F. Fornai, P. Lenzi, L. Capobianco et al., "Involvement of dopamine receptors and beta-arrestin in methamphetamine-induced inclusions formation in PC12 cells," *Journal of Neurochemistry*, vol. 105, no. 5, pp. 1939–1947, 2008.

[99] D. Wang, X. Ji, J. Liu, Z. Li, and X. Zhang, "Dopamine receptor subtypes differentially regulate autophagy," *International Journal of Molecular Sciences*, vol. 19, no. 5, p. 1540, 2018.

[100] R. Pitaksalee, Y. Sanvarida, T. Sinchai et al., "Autophagy inhibition by caffeine increases toxicity of methamphetamine in SH-SY5Y neuroblastoma cell line," *Neurotoxicity Research*, vol. 27, no. 4, pp. 421–429, 2015.

[101] L. Cao, M. Fu, S. Kumar, and A. Kumar, "Methamphetamine potentiates HIV-1 gp120-mediated autophagy via Beclin-1 and Atg5/7 as a pro-survival response in astrocytes," *Cell Death & Disease*, vol. 7, no. 10, article e2425, 2016.

[102] C. Zhao, Y. Mei, X. Chen et al., "Autophagy plays a pro-survival role against methamphetamine-induced apoptosis in H9C2 cells," *Toxicology Letters*, vol. 294, pp. 156–165, 2018.

[103] S. Chandra, G. Gallardo, R. Fernández-Chacón, O. M. Schlüter, and T. C. Südhof, "α-synuclein cooperates with CSPα in preventing neurodegeneration," *Cell*, vol. 123, no. 3, pp. 383–396, 2005.

[104] Y. Machida, T. Chiba, A. Takayanagi et al., "Common anti-apoptotic roles of parkin and α-synuclein in human dopaminergic cells," *Biochemical and Biophysical Research Communications*, vol. 332, no. 1, pp. 233–240, 2005.

[105] O. M. Schlüter, F. Fornai, M. G. Alessandrí et al., "Role of alpha-synuclein in 1-methyl-4-phenyl-1,2,3,6-tetrahydropyridine-induced parkinsonism in mice," *Neuroscience*, vol. 118, no. 4, pp. 985–1002, 2003.

[106] W. H. Song, Y. J. Yia, M. Sutovskya, S. Meyers, and P. Sutovsky, "Autophagy and ubiquitin–proteasome system contribute to sperm mitophagy after mammalian fertilization," *Proceedings of the National Academy of Sciences of the United States of America*, vol. 113, no. 36, pp. E5261–E5270, 2016.

[107] S. Akabane, K. Matsuzaki, S. Yamashita et al., "Constitutive activation of PINK1 protein leads to proteasome-mediated and non-apoptotic cell death independently of mitochondrial autophagy," *The Journal of Biological Chemistry*, vol. 291, no. 31, pp. 16162–16174, 2016.

Aberrant Metabolism in Hepatocellular Carcinoma Provides Diagnostic and Therapeutic Opportunities

Serena De Matteis,[1] Andrea Ragusa ⓘ,[2,3] Giorgia Marisi,[1] Stefania De Domenico,[4] Andrea Casadei Gardini ⓘ,[5] Massimiliano Bonafè,[1,6] and Anna Maria Giudetti ⓘ[7]

[1]Biosciences Laboratory, Istituto Scientifico Romagnolo per lo Studio e Cura dei Tumori (IRST) IRCCS, Meldola, Italy
[2]Department of Engineering for Innovation, University of Salento, Lecce, Italy
[3]CNR Nanotec, Institute of Nanotechnology, via Monteroni, 73100 Lecce, Italy
[4]Italian National Research Council, Institute of Sciences of Food Production (ISPA), Lecce 73100, Italy
[5]Department of Medical Oncology, Istituto Scientifico Romagnolo per lo Studio e Cura dei Tumori (IRST) IRCCS, Meldola, Italy
[6]Department of Experimental, Diagnostic & Specialty Medicine, Alma Mater Studiorum, University of Bologna, Bologna, Italy
[7]Department of Biological and Environmental Sciences and Technologies, University of Salento, Lecce, Italy

Correspondence should be addressed to Anna Maria Giudetti; anna.giudetti@unisalento.it

Academic Editor: Javier Egea

Hepatocellular carcinoma (HCC) accounts for over 80% of liver cancer cases and is highly malignant, recurrent, drug-resistant, and often diagnosed in the advanced stage. It is clear that early diagnosis and a better understanding of molecular mechanisms contributing to HCC progression is clinically urgent. Metabolic alterations clearly characterize HCC tumors. Numerous clinical parameters currently used to assess liver functions reflect changes in both enzyme activity and metabolites. Indeed, differences in glucose and acetate utilization are used as a valid clinical tool for stratifying patients with HCC. Moreover, increased serum lactate can distinguish HCC from normal subjects, and serum lactate dehydrogenase is used as a prognostic indicator for HCC patients under therapy. Currently, the emerging field of metabolomics that allows metabolite analysis in biological fluids is a powerful method for discovering new biomarkers. Several metabolic targets have been identified by metabolomics approaches, and these could be used as biomarkers in HCC. Moreover, the integration of different omics approaches could provide useful information on the metabolic pathways at the systems level. In this review, we provided an overview of the metabolic characteristics of HCC considering also the reciprocal influences between the metabolism of cancer cells and their microenvironment. Moreover, we also highlighted the interaction between hepatic metabolite production and their serum revelations through metabolomics researches.

1. Introduction

Hepatocellular carcinoma (HCC) is the most common type of primary liver cancer. It represents the fifth most common cancer worldwide and the second most frequent cause of cancer-related deaths [1]. HCC occurs most often in people with chronic liver diseases related to viral (chronic hepatitis B and C), toxic (alcohol and aflatoxin), metabolic (diabetes, hemochromatosis, and nonalcoholic fatty liver disease), and immune (autoimmune hepatitis and primary biliary) factors [1].

Effective management of HCC depends on early diagnosis and proper monitoring of the patients' response to therapy through the identification of pathways and mechanisms that are modulated during the process of tumorigenesis. In this context, the interest towards the concept of tumor metabolism is growing for several reasons: (i) metabolic alteration is a recognized hallmark of cancer, (ii) oncogenes drive alterations in cancer metabolism, (iii) metabolites can regulate gene and protein expressions, and (iv) metabolic proteins and/or metabolites represent diagnostic and prognostic biomarkers [2–6].

Metabolic alterations constitute a selective advantage for tumor growth, proliferation, and survival as they provide support to the crucial needs of cancer cells, such as increased energy production, macromolecular biosynthesis, and maintenance of redox balance. Although this is a common feature for all tumor types, it is still not completely clear how the tumor metabolic demand can really influence the metabolic profile and homeostasis of other tissues. Can they act as tumor bystanders or do they have an active role in supporting tumor growth? In this scenario, the liver represents a perfect metabolic model that governs body energy metabolism through the physiological regulation of different metabolites including sugars, lipids, and amino acids [7]. How can HCC metabolic alterations support tumor growth and influence systemic metabolism?

In this review, we take a detailed look at the alterations in intracellular and extracellular metabolites and metabolic pathways that are associated with HCC and describe the functional contribution on cancer progression and metabolic reprogramming of tumor microenvironment including immune cells. The analysis of circulating metabolites by metabolomics may provide us with novel data about this systemic crosstalk.

2. Reprogramming of Glucose Metabolism: Increased Uptake of Glucose and Lactate Production

In physiological conditions, the liver produces, stores, and releases glucose depending on the body's need for this substrate. After a meal, blood glucose enters the hepatocytes via the plasma membrane glucose transporter (GLUT). Human GLUT protein family includes fourteen members which exhibit different substrate specificities and tissue expression [8]. Once inside the cell, glucose is first converted, by glycolysis, into pyruvate and then completely oxidized into the mitochondrial matrix by the tricarboxylic acid (TCA) cycle and the oxidative phosphorylation. Alternatively, it can be channelled in the fatty acid synthesis pathway through the *de novo* lipogenesis (*DNL*). Glucose-6-phosphate dehydrogenase, the rate-limiting enzyme of the pentose phosphate pathway, is used in the liver to generate reduced nicotinamide adenine dinucleotide phosphate (NADPH) that is required for lipogenesis and biosynthesis of other bioactive molecules. In pathological conditions, glucose energy metabolism is altered. Important changes have been observed not only in the expression of specific transporters and enzyme isoforms but also in the flux of metabolites.

HCC tumors display a high level of glucose metabolism [9] (Figure 1). This enhanced metabolic demand is important for metabolic imaging and well supported by the ability of 18F-fludeoxyglucose (18F-FDG) positron emission tomography (PET) to correlate with unfavorable histopathologic features [10] and with the proliferative activity of tumor [11]. Moreover, high glucose levels as observed in patients with diabetes can accelerate tumorigenesis in HCC cells by generating advanced glycation

end-products and O-GlcNAcylation of the Yes-associated protein (YAP) and c-Jun [12, 13].

The common feature of these alterations is an increased glucose uptake and production of lactate even in the presence of oxygen and fully functioning mitochondria (Warburg effect) [2, 3], but it is not correlated with enhanced gluconeogenesis as the expression of phosphoenolpyruvate carboxykinases 1 and 2 and fructose 1,6-bisphosphatase 1 (FBP1), has been reported to be downregulated in HCC [14]. Overall, this metabolic reprogramming promotes growth, survival, proliferation, and long-term maintenance [15]. To respond to this metabolic requirement, HCC tumors enhance glucose uptake [16] by upregulating GLUT1 and GLUT2 isoforms [17–19]. siRNA-mediated abrogation of GLUT1 expression inhibits proliferative and migratory potential of HCC cells [20], while GLUT2 overexpression was correlated to a worse prognosis [21, 22].

Once inside the cell, glucose is converted in glucose-6-phosphate (G6P) by the hexokinase (HK), which is the first enzyme of the glycolytic pathway. Five major hexokinase isoforms are expressed in mammalian tissues and denoted as HK1, HK2, HK3, HK4, and the isoform hexokinase domain containing 1 (HKDC1). HCC tumors express high levels of the HK2 isoform, and its expression is correlated with the pathological stage of the tumor [23, 24]. In HCC, HK2 knockdown inhibited the flux of glucose to pyruvate and lactate, increased oxidative phosphorylation, and sensitized to metformin [24]. Moreover, HK2 silencing also synergized with sorafenib to inhibit tumor growth in mice [24]. Interestingly, a new member of the HK family the isoform HKDC1 was upregulated in HCC tissues compared with the adjacent normal tissues. HCC patients with high expression levels of HKDC1 had poor overall survival. Silencing HKDC1 suppressed HCC cell proliferation and migration *in vitro*, probably by the repression of the Wnt/β-catenin pathway [25].

The transition to glucose metabolism involves alterations in different glycolytic enzymes. A well-characterized example is the decreased expression of FBP1 [26]. FBP1 downregulation by promoter methylation and copy-number loss contributed to HCC progression by altering glucose metabolism [26]. An increased expression of glyceraldehyde-3-phosphate dehydrogenase (GAPDH) [27, 28] and pyruvate kinases 2 (PKM2) [9, 29, 30] was also described. The altered expression of these enzymes supports the flux of glucose in the glycolytic pathway leading to the generation of pyruvate that may be either used to generate lactate or be directed towards the TCA cycle. The high glutamine utilization and the high levels of lactate observed in HCC tissues are both in accordance with the first hypothesis, suggesting an increased TCA carbon anaplerosis in HCC cells [24, 31]. Glutamine represents the most abundant amino acid in blood and tissues and represents the major hepatic gluconeogenic substrate. A metabolic shift towards glutamine regulates tumor growth in HCC [14]. Hepatoma cells have an accelerated metabolism and net glutamine consumption, with potential implication at the systemic level [32].

Glutamine is metabolized in several distinct pathways. By glutaminolysis, glutamine can be converted to α-ketoglutarate

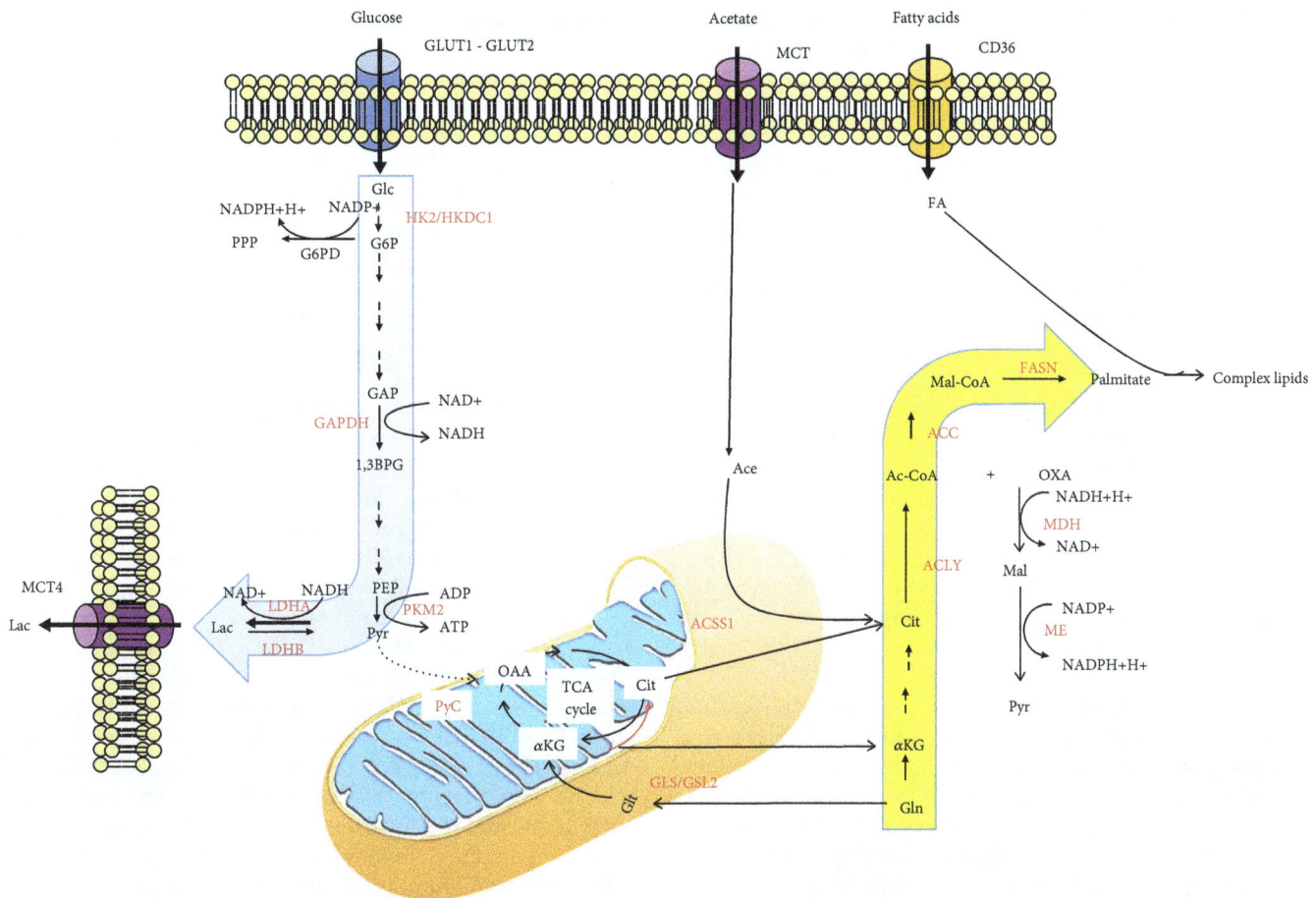

FIGURE 1: Metabolic reprogramming in HCC. Glucose enters the cancer cell via glucose transporters 1 and 2 (GLUT1 and GLUT2), and it is mainly used in the glycolytic pathway due to the overexpression of enzymes such as hexokinase 2 (HK2) and hexokinase domain containing 1 (HKDC1), glyceraldehyde-3-phosphate dehydrogenase (GAPDH), and pyruvate kinase 2 (PK2). The glycolytic pathway mainly produces, by the overexpression of lactate dehydrogenase A (LDHA) isoform, lactate (Lac) which is transported outside of the cell mainly throughout the monocarboxylate transporter isoform 4 (MCT4). Fatty acids enter cancer cells thanks to the upregulation of fatty acid translocase CD36. Nevertheless, fatty acid synthesis can also start from acetate (Ace), which is transported in the cell by MCT and converted into acetyl-CoA (Ac-CoA) by the mitochondrial isoform of acetyl-CoA synthase 1 (ACSS1). Moreover, glutamine (Gln) takes part in lipid synthesis after conversion into glutamate by mitochondrial glutaminase enzymes (GLS/GLS2). Glutamate is then converted into α-ketoglutarate (αKG) which can enter the tricarboxylic acid (TCA) cycle. Alternatively, αKG can undergo a reductive carboxylation by which it is transformed in citrate in the mitochondria (red arrow) or in the cytosol. In glutamine-free conditions, pyruvate (Pyr) can be converted into oxaloacetate (OAA) by the anaplerotic reaction catalysed by pyruvate carboxylase (PyC) enzyme. The *de novo* fatty acids synthesis is increased in cancer cells, and it is associated with a high expression of key enzymes such as acetyl-CoA carboxylase (ACC) and fatty acid synthase (FASN). This latter metabolic pathway is associated to a high production of reducing equivalents in the form of reduced nicotinamide adenine dinucleotide phosphate (NADPH) that is mainly produced in the first reaction of the pentose phosphate pathway (PPP) catalysed by glucose-6-phosphate dehydrogenase (G6PD) and by the malic enzyme (ME).

to replenish TCA cycle thus supporting energy production and providing intermediates for other biosynthetic pathways. By reductive carboxylation, glutamine moves in reverse of the TCA cycle from α-ketoglutarate to citrate to sustain lipid synthesis. So far, conflicting data have been reported on the role of glutamine in HCC. In fact, a study demonstrated that glutamine is metabolized mainly via glutaminolysis and not via reductive carboxylation to be converted into lactate [24]. Another study did not support this hypothesis as the great majority of enzymes involved in the conversion of glutamine to α-ketoglutarate were significantly downregulated in HCC compared to the normal liver [14]. This highlights the heterogeneous behaviour of this pathway that might be influenced by specific conditions of the microenvironment or its correlation to specific genetic alterations. For instance, glutamine metabolism in HCC varied in relation to the initiating lesion. Mouse liver tumors induced by MYC overexpression significantly increased both glucose and glutamine catabolism, whereas MET-induced liver tumors used glucose to produce glutamine [33].

The metabolic reaction that generates lactate from pyruvate is catalysed by lactate dehydrogenase (LDH). In humans, five active LDH isoenzymes are present and each of which is a tetrameric enzyme composed of two major subunits, M and H (formally A and B), encoded by *Ldh-A* and *Ldh-B*, respectively. The M subunit is predominantly found in the skeletal muscle, whereas the H subunit in the heart. LDHA and LDHB are upregulated in human cancers and associated with aggressive tumor outcomes [34–36].

In human HCC, LDHA expression was upregulated as a consequence of the downregulation of the microRNA-383 [37]. LDHA knockdown induced apoptosis and cell growth arrest in HCC cells and suppressed metastasis in a xenograft mouse model [38]. Serum LDH has been used as a prognostic indicator for patients with HCC treated with sorafenib, undergoing transcatheter arterial chemoembolization (TACE), or curative resection [39–42].

Lactate, the product of LDH activity, is exported in the extracellular milieu by monocarboxylate transporters (MCT). In HCC samples, an overexpression of MCT4 has been reported [43] and was also associated with Ki-67 expression [44]. Basigin, a transmembrane glycoprotein also called CD147, was found to be involved in the reprogramming of glucose metabolism in HCC cells. In particular, CD147 promoted glycolysis and facilitated the cell surface expression of MCT1 and lactate export [45]. Interestingly, blocking CD147 and/or MCT1 was reported to suppress HCC proliferation [45].

At a metabolic level, a high level of lactate with a low level of glucose was detected by nuclear magnetic resonance analysis in HCC samples [46]. This confirms the glycolytic shift toward lactate and provides a correlation between enzymatic alterations and metabolite expression [46]. The increased lactate concentration observed in the serum of HCC patients, compared to normal subjects, seems to be a consequence of this metabolic change [47]. However, the role of this secreted lactate still remains largely unclear. Nevertheless, increased lactate production was observed in patients with steatosis and steatohepatitis (NASH) compared to normal patients suggesting that the shift toward and anaerobic glucose metabolism can be involved in the first steps of liver carcinogenesis [48].

3. Altered Anabolic and Catabolic Lipid Pathways in HCC

The liver plays a key role in the metabolism of lipids and lipoproteins, and the anomalies in these metabolic pathways underlie HCC pathogenesis as demonstrated by increased risks observed in patients with obesity [49], diabetes [50], and hepatic steatosis [51]. After a carbohydrate reach meal, fatty acids can be synthetized from glycolytic pyruvate by DNL. Thus, entering the mitochondria, pyruvate is converted into acetyl-CoA by the pyruvate dehydrogenase enzyme. In the mitochondrial matrix, acetyl-CoA condensates with oxaloacetate to form citrate which, in conditions of high energetic charge, is conveyed to the cytoplasm throughout the citrate carrier for lipid synthesis. Key enzymes of cytosolic DNL are acetyl-CoA carboxylase (ACC), which catalyses the ATP-dependent carboxylation of acetyl-CoA to malonyl-CoA, and the multifunctional enzyme fatty acid synthase (FASN), which utilizes malonyl-CoA for synthesizing palmitoyl-CoA [52]. DNL also needs reducing power in the form of NADPH + H$^+$, which is mainly generated through the glucose metabolism

in the pentose phosphate pathway and in the malic enzyme reaction. DNL alterations were observed in HCC samples [53] and in other liver diseases, including nonalcoholic fatty liver disease (NAFLD) [54]. A combinatorial network-based analysis revealed that many enzymes involved in DNL, as well as enzymes related to NADPH production, such as glucose-6-phosphate dehydrogenase and malic enzyme, were upregulated in HCC with respect to the noncancerous liver samples [14].

During cancer progression, an overexpression of FASN is important for promoting tumor cell survival and proliferation [54], and it was also associated with poor patient prognosis [55]. In line with what observed in other types of tumors, recent studies described a functional association among lipogenesis, FASN, sterol regulatory element-binding protein-1 (SREBP-1), a transcription factor regulating FASN expression, and HCC [56–64]. The therapeutic effects of targeting FASN were investigated in several works. For instance, HCC induced by AKT/c-Met was fully inhibited in FASN knockout mice [65].

Alternative carbon sources can support the generation of acetyl-CoA required for DNL. This can derive from exogenous acetate, which is transported into cells by members of the MCT family and then converted to acetyl-CoA by acetyl-CoA synthase enzymes (mitochondrial ACSS1 and ACSS3 or cytosolic ACSS2) to fuel fatty acid synthesis (Figure 1). Mitochondrial ACSS1 expression, but not ACSS2 or ACSS3 ones, is significantly upregulated in HCC compared to noncancerous liver and associated with increased tumor growth and malignancy under hypoxic conditions [14].

Tumors can be addicted or independent from DNL by the activation of complementary pathways. In fact, both de novo synthetized and exogenous fatty acids can support the growth of HCC tumors [66]. The studies performed on animal models demonstrated that the inhibition of lipogenesis via genetic deletion of ACC genes increased susceptibility to tumorigenesis in mice treated with the hepatocellular carcinogen diethylnitrosamine, demonstrating that lipogenesis is essential for liver tumorigenesis [67].

The liver is able to take up nonesterified fatty acids from the blood, in proportion to their concentration, either via specific transporters (fatty acid transport protein (FATP) or fatty acid translocase/CD36) or by diffusion. The activation of the CD36 pathway has been associated with tumor aggressiveness by the induction of the epithelial-mesenchymal transition (EMT) program [68], which is a process that contributes to cancer progression [69, 70]. This is mediated through the involvement of specific pathways. The analysis of the Cancer Genome Atlas (TGCA) dataset revealed a significant association between CD36 and EMT markers, potentially by the activation of Wnt and TGF-β signaling pathways [71].

The liver is able to oxidize fatty acids by both mitochondrial and peroxisomal β-oxidation. The entry of fatty acids into the mitochondria is regulated by the activity of the enzyme carnitine palmitoyltransferase-I (CPT-I) [72], which catalyses the synthesis of acylcarnitines from very long acyl-CoA and carnitine, thus allowing the entry of polar fatty acids in the mitochondrial matrix. In a rat model of NASH, a decreased mitochondrial CPT-I activity [73] and dysfunction of both complex I and II of the mitochondrial respiratory chain [74] have been demonstrated. Moreover, deregulation of mitochondrial β-oxidation with downregulation of many enzymes involved in fatty acid oxidation has been reported in HCC patients [14]. Accordingly, the urinary level of short- and medium-chain acylcarnitines was found to be different in HCC vs. cirrhosis, and butyrylcarnitine (carnitine C4:0) was defined as a potential marker for distinguishing between HCC and cirrhosis [75]. All together, these data indicate that mitochondrial alterations can represent an early determinant in HCC.

The liver represents also a major site of synthesis and metabolism of endogenous cholesterol. The pool of cholesterol is tightly regulated, and it reflects the input of cholesterol from the diet, its biosynthesis, the secretion and uptake of cholesterol from plasma lipoproteins, the conversion of cholesterol into bile, and the reuptake of biliary cholesterol and bile acids from the intestine to the liver. The rate-limiting enzyme in the cholesterol synthesis is the 3-hydroxy-3-methylglutaryl-CoA reductase, which catalyses the synthesis of mevalonate.

There is increasing evidence that the mevalonate pathway is implicated in the pathogenesis of HCC [76, 77]. To this respect, clinical studies demonstrated that statins, widely used to reduce cholesterol levels, were able to reduce the risk of HCC [78] and showed antiproliferative effects in vitro on HepG2 cells and in vivo on rats with HCC [79]. Data from a meta-analysis report that the use of statins could significantly cut the risk of liver cancer and that fluvastatin is the most effective drug for reducing HCC risk compared to other statin interventions [80].

Cholesterol is also used in the liver for the synthesis of bile acids, which are hydroxylated steroids that, once secreted in the intestine, provide for solubilisation of dietary cholesterol, lipids, fat-soluble vitamins, and other essential nutrients, thus promoting their delivery to the liver. Primary bile acids, such as cholic acid and chenodeoxycholic acid, are synthesized in hepatocytes and can be conjugated to glycine or taurine [81]. Cholic acid conjugated to glycine, in the form of glycocholic acid, represents a secondary bile acid that is synthesized by microbiota in the small intestine [81]. It has been reported that intrahepatic bile acid may have a stimulatory effect of hepatic tumorigenesis [82] and abnormal bile acid metabolism has been correlated with HCC [83–86]. The hepatic deregulation of bile acid metabolism can result in increased serum level of glycolic acid, as reported by Guo and collaborators [87].

Modification in the activity of enzymes related to phospholipid remodelling has been reported in a rat model of cirrhosis [88]. Moreover, an altered lipid metabolism, including phospholipids, fatty acids, and bile metabolites, was observed in serum samples from HCC patients [89, 90]. In particular, higher phosphatidylcholines (PC) concentrations were observed in HCC patients at early and late stage compared to cirrhotic and control subjects, indicating a disturbance of the phospholipid catabolism [85]. This result significantly correlated with higher levels of PC observed at tissue level [91].

4. Alterations in Amino Acid and Protein Metabolism Underlying HCC

The liver carries out many functions in protein metabolism. A broad spectrum of proteins responsible for the maintenance of hemostasis, oncotic pressure, hormone, lipid transport, and acute phase reactions are synthetized in the liver. Among these proteins, albumin is synthesized almost exclusively by the liver, and alone, it accounts for 40% of hepatic protein synthesis. Moreover, the liver is also able to synthetize thyroid-binding globulin, VLDL apoB 100, and complement.

A very recent work reports that patients with lower serum albumin levels have significantly larger maximum tumor diameters, greater prevalence of portal vein thrombosis, increased tumor multifocality, and higher α-fetoprotein levels with respect to patients with higher albumin levels. These data indicate that decreased serum albumin correlates with increased parameters of HCC aggressiveness, therefore, having a role in HCC aggressiveness [92].

In the liver, the synthetized nonessential amino acids (AA) play a pivotal role in the maintenance of diverse homeostatic functions such as gluconeogenesis. Both synthetized amino acids and those derived from the diet are utilized either for protein synthesis or catabolized (except branched chain amino acids) by transamination or oxidative deamination reactions. These processes produce keto acids that can be oxidized to produce energy in the form of ATP. Several enzymes used in these pathways (for example, alanine transaminase and aspartate transaminase) are commonly assayed in serum to assess liver damage. Moreover, the oxidative deamination of amino acids produces ammonium ions, a toxic product whose detoxification can either occur in extrahepatic tissues, throughout the synthesis of glutamine when combined with glutamate, or in the liver, to make urea which is then transported to the kidneys where it can be directly excreted in urine.

An increased AA metabolism is generally observed in human tumors, in line with the role of AA and enzymes responsible for their production in cancer initiation and progression [93–96]. The shift toward an increased amino acid production is considered as a consequence of the described altered glucose metabolism. In the condition of increased consumption of glucose by aerobic glycolysis, amino acids can be used as glucose precursors or activators of glycolytic enzymes [97].

An altered AA metabolism characterizes HCC compared to other liver diseases. For instance, serum levels of alanine, serine, glycine, cysteine, aspartic acid, lysine, methionine, tyrosine, phenylalanine, tryptophan, and glutamic acid were dramatically increased in HCC compared with healthy subjects, together with a lower ratio of branched-chain amino acids (valine, leucine, and isoleucine) to aromatic amino acids (tyrosine, phenylalanine, and tryptophan) [98, 99].

Furthermore, AA bioavailability not only contributes to anabolic and catabolic pathways but it is also essential during HCC pathogenesis by supporting cellular hypoxic responses [100].

5. Oxidative Metabolism Imbalance in HCC

Oxidative stress occurs when reactive oxygen species (ROS) production overwhelms the normal antioxidant capacity of cells [101]. ROS are short-lived and very reactive molecules that rapidly react with cellular biomolecules yielding oxidatively modified products that eventually lead to cell injury and death. Due to the high instability of ROS, they cannot be easily detected, and protein carbonyls, 8-hydroxydeoxyguanosine, and 4-hydroxynonenal (which are oxidatively modified products of proteins, DNA, and lipids, respectively) have been widely used as markers for oxidative stress [102].

Accumulating evidence suggests that many types of cancer cells have increased levels of oxidative stress and ROS production with respect to normal cells [103]. As a consequence of this, redox homeostasis is finely regulated in cancer cells with an underappreciated role in the control of cell signaling and metabolism. For instance, ROS-mediated inhibition of PKM2 allows cancer cells to sustain antioxidant responses by diverting glucose flux into the pentose phosphate pathway and increasing the production of reducing equivalents for ROS detoxification [104]. Understanding the mechanisms at the basis of ROS homeostasis might have therapeutic implications.

Oxidative damage is considered a key pathway in HCC progression and increases patient vulnerability for HCC recurrence [105]. Oxidative stress closely correlates with HCV- and NASH-related HCC, but relatively weakly with HBV-related HCC [106]. Moreover, it has been reported that NASH-related HCC patients had a diminished serum antioxidative function compared with nonalcoholic fatty liver disease patients [107].

Glutathione is a nonenzymatic tripeptide that plays a central role in the cellular antioxidant defense system, and it represents the most abundant antioxidant in hepatocytes. Glutathione is synthesized intracellularly from cysteine, glycine, and glutamate, and it is abundantly found in the cytosol and mitochondria and in a smaller percentage in the endoplasmic reticulum [108]. During glutathione antioxidant function, the reduced form of glutathione (GSH) is oxidized to the glutathione disulfide dimer (GSSG). The regeneration of the reduced form requires the enzymatic action of glutathione reductase and reducing equivalents in the form of $NADPH + H^+$. A significant increase in all amino acids related to the GSH synthesis, including 5-oxoproline, was observed in the serum of HCC patients, and an increase of G6P that represents an important source of NADPH for the generation of GSH has been also reported [109]. Moreover, signs of DNA and lipid oxidative damages were found in HCC. Indeed, an increased level of 8-hydroxydeoxy guanosine was found in chronic hepatitis, corresponding to an increased risk of HCC [110, 111]. In addition, a mass spectrometry study highlighted an increased level of 4-hydroxynonenal in human tissues of HCC compared to peripheral noncancerous tissues [112].

The GSH:GSSG ratio is considered an important indicator of the redox balance in cells, with a higher ratio representing low oxidative stress [107]. Upon depletion of GSH, ROS induce oxidative stress which causes liver damage, and reduced GSH levels have been reported in various liver diseases [113]. By-products of GSH synthesis are represented by γ-glutamyl peptides that are biosynthesized through a reaction of ligation of glutamate with various amino acids and amines by the action of γ-glutamylcysteine synthetase. Serum level of γ-glutamyl peptides, measured by capillary chromatography-MS/MS, was increased in patients with virus-related HCC [114, 115], and it was considered a reliable potential biomarker for this pathology [115]. The 2-hydroxybutyric acid is another compound considered in relation to GSH metabolism. It is primarily produced in mammalian hepatic tissues, which catabolize threonine or synthesize glutathione. Under conditions of intense oxidative stress, hepatic glutathione synthesis is increased, and there is a high demand for cysteine. In such cases, homocysteine is diverted from the transmethylation pathway and instead it is used to produce cystathionine, which is then cleaved into cysteine and finally incorporated into glutathione. 2-Hydroxybutyric acid is then produced from reduction of α-ketobutyrate, which is released as a by-product of the cystathionine conversion to cysteine. An increased serum concentration of 2-hydroxybutyric acid as well as of xanthine, an intermediate in the purine degradation process producing H_2O_2, and several γ-glutamyl peptides, were found in HCC with respect to control subjects [116, 117].

6. Metabolic Reprogramming of HCC Microenvironment

HCC microenvironment consists of stromal cells, hepatic stellate cells, and endothelial and immune cells. The crosstalk between tumor cells and their surrounding microenvironment is required for sustaining HCC development by promoting angiogenesis, EMT, or by modulating the polarization of immune cells. Tumor-associated macrophages (TAM) and myeloid-derived suppressor cells (MDSC) are the major components of tumor-infiltrate and are abundant in HCC microenvironment (Figure 2) [118–120]. Metabolites released from tumor cells can have an impact on immune cells.

Inflammatory stimuli promote the switching of macrophages towards an M1-like phenotype characterized by the production of inflammatory cytokines. On the contrary, anti-inflammatory stimuli induce these cells to acquire an M2-like phenotype with immunosuppressive functions [121]. Thus, during chronic inflammation, macrophages predispose a given tissue to tumor initiation by releasing themselves factors that promote neoplastic transformation. In the successive phases of inflammation, the macrophage phenotype shifts more toward one that is immunosuppressive and supports tumor growth, angiogenesis, and metastasis [122]. In this respect, both epidemiological and clinical studies have demonstrated that various chronic

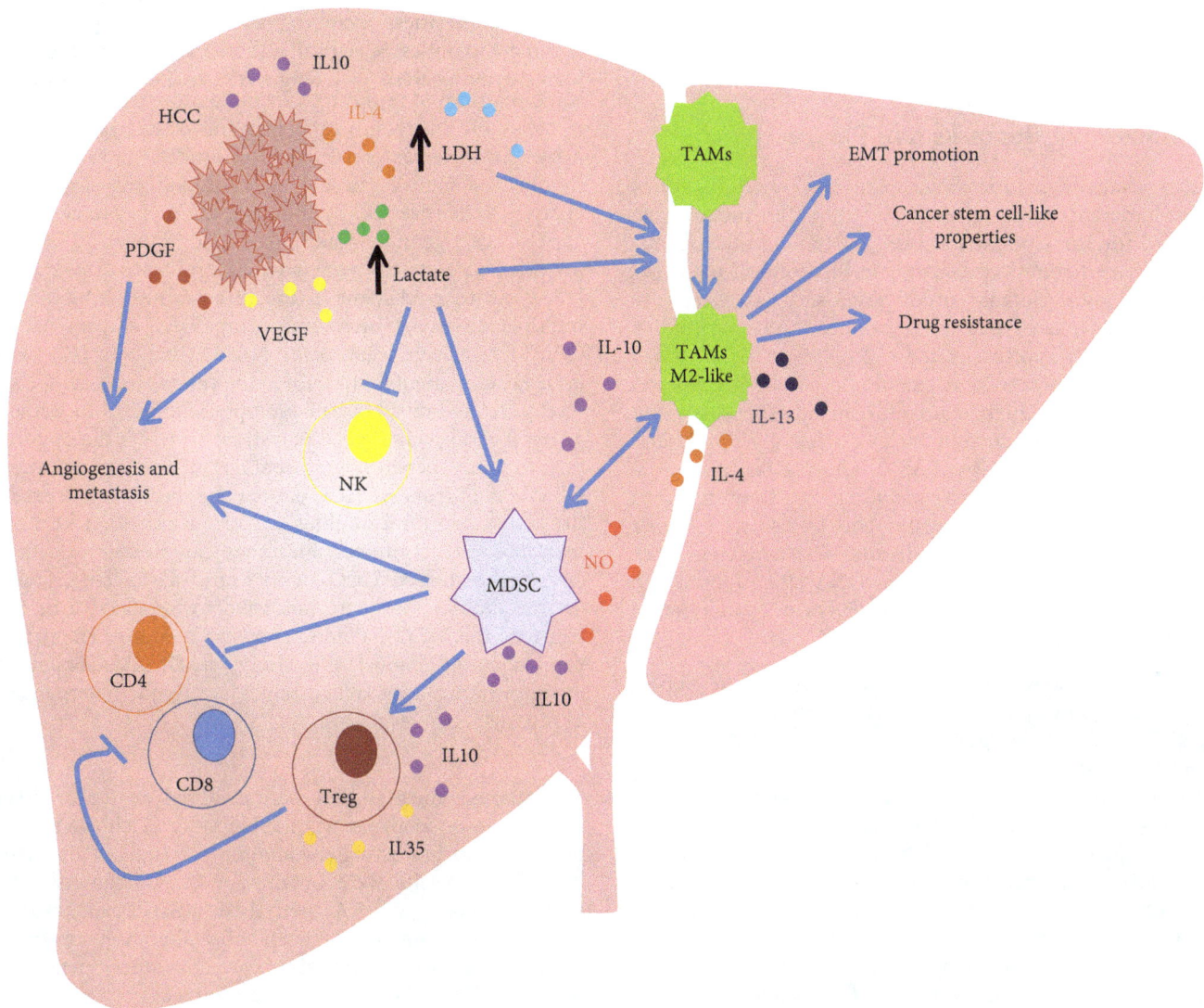

FIGURE 2: Metabolic connections between HCC and immune cells. Tumor-associated macrophages (TAM) and myeloid-derived suppressor cells (MDSC) are the major components of tumor-infiltrate and are abundant in HCC microenvironment, with a key role in supporting tumor initiation, progression, angiogenesis, metastasis, and drug resistance. HCC cells acquire an altered metabolism resulting in increased levels of LDH and lactate that, on the one hand, promote TAM polarization in M2-like phenotype, favoring the EMT, cancer stem cell-like properties, and drug resistance, and, on the other hand, increase the number of MDSC and inhibit NK cell function.

inflammatory diseases can predispose to increased risk of cancer at the same site of inflammation, and HCC is a clear example of inflammation-related cancer.

TAM originate from circulating monocytic precursors, and they are recruited to tumor cells by tumor-derived signals. It has been reported that, in the early phase of the tumor, TAM acquire an inflammatory phenotype and shift their metabolism toward an anaerobic glycolytic pathway [122, 123]. This allows polarized macrophages to rapidly fuel themselves with energy and to cope with hypoxic tissue microenvironment. The interplay between M2-like TAM and cancer is complex, and it is involved in each step of HCC development. It has been demonstrated that this TAM subset promotes migration and EMT. It also induces cancer stem cell-like properties and drug resistance in human HCC, thus highlighting the importance of targeting

the immune microenvironment as a mechanism to inhibit HCC recurrence and metastasis (Figure 2) [124]. Moreover, it has been shown that an increase in the M2-macrophage population is associated with poor prognosis in HCC [125]. TAM can use metabolites released from cancer cells to modulate their polarization status. This is supported by the findings that demonstrated that tumor-released lactate is utilized by TAM to increase the expression of vascular endothelial growth factor and to induce an M2-like status [126]. Lactate can also have effects on other cell types by increasing the number of MDSC, thus inhibiting NK cell function (Figure 2) [127]. The immunosuppressive functions of MDSC can also be regulated by other metabolites, including fatty acids. In MDSC, increased fatty acid uptake and fatty acid oxidation are induced by a STAT3/STAT5-mediated pathway leading to an increased expression of CD36. Accumulation of lipids increases the oxidative metabolism of MDSC and activates their immunosuppressive mechanisms [128].

7. Concluding Remarks and Perspectives

Global changes in metabolic pathways were identified across different tumor types [129, 130]. The picture that emerged for the comparison between tumors and normal tissue revealed common demands in biochemical pathways associated with biomass production, such as glycolysis, pentose phosphate pathway, purine, and pyrimidine biosynthesis, irrespective of the cell of origin. This cancer tissue-specific metabolic signature is well defined in HCC, where the high glucose demand supports PPP pathway, lactate production by anaerobic glycolysis, and fatty acid production by FASN. Glucose utilization is regulated at multiple levels, including the transcriptional regulation of metabolic enzymes and transporters whose expression is altered in HCC tissues, and consistent with the identification of mitochondrial DNA alterations which was associated with a reduced oxidative phosphorylation and enhanced glycolysis [131].

HCC cells also rely on other carbon substrates to support anaplerotic pathways. A role for glutamine and acetate in sustaining HCC bioenergetics has been proposed. Alternative anaplerotic pathways exist that rely on the transformation of pyruvate to oxaloacetate by pyruvate carboxylase to support the growth of HCC cells in glutamine-free conditions [132]. The dependence of HCC cells from lipid uptake should be also considered, suggesting the existence of a metabolic flexibility and of a possible cross-talk between metabolic pathways that might result by changes imposed by the tumor microenvironment or by the activation of specific signaling pathways. HCC cells can, for instance, modulate fatty acids uptake by the upregulation of CD36 and caveolin 1 that is mediated by the activation of Wnt and TGF-β pathways.

More unique metabolic features were also defined by TGCA studies where significant alterations by mutation or downregulation by hypermethylation in albumin, apolipoprotein B, and carbamoyl phosphate synthase I metabolic genes were observed in HCC [71].

Overall, this metabolic program seems to be essential for HCC biology to sustain tumor growth and progression, and targeting of these pathways might have significant clinical implications. For instance, clinical effects of dexamethasone are explicated *in vivo* by restoring gluconeogenesis [133], inhibition of proline production and targeting of transketolase significantly enhances the cytotoxic effect of sorafenib *in vivo* [134], and insights into nucleotide and lipid metabolism of HCC may provide novel clinical opportunities [135].

However, the design of therapeutic metabolic targeted strategies should be carefully evaluated taking into account tumor heterogeneity and tumor interaction with the microenvironment. Several approaches were applied to address these complexities, including computational, proteomics, and metabolomics. Specifically, these methods tried to move forward the analysis of a single metabolite to obtain not a static snapshot of tumor biology but a more dynamic picture of metabolic changes in cancer. In this context, the field has expanded to bypass some classical limitations as the small number of samples to be analyzed and the number of analytes to be revealed. By the integration of different omics approaches, genome-scale metabolic models (GEMM) provided a way to study metabolic pathways at systems level [136] and to predict the action of a pathway inhibition at multiple layers of biological complexity. A personalized GEMM has been realized for NAFLD patients [137, 138] and HCC patients [14, 139] to characterize a specific disease-related metabolic phenotype. Moreover, the detailed analysis of a specific metabolic status provides the opportunity to study network perturbations after drug treatment. GEMM built from six HCC patients has been used to predict the action of antimetabolites on cancer growth. The model identified 147 antimetabolites that can inhibit growth in any of the studied HCC tumors, and a smaller group of antimetabolites that were predicted to be effective in only some of the HCC patients, showing a more personalized mechanism of action [139]. Moreover, GEMM has become an informative approach to elucidate tumor heterogeneity at the metabolic level [14].

Although most studies were centered on tumor tissue, metabolomics analyses at the blood level showed to be promising in predicting metabolic alterations at the tissue level. Solid results were obtained with some metabolites, such as lactate and AA, and their altered expression in serum clearly mirrors a metabolic alteration of tumor tissue. The same is probably true for other metabolites such as fatty acids but not yet clarified.

References

[1] A. Forner, M. Reig, and J. Bruix, "Hepatocellular carcinoma," *The Lancet*, vol. 391, no. 10127, pp. 1301–1314, 2018.

[2] N. N. Pavlova and C. B. Thompson, "The emerging hallmarks of cancer metabolism," *Cell Metabolism*, vol. 23, no. 1, pp. 27–47, 2016.

[3] R. J. DeBerardinis and N. S. Chandel, "Fundamentals of cancer metabolism," *Science Advances*, vol. 2, no. 5, article e1600200, 2016.

[4] A. J. Wolpaw and C. V. Dang, "Exploiting metabolic vulnerabilities of cancer with precision and accuracy," *Trends in Cell Biology*, vol. 28, no. 3, pp. 201–212, 2018.

[5] D. Vergara, E. Stanca, F. Guerra et al., "β-Catenin knockdown affects mitochondrial biogenesis and lipid metabolism in breast cancer cells," *Frontiers in Physiology*, vol. 8, p. 544, 2017.

[6] C. Agostinelli, S. Carloni, F. Limarzi et al., "The emerging role of GSK-3β in the pathobiology of classical Hodgkin lymphoma," *Histopathology*, vol. 71, no. 1, pp. 72–80, 2017.

[7] L. Rui, "Energy metabolism in the liver," *Comprehensive Physiology*, vol. 4, no. 1, pp. 177–197, 2014.

[8] C. C. Barron, P. J. Bilan, T. Tsakiridis, and E. Tsiani, "Facilitative glucose transporters: implications for cancer detection, prognosis and treatment," *Metabolism*, vol. 65, no. 2, pp. 124–139, 2016.

[9] R. Z. Shang, S. B. Qu, and D. S. Wang, "Reprogramming of glucose metabolism in hepatocellular carcinoma: progress and prospects," *World Journal of Gastroenterology*, vol. 22, no. 45, pp. 9933–9943, 2016.

[10] A. Kornberg, M. Freesmeyer, E. Bärthel et al., "18F-FDG-uptake of hepatocellular carcinoma on PET predicts microvascular tumor invasion in liver transplant patients," *American Journal of Transplantation*, vol. 9, no. 3, pp. 592–600, 2009.

[11] K. Kitamura, E. Hatano, T. Higashi et al., "Proliferative activity in hepatocellular carcinoma is closely correlated with glucose metabolism but not angiogenesis," *Journal of Hepatology*, vol. 55, no. 4, pp. 846–857, 2011.

[12] X. Zhang, Y. Qiao, Q. Wu et al., "The essential role of YAP O-GlcNAcylation in high-glucose-stimulated liver tumorigenesis," *Nature Communications*, vol. 8, article 15280, 2017.

[13] Y. Qiao, X. Zhang, Y. Zhang et al., "High glucose stimulates tumorigenesis in hepatocellular carcinoma cells through AGER-dependent O-GlcNAcylation of c-Jun," *Diabetes*, vol. 65, no. 3, pp. 619–632, 2016.

[14] E. Björnson, B. Mukhopadhyay, A. Asplund et al., "Stratification of hepatocellular carcinoma patients based on acetate utilization," *Cell Reports*, vol. 13, no. 9, pp. 2014–2026, 2015.

[15] N. Hay, "Reprogramming glucose metabolism in cancer: can it be exploited for cancer therapy?," *Nature Reviews Cancer*, vol. 16, no. 10, pp. 635–649, 2016.

[16] U. Parikh, C. Marcus, R. Sarangi, M. Taghipour, and R. M. Subramaniam, "FDG PET/CT in pancreatic and hepatobiliary carcinomas: value to patient management and patient outcomes," *PET Clinics*, vol. 10, no. 3, pp. 327–343, 2015.

[17] T. Yamamoto, Y. Seino, H. Fukumoto et al., "Over-expression of facilitative glucose transporter genes in human cancer," *Biochemical and Biophysical Research Communications*, vol. 170, no. 1, pp. 223–230, 1990.

[18] R. Grobholz, H. J. Hacker, B. Thorens, and P. Bannasch, "Reduction in the expression of glucose transporter protein GLUT 2 in preneoplastic and neoplastic hepatic lesions and reexpression of GLUT 1 in late stages of hepatocarcinogenesis," *Cancer Research*, vol. 53, no. 18, pp. 4204–4211, 1993.

[19] T. S. Su, T. F. Tsai, C. W. Chi, S. H. Han, and C. K. Chou, "Elevation of facilitated glucose-transporter messenger RNA in human hepatocellular carcinoma," *Hepatology*, vol. 11, no. 1, pp. 118–122, 1990.

[20] T. Amann and C. Hellerbrand, "GLUT1 as a therapeutic target in hepatocellular carcinoma," *Expert Opinion on Therapeutic Targets*, vol. 13, no. 12, pp. 1411–1427, 2009.

[21] K. Daskalow, D. Pfander, W. Weichert et al., "Distinct temporospatial expression patterns of glycolysis-related proteins in human hepatocellular carcinoma," *Histochemistry and Cell Biology*, vol. 132, no. 1, pp. 21–31, 2009.

[22] Y. H. Kim, D. C. Jeong, K. Pak et al., "SLC2A2 (GLUT2) as a novel prognostic factor for hepatocellular carcinoma," *Oncotarget*, vol. 8, no. 40, pp. 68381–68392, 2017.

[23] L. Gong, Z. Cui, P. Chen, H. Han, J. Peng, and X. Leng, "Reduced survival of patients with hepatocellular carcinoma expressing hexokinase II," *Medical Oncology*, vol. 29, no. 2, pp. 909–914, 2012.

[24] D. DeWaal, V. Nogueira, A. R. Terry et al., "Hexokinase-2 depletion inhibits glycolysis and induces oxidative phosphorylation in hepatocellular carcinoma and sensitizes to metformin," *Nature Communications*, vol. 9, no. 1, p. 446, 2018.

[25] Z. Zhang, S. Huang, H. Wang et al., "High expression of hexokinase domain containing 1 is associated with poor prognosis and aggressive phenotype in hepatocarcinoma," *Biochemical and Biophysical Research Communications*, vol. 474, no. 4, pp. 673–679, 2016.

[26] H. Hirata, K. Sugimachi, H. Komatsu et al., "Decreased expression of fructose-1,6-bisphosphatase associates with glucose metabolism and tumor progression in hepatocellular carcinoma," *Cancer Research*, vol. 76, no. 11, pp. 3265–3276, 2016.

[27] S. Liu, Y. Sun, M. Jiang et al., "Glyceraldehyde-3-phosphate dehydrogenase promotes liver tumorigenesis by modulating phosphoglycerate dehydrogenase," *Hepatology*, vol. 66, no. 2, pp. 631–645, 2017.

[28] S. Ganapathy-Kanniappan, R. Kunjithapatham, and J. F. Geschwind, "Glyceraldehyde-3-phosphate dehydrogenase: a promising target for molecular therapy in hepatocellular carcinoma," *Oncotarget*, vol. 3, no. 9, pp. 940–953, 2012.

[29] C. C.-L. Wong, S. L.-K. Au, A. P.-W. Tse et al., "Switching of pyruvate kinase isoform L to M2 promotes metabolic reprogramming in hepatocarcinogenesis," *PLoS One*, vol. 9, no. 12, article e115036, 2014.

[30] K. Nakao, H. Miyaaki, and T. Ichikawa, "Antitumor function of microRNA-122 against hepatocellular carcinoma," *Journal of Gastroenterology*, vol. 49, no. 4, pp. 589–593, 2014.

[31] A. A. Cluntun, M. J. Lukey, R. A. Cerione, and J. W. Locasale, "Glutamine metabolism in cancer: understanding the heterogeneity," *Trends in Cancer*, vol. 3, no. 3, pp. 169–180, 2017.

[32] B. P. Bode and W. W. Souba, "Glutamine transport and human hepatocellular transformation," *Journal of Parenteral and Enteral Nutrition*, vol. 23, 5_Supplement, pp. S33–S37, 1999.

[33] M. O. Yuneva, T. W. M. Fan, T. D. Allen et al., "The metabolic profile of tumors depends on both the responsible genetic lesion and tissue type," *Cell Metabolism*, vol. 15, no. 2, pp. 157–170, 2012.

[34] H. Xie, J. I. Hanai, J. G. Ren et al., "Targeting lactate dehydrogenase-A inhibits tumorigenesis and tumor progression in mouse models of lung cancer and impacts tumor-initiating cells," *Cell Metabolism*, vol. 19, no. 5, pp. 795–809, 2014.

[35] D. Vergara, P. Simeone, P. del Boccio et al., "Comparative proteome profiling of breast tumor cell lines by gel electrophoresis and mass spectrometry reveals an epithelial mesenchymal transition associated protein signature," *Molecular BioSystems*, vol. 9, no. 6, pp. 1127–1138, 2013.

[36] L. Brisson, P. Bański, M. Sboarina et al., "Lactate dehydrogenase B controls lysosome activity and autophagy in cancer," *Cancer Cell*, vol. 30, no. 3, pp. 418–431, 2016.

[37] Z. Fang, L. He, H. Jia, Q. Huang, D. Chen, and Z. Zhang, "The miR-383-LDHA axis regulates cell proliferation, invasion and glycolysis in hepatocellular cancer," *Iranian Journal of Basic Medical Sciences*, vol. 20, no. 2, pp. 187–192, 2017.

[38] S. L. Sheng, J. J. Liu, Y. H. Dai, X. G. Sun, X. P. Xiong, and G. Huang, "Knockdown of lactate dehydrogenase A suppresses tumor growth and metastasis of human

hepatocellular carcinoma," *FEBS Journal*, vol. 279, no. 20, pp. 3898–3910, 2012.

[39] L. Faloppi, M. Scartozzi, M. Bianconi et al., "The role of LDH serum levels in predicting global outcome in HCC patients treated with sorafenib: implications for clinical management," *BMC Cancer*, vol. 14, no. 1, p. 110, 2014.

[40] M. Scartozzi, L. Faloppi, M. Bianconi et al., "The role of LDH serum levels in predicting global outcome in HCC patients undergoing TACE: implications for clinical management," *PLoS One*, vol. 7, no. 3, article e32653, 2012.

[41] J. P. Zhang, H. B. Wang, Y. H. Lin et al., "Lactate dehydrogenase is an important prognostic indicator for hepatocellular carcinoma after partial hepatectomy," *Translational Oncology*, vol. 8, no. 6, pp. 497–503, 2015.

[42] L. Faloppi, M. Bianconi, R. Memeo et al., "Lactate dehydrogenase in hepatocellular carcinoma: something old, something new," *BioMed Research International*, vol. 2016, Article ID 7196280, 7 pages, 2016.

[43] H. J. Gao, M. C. Zhao, Y. J. Zhang et al., "Monocarboxylate transporter 4 predicts poor prognosis in hepatocellular carcinoma and is associated with cell proliferation and migration," *Journal of Cancer Research and Clinical Oncology*, vol. 141, no. 7, pp. 1151–1162, 2015.

[44] V. A. Alves, C. Pinheiro, F. Morais-Santos, A. Felipe-Silva, A. Longatto-Filho, and F. Baltazar, "Characterization of monocarboxylate transporter activity in hepatocellular carcinoma," *World Journal of Gastroenterology*, vol. 20, no. 33, pp. 11780–11787, 2014.

[45] Q. Huang, J. Li, J. Xing et al., "CD147 promotes reprogramming of glucose metabolism and cell proliferation in HCC cells by inhibiting the p53-dependent signaling pathway," *Journal of Hepatology*, vol. 61, no. 4, pp. 859–866, 2014.

[46] C. Teilhet, D. Morvan, J. Joubert-Zakeyh et al., "Specificities of human hepatocellular carcinoma developed on non-alcoholic fatty liver disease in absence of cirrhosis revealed by tissue extracts ^{1}H-NMR spectroscopy," *Metabolites*, vol. 7, no. 4, p. 49, 2017.

[47] Y. Chen, J. Zhou, J. Li, J. Feng, Z. Chen, and X. Wang, "Plasma metabolomic analysis of human hepatocellular carcinoma: diagnostic and therapeutic study," *Oncotarget*, vol. 7, no. 30, pp. 47332–47342, 2016.

[48] S. C. Kalhan, L. Guo, J. Edmison et al., "Plasma metabolomic profile in nonalcoholic fatty liver disease," *Metabolism*, vol. 60, no. 3, pp. 404–413, 2011.

[49] L. Gan, Z. Liu, and C. Sun, "Obesity linking to hepatocellular carcinoma: a global view," *Biochimica et Biophysica Acta (BBA) - Reviews on Cancer*, vol. 1869, no. 2, pp. 97–102, 2018.

[50] X. Li, X. Wang, and P. Gao, "Diabetes mellitus and risk of hepatocellular carcinoma," *BioMed Research International*, vol. 2017, Article ID 5202684, 10 pages, 2017.

[51] A. Borrelli, P. Bonelli, F. M. Tuccillo et al., "Role of gut microbiota and oxidative stress in the progression of non-alcoholic fatty liver disease to hepatocarcinoma: current and innovative therapeutic approaches," *Redox Biology*, vol. 15, pp. 467–479, 2018.

[52] S. Smith, A. Witkowski, and A. K. Joshi, "Structural and functional organization of the animal fatty acid synthase," *Progress in Lipid Research*, vol. 42, no. 4, pp. 289–317, 2003.

[53] D. F. Calvisi, "De novo lipogenesis: role in hepatocellular carcinoma," *Der Pathologe*, vol. 32, no. S2, pp. 174–180, 2011.

[54] K. L. Donnelly, C. I. Smith, S. J. Schwarzenberg, J. Jessurun, M. D. Boldt, and E. J. Parks, "Sources of fatty acids stored in liver and secreted via lipoproteins in patients with nonalcoholic fatty liver disease," *The Journal of Clinical Investigation*, vol. 115, no. 5, pp. 1343–1351, 2005.

[55] C. Mounier, L. Bouraoui, and E. Rassart, "Lipogenesis in cancer progression (review)," *International Journal of Oncology*, vol. 45, no. 2, pp. 485–492, 2014.

[56] L. Li, L. Che, C. Wang et al., "[^{11}C]acetate PET imaging is not always associated with increased lipogenesis in hepatocellular carcinoma in mice," *Molecular Imaging and Biology*, vol. 18, no. 3, pp. 360–367, 2016.

[57] Y. Gao, L. P. Lin, C. H. Zhu, Y. Chen, Y. T. Hou, and J. Ding, "Growth arrest induced by C75, a fatty acid synthase inhibitor, was partially modulated by p38 MAPK but not by p53 in human hepatocellular carcinoma," *Cancer Biology & Therapy*, vol. 5, no. 8, pp. 978–985, 2006.

[58] D. F. Calvisi, C. Wang, C. Ho et al., "Increased lipogenesis, induced by AKT-mTORC1-RPS6 signaling, promotes development of human hepatocellular carcinoma," *Gastroenterology*, vol. 140, no. 3, pp. 1071–1083.e5, 2011.

[59] T. Y. Na, Y. K. Shin, K. J. Roh et al., "Liver X receptor mediates hepatitis B virus X protein-induced lipogenesis in hepatitis B virus-associated hepatocellular carcinoma," *Hepatology*, vol. 49, no. 4, pp. 1122–1131, 2009.

[60] X. Zhu, X. Qin, M. Fei et al., "Combined phosphatase and tensin homolog (PTEN) loss and fatty acid synthase (FAS) overexpression worsens the prognosis of Chinese patients with hepatocellular carcinoma," *International Journal of Molecular Sciences*, vol. 13, no. 8, pp. 9980–9991, 2012.

[61] L. Che, M. G. Pilo, A. Cigliano et al., "Oncogene dependent requirement of fatty acid synthase in hepatocellular carcinoma," *Cell Cycle*, vol. 16, no. 6, pp. 499–507, 2017.

[62] Q. Wang, W. Zhang, Q. Liu et al., "A mutant of hepatitis B virus X protein (HBxDelta127) promotes cell growth through a positive feedback loop involving 5-lipoxygenase and fatty acid synthase," *Neoplasia*, vol. 12, no. 2, pp. 103–IN3, 2010.

[63] T. Yamashita, M. Honda, H. Takatori et al., "Activation of lipogenic pathway correlates with cell proliferation and poor prognosis in hepatocellular carcinoma," *Journal of Hepatology*, vol. 50, no. 1, pp. 100–110, 2009.

[64] C. Li, W. Yang, J. Zhang et al., "SREBP-1 has a prognostic role and contributes to invasion and metastasis in human hepatocellular carcinoma," *International Journal of Molecular Sciences*, vol. 15, no. 5, pp. 7124–7138, 2014.

[65] J. Hu, L. Che, L. Li et al., "Co-activation of AKT and c-Met triggers rapid hepatocellular carcinoma development via the mTORC1/FASN pathway in mice," *Scientific Reports*, vol. 6, no. 1, article 20484, 2016.

[66] D. Cao, X. Song, L. Che et al., "Both de novo synthetized and exogenous fatty acids support the growth of hepatocellular carcinoma cells," *Liver International*, vol. 37, no. 1, pp. 80–89, 2017.

[67] M. E. Nelson, S. Lahiri, J. D. Y. Chow et al., "Inhibition of hepatic lipogenesis enhances liver tumorigenesis by increasing antioxidant defence and promoting cell survival," *Nature Communications*, vol. 8, article 14689, 2017.

[68] A. Nath, I. Li, L. R. Roberts, and C. Chan, "Elevated free fatty acid uptake via CD36 promotes epithelial-mesenchymal transition in hepatocellular carcinoma," *Scientific Reports*, vol. 5, no. 1, article 14752, 2015.

[69] G. Giannelli, P. Koudelkova, F. Dituri, and W. Mikulits, "Role of epithelial to mesenchymal transition in hepatocellular carcinoma," *Journal of Hepatology*, vol. 65, no. 4, pp. 798–808, 2016.

[70] D. D. Stefania and D. Vergara, "The many-faced program of epithelial-mesenchymal transition: a system biology-based view," *Frontiers in Oncology*, vol. 7, p. 274, 2017.

[71] A. Ally, M. Balasundaram, R. Carlsen et al., "Comprehensive and integrative genomic characterization of hepatocellular carcinoma," *Cell*, vol. 169, no. 7, pp. 1327–1341.e23, 2017.

[72] J. Kerner and C. Hoppel, "Fatty acid import into mitochondria," *Biochimica et Biophysica Acta (BBA) - Molecular and Cell Biology of Lipids*, vol. 1486, no. 1, pp. 1–17, 2000.

[73] G. Serviddio, A. M. Giudetti, F. Bellanti et al., "Oxidation of hepatic carnitine palmitoyl transferase-I (CPT-I) impairs fatty acid beta-oxidation in rats fed a methionine-choline deficient diet," *PLoS One*, vol. 6, no. 9, article e24084, 2011.

[74] G. Serviddio, F. Bellanti, R. Tamborra et al., "Alterations of hepatic ATP homeostasis and respiratory chain during development of non-alcoholic steatohepatitis in a rodent model," *European Journal of Clinical Investigation*, vol. 38, no. 4, pp. 245–252, 2008.

[75] Y. Shao, B. Zhu, R. Zheng et al., "Development of urinary pseudotargeted LC-MS-based metabolomics method and its application in hepatocellular carcinoma biomarker discovery," *Journal of Proteome Research*, vol. 14, no. 2, pp. 906–916, 2015.

[76] A. Wada, K. Fukui, Y. Sawai et al., "Pamidronate induced anti-proliferative, apoptotic, and anti-migratory effects in hepatocellular carcinoma," *Journal of Hepatology*, vol. 44, no. 1, pp. 142–150, 2006.

[77] Y. Honda, H. Aikata, F. Honda et al., "Clinical outcome and prognostic factors in hepatocellular carcinoma patients with bone metastases medicated with zoledronic acid," *Hepatology Research*, vol. 47, no. 10, pp. 1053–1060, 2017.

[78] S. Singh, P. P. Singh, A. G. Singh, M. H. Murad, and W. Sanchez, "Statins are associated with a reduced risk of hepatocellular cancer: a systematic review and meta-analysis," *Gastroenterology*, vol. 144, no. 2, pp. 323–332, 2013.

[79] E. Ridruejo, G. Romero-Caími, M. J. Obregón, D. Kleiman de Pisarev, and L. Alvarez, "Potential molecular targets of statins in the prevention of hepatocarcinogenesis," *Annals of Hepatology*, vol. 17, no. 3, pp. 490–500, 2018.

[80] Y. Y. Zhou, G. Q. Zhu, Y. Wang et al., "Systematic review with network meta-analysis: statins and risk of hepatocellular carcinoma," *Oncotarget*, vol. 7, no. 16, pp. 21753–21762, 2016.

[81] J. Y. L. Chiang, "Bile acids: regulation of synthesis," *Journal of Lipid Research*, vol. 50, no. 10, pp. 1955–1966, 2009.

[82] E. Lozano, L. Sanchez-Vicente, M. J. Monte et al., "Cocarcinogenic effects of intrahepatic bile acid accumulation in cholangiocarcinoma development," *Molecular Cancer Research*, vol. 12, no. 1, pp. 91–100, 2014.

[83] T. Takahashi, U. Deuschle, S. Taira et al., "Tsumura-Suzuki obese diabetic mice-derived hepatic tumors closely resemble human hepatocellular carcinomas in metabolism-related genes expression and bile acid accumulation," *Hepatology International*, vol. 12, no. 3, pp. 254–261, 2018.

[84] S. Yamada, Y. Takashina, M. Watanabe et al., "Bile acid metabolism regulated by the gut microbiota promotes non-alcoholic steatohepatitis-associated hepatocellular carcinoma in mice," *Oncotarget*, vol. 9, no. 11, pp. 9925–9939, 2018.

[85] S. H. Jee, M. Kim, M. Kim et al., "Metabolomics profiles of hepatocellular carcinoma in a Korean prospective cohort: the Korean cancer prevention study-II," *Cancer Prevention Research*, vol. 11, no. 5, pp. 303–312, 2018.

[86] W. Jia, G. Xie, and W. Jia, "Bile acid-microbiota crosstalk in gastrointestinal inflammation and carcinogenesis," *Nature Reviews Gastroenterology & Hepatology*, vol. 15, no. 2, pp. 111–128, 2018.

[87] C. Guo, C. Xie, P. Ding et al., "Quantification of glycocholic acid in human serum by stable isotope dilution ultra performance liquid chromatography electrospray ionization tandem mass spectrometry," *Journal of Chromatography B*, vol. 1072, pp. 315–319, 2018.

[88] E. Stanca, G. Serviddio, F. Bellanti, G. Vendemiale, L. Siculella, and A. M. Giudetti, "Down-regulation of LPCAT expression increases platelet-activating factor level in cirrhotic rat liver: potential antiinflammatory effect of silybin," *Biochimica et Biophysica Acta (BBA) - Molecular Basis of Disease*, vol. 1832, no. 12, pp. 2019–2026, 2013.

[89] Y. Liu, Z. Hong, G. Tan et al., "NMR and LC/MS-based global metabolomics to identify serum biomarkers differentiating hepatocellular carcinoma from liver cirrhosis," *International Journal of Cancer*, vol. 135, no. 3, pp. 658–668, 2014.

[90] T. Chen, G. Xie, X. Wang et al., "Serum and urine metabolite profiling reveals potential biomarkers of human hepatocellular carcinoma," *Molecular & Cellular Proteomics*, vol. 10, no. 7, article M110.004945, 2011.

[91] Q. Huang, Y. Tan, P. Yin et al., "Metabolic characterization of hepatocellular carcinoma using nontargeted tissue metabolomics," *Cancer Research*, vol. 73, no. 16, pp. 4992–5002, 2013.

[92] B. I. Carr and V. Guerra, "Serum albumin levels in relation to tumor parameters in hepatocellular carcinoma patients," *The International Journal of Biological Markers*, vol. 32, no. 4, pp. e391–e396, 2017.

[93] J. Luo, "Cancer's sweet tooth for serine," *Breast Cancer Research*, vol. 13, no. 6, p. 317, 2011.

[94] J. W. Locasale, A. R. Grassian, T. Melman et al., "Phosphoglycerate dehydrogenase diverts glycolytic flux and contributes to oncogenesis," *Nature Genetics*, vol. 43, no. 9, pp. 869–874, 2011.

[95] R. Possemato, K. M. Marks, Y. D. Shaul et al., "Functional genomics reveal that the serine synthesis pathway is essential in breast cancer," *Nature*, vol. 476, no. 7360, pp. 346–350, 2011.

[96] M. Jain, R. Nilsson, S. Sharma et al., "Metabolite profiling identifies a key role for glycine in rapid cancer cell proliferation," *Science*, vol. 336, no. 6084, pp. 1040–1044, 2012.

[97] B. Chaneton, P. Hillmann, L. Zheng et al., "Serine is a natural ligand and allosteric activator of pyruvate kinase M2," *Nature*, vol. 491, no. 7424, pp. 458–462, 2012.

[98] R. Gao, J. Cheng, C. Fan et al., "Serum metabolomics to identify the liver disease-specific biomarkers for the progression of hepatitis to hepatocellular carcinoma," *Scientific Reports*, vol. 5, no. 1, article 18175, 2016.

[99] M. Stepien, T. Duarte-Salles, V. Fedirko et al., "Alteration of amino acid and biogenic amine metabolism in hepatobiliary cancers: findings from a prospective cohort study," *International Journal of Cancer*, vol. 138, no. 2, pp. 348–360, 2016.

[100] L. Tang, J. Zeng, P. Geng et al., "Global metabolic profiling identifies a pivotal role of proline and hydroxyproline metabolism in supporting hypoxic response in hepatocellular carcinoma," *Clinical Cancer Research*, vol. 24, no. 2, pp. 474–485, 2018.

[101] P. Muriel, "Role of free radicals in liver diseases," *Hepatology International*, vol. 3, no. 4, pp. 526–536, 2009.

[102] J. Arauz, E. Ramos-Tovar, and P. Muriel, "Redox state and methods to evaluate oxidative stress in liver damage: from bench to bedside," *Annals of Hepatology*, vol. 15, no. 2, pp. 160–173, 2016.

[103] G. Y. Liou and P. Storz, "Reactive oxygen species in cancer," *Free Radical Research*, vol. 44, no. 5, pp. 479–496, 2010.

[104] D. Anastasiou, G. Poulogiannis, J. M. Asara et al., "Inhibition of pyruvate kinase M2 by reactive oxygen species contributes to cellular antioxidant responses," *Science*, vol. 334, no. 6060, pp. 1278–1283, 2011.

[105] A. I. Fitian and R. Cabrera, "Disease monitoring of hepatocellular carcinoma through metabolomics," *World Journal of Hepatology*, vol. 9, no. 1, pp. 1–17, 2017.

[106] A. Takaki and K. Yamamoto, "Control of oxidative stress in hepatocellular carcinoma: helpful or harmful?," *World Journal of Hepatology*, vol. 7, no. 7, pp. 968–979, 2015.

[107] Y. Shimomura, A. Takaki, N. Wada et al., "The serum oxidative/anti-oxidative stress balance becomes dysregulated in patients with non-alcoholic steatohepatitis associated with hepatocellular carcinoma," *Internal Medicine*, vol. 56, no. 3, pp. 243–251, 2017.

[108] S. C. Lu, "Glutathione synthesis," *Biochimica et Biophysica Acta (BBA) - General Subjects*, vol. 1830, no. 5, pp. 3143–3153, 2013.

[109] L. Andrisic, D. Dudzik, C. Barbas, L. Milkovic, T. Grune, and N. Zarkovic, "Short overview on metabolomics approach to study pathophysiology of oxidative stress in cancer," *Redox Biology*, vol. 14, pp. 47–58, 2018.

[110] S. Tanaka, K. Miyanishi, M. Kobune et al., "Increased hepatic oxidative DNA damage in patients with nonalcoholic steatohepatitis who develop hepatocellular carcinoma," *Journal of Gastroenterology*, vol. 48, no. 11, pp. 1249–1258, 2013.

[111] N. Nishida, T. Arizumi, M. Takita et al., "Reactive oxygen species induce epigenetic instability through the formation of 8-hydroxydeoxyguanosine in human hepatocarcinogenesis," *Digestive Diseases*, vol. 31, no. 5-6, pp. 459–466, 2013.

[112] M. Xiao, H. Zhong, L. Xia, Y. Tao, and H. Yin, "Pathophysiology of mitochondrial lipid oxidation: role of 4-hydroxynonenal (4-HNE) and other bioactive lipids in mitochondria," *Free Radical Biology and Medicine*, vol. 111, pp. 316–327, 2017.

[113] S. Li, H.-Y. Tan, N. Wang et al., "The role of oxidative stress and antioxidants in liver diseases," *International Journal of Molecular Sciences*, vol. 16, no. 11, pp. 26087–26124, 2015.

[114] T. Soga, M. Sugimoto, M. Honma et al., "Serum metabolomics reveals γ-glutamyl dipeptides as biomarkers for discrimination among different forms of liver disease," *Journal of Hepatology*, vol. 55, no. 4, pp. 896–905, 2011.

[115] T. Saito, M. Sugimoto, K. Okumoto et al., "Serum metabolome profiles characterized by patients with hepatocellular carcinoma associated with hepatitis B and C," *World Journal of Gastroenterology*, vol. 22, no. 27, pp. 6224–6234, 2016.

[116] J. Zeng, P. Yin, Y. Tan et al., "Metabolomics study of hepatocellular carcinoma: discovery and validation of serum potential biomarkers by using capillary electrophoresis-mass spectrometry," *Journal of Proteome Research*, vol. 13, no. 7, pp. 3420–3431, 2014.

[117] A. I. Fitian, D. R. Nelson, C. Liu, Y. Xu, M. Ararat, and R. Cabrera, "Integrated metabolomic profiling of hepatocellular carcinoma in hepatitis C cirrhosis through GC/MS and UPLC/MS-MS," *Liver International*, vol. 34, no. 9, pp. 1428–1444, 2014.

[118] S. K. Biswas, P. Allavena, and A. Mantovani, "Tumor-associated macrophages: functional diversity, clinical significance, and open questions," *Seminars in Immunopathology*, vol. 35, no. 5, pp. 585–600, 2013.

[119] B. Z. Qian and J. W. Pollard, "Macrophage diversity enhances tumor progression and metastasis," *Cell*, vol. 141, no. 1, pp. 39–51, 2010.

[120] T. Kapanadze, J. Gamrekelashvili, C. Ma et al., "Regulation of accumulation and function of myeloid derived suppressor cells in different murine models of hepatocellular carcinoma," *Journal of Hepatology*, vol. 59, no. 5, pp. 1007–1013, 2013.

[121] S. K. Biswas and A. Mantovani, "Macrophage plasticity and interaction with lymphocyte subsets: cancer as a paradigm," *Nature Immunology*, vol. 11, no. 10, pp. 889–896, 2010.

[122] S. K. Biswas and A. Mantovani, "Orchestration of metabolism by macrophages," *Cell Metabolism*, vol. 15, no. 4, pp. 432–437, 2012.

[123] S. K. Biswas, A. Sica, and C. E. Lewis, "Plasticity of macrophage function during tumor progression: regulation by distinct molecular mechanisms," *Journal of Immunology*, vol. 180, no. 4, pp. 2011–2017, 2008.

[124] S. Wan, E. Zhao, I. Kryczek et al., "Tumor-associated macrophages produce interleukin 6 and signal via STAT3 to promote expansion of human hepatocellular carcinoma stem cells," *Gastroenterology*, vol. 147, no. 6, pp. 1393–1404, 2014.

[125] A. Budhu, M. Forgues, Q. H. Ye et al., "Prediction of venous metastases, recurrence, and prognosis in hepatocellular carcinoma based on a unique immune response signature of the liver microenvironment," *Cancer Cell*, vol. 10, no. 2, pp. 99–111, 2006.

[126] O. R. Colegio, N. Q. Chu, A. L. Szabo et al., "Functional polarization of tumour-associated macrophages by tumour-derived lactic acid," *Nature*, vol. 513, no. 7519, pp. 559–563, 2014.

[127] Z. Husain, Y. Huang, P. Seth, and V. P. Sukhatme, "Tumor-derived lactate modifies antitumor immune response: effect on myeloid-derived suppressor cells and NK cells," *Journal of Immunology*, vol. 191, no. 3, pp. 1486–1495, 2013.

[128] A. A. Al-Khami, L. Zheng, L. Del Valle et al., "Exogenous lipid uptake induces metabolic and functional reprogramming of tumor-associated myeloid-derived suppressor cells," *OncoImmunology*, vol. 6, no. 10, article e1344804, 2017.

[129] J. Hu, J. W. Locasale, J. H. Bielas et al., "Heterogeneity of tumor-induced gene expression changes in the human metabolic network," *Nature Biotechnology*, vol. 31, no. 6, pp. 522–529, 2013.

[130] E. Gaude and C. Frezza, "Tissue-specific and convergent metabolic transformation of cancer correlates with metastatic potential and patient survival," *Nature Communications*, vol. 7, article 13041, 2016.

[131] C. C. Hsu, H. C. Lee, and Y. H. Wei, "Mitochondrial DNA alterations and mitochondrial dysfunction in the progression

of hepatocellular carcinoma," *World Journal of Gastroenterology*, vol. 19, no. 47, pp. 8880–8886, 2013.

[132] T. Cheng, J. Sudderth, C. Yang et al., "Pyruvate carboxylase is required for glutamine-independent growth of tumor cells," *Proceedings of the National Academy of Sciences of the United States of America*, vol. 108, no. 21, pp. 8674–8679, 2011.

[133] R. Ma, W. Zhang, K. Tang et al., "Switch of glycolysis to gluconeogenesis by dexamethasone for treatment of hepatocarcinoma," *Nature Communications*, vol. 4, no. 1, article 2508, 2013.

[134] I. M.-J. Xu, R. K.-H. Lai, S.-H. Lin et al., "Transketolase counteracts oxidative stress to drive cancer development," *Proceedings of the National Academy of Sciences of the United States of America*, vol. 113, no. 6, pp. E725–E734, 2016.

[135] M. J. Kim, Y. K. Choi, S. Y. Park et al., "PPARδ reprograms glutamine metabolism in sorafenib-resistant HCC," *Molecular Cancer Research*, vol. 15, no. 9, pp. 1230–1242, 2017.

[136] C. Zhang and Q. Hua, "Applications of genome-scale metabolic models in biotechnology and systems medicine," *Frontiers in Physiology*, vol. 6, p. 413, 2016.

[137] A. Mardinoglu, R. Agren, C. Kampf, A. Asplund, M. Uhlen, and J. Nielsen, "Genome-scale metabolic modelling of hepatocytes reveals serine deficiency in patients with nonalcoholic fatty liver disease," *Nature Communications*, vol. 5, no. 1, article 3083, 2014.

[138] A. Mardinoglu, E. Bjornson, C. Zhang et al., "Personal model-assisted identification of NAD^+ and glutathione metabolism as intervention target in NAFLD," *Molecular Systems Biology*, vol. 13, no. 3, p. 916, 2017.

[139] R. Agren, A. Mardinoglu, A. Asplund, C. Kampf, M. Uhlen, and J. Nielsen, "Identification of anticancer drugs for hepatocellular carcinoma through personalized genome-scale metabolic modeling," *Molecular Systems Biology*, vol. 10, no. 3, p. 721, 2014.

5

Combination of Coenzyme Q$_{10}$ Intake and Moderate Physical Activity Counteracts Mitochondrial Dysfunctions in a SAMP8 Mouse Model

C. Andreani[ID],[1] C. Bartolacci,[1] M. Guescini[ID],[2] M. Battistelli,[2] V. Stocchi,[2] F. Orlando,[3] M. Provinciali,[3,4] A. Amici,[1] C. Marchini,[1] L. Tiano[ID],[5] P. Orlando[ID],[5] and S. Silvestri[5,6]

[1]University of Camerino, via Gentile III da Varano, 62032 Camerino, Italy
[2]University of Urbino, via Aurelio Saffi, 61029 Urbino, Italy
[3]Experimental Animal Models for Aging Unit Scientific Technological Area, IRCCS INRCA, via del Fossatello, 60127 Ancona, Italy
[4]Advanced Technological Center for Aging Research Scientific Technological Area, IRCCS INRCA, via Birarelli 8, 60121 Ancona, Italy
[5]Polytechnic University of Marche, Department of Life and Environmental Sciences (DISVA), via Brecce Bianche, Ancona, Italy
[6]Biomedfood srl, Spinoff of Polytechnic University of Marche, via Brecce Bianche, 60131 Ancona, Italy

Correspondence should be addressed to P. Orlando; p.orlando@univpm.it

Academic Editor: Carine Smith

Aging skeletal muscles are characterized by a progressive decline in muscle mass and muscular strength. Such muscular dysfunctions are usually associated with structural and functional alterations of skeletal muscle mitochondria. The senescence-accelerated mouse-prone 8 (SAMP8) model, characterized by premature aging and high degree of oxidative stress, was used to investigate whether a combined intervention with mild physical exercise and ubiquinol supplementation was able to improve mitochondrial function and preserve skeletal muscle health during aging. 5-month-old SAMP8 mice, in a presarcopenia phase, have been randomly divided into 4 groups ($n = 10$): untreated controls and mice treated for two months with either physical exercise (0.5 km/h, on a 5% inclination, for 30 min, 5/7 days per week), ubiquinol 10 (500 mg/kg/day), or a combination of exercise and ubiquinol. Two months of physical exercise significantly increased mitochondrial damage in the muscles of exercised mice when compared to controls. On the contrary, ubiquinol and physical exercise combination significantly improved the overall status of the skeletal muscle, preserving mitochondrial ultrastructure and limiting mitochondrial depolarization induced by physical exercise alone. Accordingly, combination treatment while promoting mitochondrial biogenesis lowered autophagy and caspase 3-dependent apoptosis. In conclusion, the present study shows that ubiquinol supplementation counteracts the deleterious effects of physical exercise-derived ROS improving mitochondrial functionality in an oxidative stress model, such as SAMP8 in the presarcopenia phase.

1. Introduction

Aging is characterized by a progressive decline in skeletal muscle mass and muscular strength [1–3]. In healthy people, there is a 1% per year decline in muscle mass between 20 and 30 years of age. This decline is accelerated above 50 years of age [4, 5]. The progressive decline in muscle mass and strength with aging is known as sarcopenia [1, 6–8]. Sarcopenia is defined as a geriatric syndrome characterized by age-related muscular loss and dysfunction that cause physical

disability, a poor quality of life, and death. The prevalence of this pathology in adults under the age of 70 is about 25% but increases up to 40% in 80-year-old or older people [9, 10]. This condition can lead to decreased physical activity increasing the risk of falls in aged individuals [11]. Understanding the mechanisms underneath aging-induced skeletal muscle atrophy and promoting health and mobility in the elderly are crucially important goals in order to develop therapeutic strategies [12]. Several studies pointed towards a critical role of mitochondria and their implication in age-related degenerative processes, and many therapeutic attempts have been focused on mitochondria [13]. Indeed, these organelles play a key role in cellular bioenergetics and represent a sensitive target in muscle cells [14, 15]. Moreover, metabolism of reactive oxygen species (ROS), Ca^{2+} homeostasis, and apoptosis are controlled by mitochondria [16]. Aging of skeletal muscle determines the alteration of the structure and function of these organelles leading to mitochondrial dysfunction [17]. In this context, a growing body of evidence has highlighted a major role of oxidative stress and inflammation in promoting aging of skeletal muscle [18]. Accordingly, it has been recently reported that excessive production of mitochondrial ROS in skeletal muscle is strongly associated with sarcopenia and the impairment of energy homeostasis [19]. In fact, the physiologic equilibrium between ROS production and antioxidant defense is disrupted in aging subjects, and the accumulation of ROS during mitochondrial respiration can cause mutations in mitochondrial DNA (mtDNA) [20] which in turn lead, through a vicious cycle, to further impaired mitochondrial functionality. Moreover, many studies have reported that a decline in mitochondria content may also account for the loss of skeletal muscle mass [18], further impairing oxidative phosphorylation and ATP production [21, 22]. Mitochondrial biogenesis is regulated by the expression of nuclear and mitochondrial genes, controlled by the transcriptional coactivator peroxisome proliferator gamma coactivator-1α (PGC-1α) [23]. Vainshtein et al. [24] suggested a role of this coactivator also in the regulation of autophagy and mitophagy in skeletal muscle. These two are distinct but interconnected degradation processes aimed at eliminating damaged cellular components in response to stress stimuli. Both mitophagy and autophagy are regulated by autophagy-related genes (Atgs) including Beclin-1 and LC3 [25].

During aging, skeletal muscle fibers gradually lose the capability to remove dysfunctional mitochondria [13]. This condition could further impair mitochondrial respiration and enhance ROS production [26] contributing to the onset of sarcopenia. Previous studies suggested that an appropriate physical activity regimen can counterbalance age-associated muscular deficits by promoting mitochondrial biogenesis [27–29]. Exercise training has been reported to modulate skeletal muscle metabolism, regulating intracellular signaling pathways and thus mediating mitochondrial homeostasis [30, 31]. However, some authors raised doubts regarding the beneficial role of exercise in the elderly, claiming that physical activity-dependent ROS production could exacerbate oxidative damage inside aged skeletal muscles [32–34]. In this scenario, association of physical activity with antioxidant therapies might be an effective strategy to prevent the adverse effects of exercise in the elderly. Coenzyme Q_{10} represents a valuable candidate for oxidative stress prevention and for supporting muscle functionality [35–39]. Coenzyme Q (CoQ) consists of a quinone head which, in mammalian cells, is attached to a chain of 9 (CoQ_9) or 10 isoprene units CoQ_{10} [40]. In human tissues, the most abundant form is coenzyme Q_{10}, while in mice and rats it is coenzyme Q_9, although CoQ_{10} represents a significant proportion of total CoQ and its level is able to increase following oral supplementation [41–46]. As part of the mitochondrial electron transport chain (ETC), CoQ actively participates in oxidative phosphorylation and plays a key role in energy and redox state balance [47]. In addition, CoQ has been found in other subcellular localizations and in circulating plasma lipoproteins, where it acts as an endogenous lipophilic antioxidant in synergism with vitamin E [48]. Endogenous CoQ_{10} synthesis, the principal source of CoQ [49], has been shown to significantly decrease during aging and in certain degenerative diseases [50, 51], thus triggering cellular dysfunctionality. These evidences underlie the rationale for CoQ use in clinical practice and as a food supplement. CoQ exists in three states of oxidation: ubiquinone (CoQ), the fully oxidized form; ubisemiquinone (CoQH·), the partially reduced form; and ubiquinol ($CoQH_2$), the fully reduced form. In particular, the $CoQH_2$ form has several advantages being more bioavailable and readily usable by the organism not requiring reductive steps [52]. This is of particular relevance in conditions when reductive systems might be less efficient such as during aging or following intense physical exercise. Here, we investigated the effect of a combined approach of mild physical exercise and ubiquinol supplementation on the senescence-accelerated mouse-prone 8 (SAMP8) model in a presarcopenia phase [53, 54]. SAMP strains derived from AKR/J series [55] show senescence acceleration and age-related pathological phenotypes, similar to aging disorders seen in humans. In particular, we focused on SAMP8 mice since they exhibit the most striking features among SAMP strains in terms of life span, fast aging progression due to high oxidative stress status [56, 57], dramatic decrease in muscle mass and contractility [58, 59], and a huge reduction in type II muscle fiber size [60, 61]. The aim of this study is to develop prevention strategies able to preserve skeletal muscle health during aging by maintaining mitochondrial function through regular physical exercise and antioxidant supplementation using a senescence-accelerated mouse-prone model (SAMP8).

2. Materials and Methods

2.1. SAMP8 Housing and Treatment. Senescence-accelerated mice (SAMP8, Harlan) [58, 59, 62], aged 5 months, have been randomly divided into 4 groups ($n = 10$) as summarized hereafter: untreated controls (SED), trained (PHY), ubiquinol 10-administered (QH_2), and both trained and ubiquinol 10-supplemented (QH_2 + PHY). The PHY and QH_2 + PHY groups underwent treadmill running at 0.5 km/h, on a 5% inclination, for 30 min, 5 days per week, for 2 months up to 7 months of age [63, 64] (Figure 1). The QH_2 and QH_2 + PHY groups were supplemented with ubiquinol 10 (Kaneka) (500 mg/kg body weight/day in sunflower seed oil) via oral administration. Such QH_2 formulation was previously prepared and stored at −80°C in 500 μL aliquots to avoid repeated freezing-thawing cycles. An aliquot was thawed daily in a water bath at 60°C in the dark just prior to administration. An equal amount of sunflower seed oil was given to SED and PHY mouse groups. The animals were bred and housed under controlled temperature (20°C) and a circadian cycle (12-hour light/12-hour dark). The animals

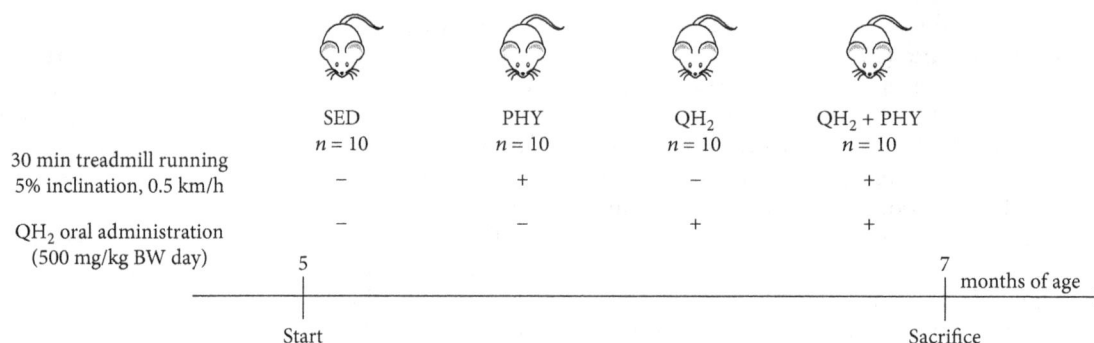

FIGURE 1: Scheme of SAMP8 mouse study.

were fed on chow diet and water *ad libitum*. Male mice were used for all experiments. The animal procedures followed the 2010/63/EU directive on the protection of animals used for scientific purposes and were approved by the Ethic Committee on Animal Use of the University of Camerino (protocol number 14/2012).

2.2. Tissue Collection and Analysis. Mice were rapidly sacrificed by isoflurane inhalation followed by cervical dislocation, two days after the last exercise/administration session, to avoid possible metabolic effects of the last exercise/administration bout. *Gastrocnemius* (GA), *tibialis anterior* (TA), *soleus* (SO) muscle, and cardiac muscle were carefully excised. GA samples were either immediately used for flow cytometry (FACS) analysis or preserved in liquid nitrogen for mtDNA quantification or mRNA extraction. TA and cardiac muscles were used for CoQ_9 and CoQ_{10} (total and oxidized form) quantification. TA muscles were used also for protein extraction and Western blot analysis, while SO samples were fixed in 3% glutaraldehyde for 4 hours, to be analyzed for fiber morphology, number, and ultrastructure of mitochondria by electron microscopy. Other tissues including liver, spleen, and kidneys were recovered for eventual future applications and preserved at −80°C.

2.3. Coenzyme Q_9 and Q_{10} Extraction and Quantification. TA and cardiac muscles were mechanically homogenized (two bouts at 30 Hz for 5 min) in propanol (Sigma) using 7 mm steel beads (Qiagen) and TissueLyser II (Qiagen). After centrifugation (2 min at 20,000 g, 4°C), 40 μL of the supernatant was injected into a high-performance liquid chromatography (HPLC) apparatus with an electrochemical detector (ECD), model 3016 by Shiseido Co. Ltd, to measure total coenzymes Q_9 and Q_{10} and Q_9 oxidative status. The mobile phase was 50 mM sodium perchlorate in methanol/distilled water (95/5 v/v) with a flow rate of 0.2 mL/min. Using a column-switching system, coenzymes were eluted from the concentrating column by mobile phase 2, 50 mM sodium perchlorate in methanol/isopropanol (70/30 v/v) with a flow rate of 0.08 mL/min. The column oven was set at 40°C. Pumps one and two of model 3001, autosampler model 3033, and switch valve model 3012; concentration column CQC (C8 DD; 10 mm × 4.0 mm ID); and separation column CQS (C18 AQ; 150 mm × 2.0 mm ID, particle size at 3 μm diameter) were used, all from Shiseido Co. Ltd. A peculiarity of the

system was the use of a postseparation reduction column (Shiseido CQR) capable of fully reducing the peak of ubiquinone. CoQ_9 and CoQ_{10} standard solutions were previously prepared in ethanol and stored at −80°C. The oxidation potential for ECD was 650 mV. TA and cardiac muscle contents of CoQ_9 and CoQ_{10} were expressed as μg/g muscle and the oxidized form as percentage of total CoQ_9.

2.4. Electron Microscope Analysis. Control and treated SO samples were washed and immediately fixed with 2.5% glutaraldehyde in 0.1 M phosphate buffer for 1 hour, postfixed with 1% of osmium tetroxide (OsO_4) in the same buffer for 2 hours, and embedded in araldite, as previously reported [65, 66]. The sections were collected on 400-mesh nickel grids, stained with uranyl acetate, lead citrate and finally analyzed with an electron microscope at 80 kV.

2.5. Flow Cytometry Analysis

2.5.1. Skeletal Muscle Dissociation. GA muscles were dissociated into single-cell suspensions using a skeletal muscle dissociation kit (Miltenyi Biotec) according to the manufacturer's instructions. Mechanical disaggregation was performed via gentleMACS Dissociator using the m_muscle_01 program (Miltenyi Biotec).

2.5.2. Cell Viability and Cell Count. Cell viability and cell count of the obtained single-cell suspensions were evaluated using Guava ViaCount® Reagent Kit (Millipore) that discriminates among viable, apoptotic, and dead cells. Briefly, the assay exploits a mixture of cell membrane-permeable (red) and cell membrane-impermeable (yellow) DNA-binding fluorescent probes, diluted 1 : 10 in PBS, and used to stain cells immediately before reading. Cells were incubated with reagent for 5 min in the dark, and the analysis of the distribution allows the discrimination of the percentage of cell debris (R−/Y−), live cells (R+/Y−), and dead cells (R+/Y+) with Guava ViaCount software using a Guava easyCyte™ flow cytometer (Millipore).

2.5.3. Mitochondrial Membrane Depolarization. Mitochondrial membrane depolarization was measured by incubating 2.5×10^5 viable muscle cells with MitoProbe™ DiIC1(5) (Life Technologies) (40 nM final concentration) at 37°C for 20 min in the dark. During the experimental setup, a suspension of control cells, before staining, was incubated with 1 μL

TABLE 1: pRT-PCR primers for nDNA and mtDNA.

Target	Primer sequence_forward	Primer sequence_reverse
36B4	5′-CGACCTGGAAGTCCAACTAC-3′	5′-ATCTGCTGCATCTGCTTG-3′
COX1	5′-TCTACTATTCGGAGCCTGAGC-3′	5′-CAAAAGCATGGGCAGTTACG-3′

TABLE 2: Summary of used antibodies.

Primary antibodies			
Antigen	Antibody	Dilution	Brand
PGC-1α	Mouse monoclonal anti-PGC-1α	1 : 1000	Millipore
TFAM	Rabbit monoclonal anti-TFAM	1 : 2000	Abcam
VDAC1	Mouse monoclonal anti-VDAC1	1 : 1000	Abcam
H2B	Rabbit polyclonal anti-H2B	1 : 1000	Abcam
β-Actin	Mouse monoclonal anti-β-actin	1 : 1000	Cell Signaling Technology
Caspase 3	Rabbit polyclonal anti-caspase 3	1 : 1000	Cell Signaling Technology
Cleaved caspase 3	Rabbit polyclonal anti-cleaved caspase 3 (Asp175)	1 : 1000	Cell Signaling Technology
SIRT5	Rabbit monoclonal anti-SIRT5	1 : 1000	Cell Signaling Technology
Secondary antibodies			
Antibody		Dilution	Brand
HRP-conjugated goat anti-mouse IgG (H&L)		1 : 3000	Calbiochem
HRP-conjugated goat anti-rabbit IgG (H&L)		1 : 20000	Sigma-Aldrich

of carbonyl cyanide 3-chlorophenylhydrazone (CCCP) 50 mM for 5 min at 37°C in the dark. After washing with phosphate-buffered saline (PBS), cells were centrifuged at 300 g for 5 min at room temperature and finally resuspended in PBS and analyzed using the Guava easyCyte™ flow cytometer (Millipore), equipped with a red laser at 633 nm. Using the Guava InCyte software, a gate relative to cells containing depolarized mitochondria was arbitrarily set using as a reference CCCP-treated cells assuming that in this condition 90% of the cells contained depolarized mitochondria. This gate was subsequently used for all further analyses.

2.6. Mitochondrial DNA (mtDNA) Quantification. To assess mtDNA content, DNA was extracted from GA muscle using QIAamp DNA Mini kit (Qiagen) and then used for quantitative real-time PCR (qRT-PCR) on the StepOne Plus system (Applied Biosystems). The 36B4 gene was used as a nuclear DNA (nDNA) marker while the COX1 gene was used for mtDNA. The primers used are summarized in Table 1. Briefly, 10 ng of DNA was amplified using 1x SYBR Select Master Mix (Applied Biosystems), using the following protocol: 10 min denaturation at 95°C, followed by 45 cycles (95°C for 15 sec, 60°C for 15 sec, and 72°C for 30 sec) and melting curve (95°C for 15 sec, 60°C for 30 sec, and 95°C for 15 sec). Relative copy number quantification was carried out using the $\Delta\Delta$Ct method.

2.7. Western Blot Assay. TA muscle samples were mechanically homogenized in RIPA buffer (0.1% SDS, 1% NP40, and 0.5% CHAPS) supplemented with protease inhibitors aprotinin, sodium orthovanadate, and phenylmethylsulfonyl fluoride (Sigma-Aldrich). Lysates were incubated on ice for 30 min and then centrifuged at 16.000 g, 4°C, for 20 min.

The supernatant was collected, quantified via Bradford method (Bio-Rad), and stored in aliquots at −80°C to avoid repeated freezing-thawing cycles. For Western blot analysis, an equal amount of protein lysates (20–40 μg depending on the protein assayed) were separated onto Criterion™ TGX™ precast gels (Bio-Rad) and transferred to a polyvinylidene difluoride (PVDF) membrane (Millipore) using Criterion™ Blotter (Bio-Rad). Membranes were blocked with 5% BSA-TBS-T and then overnight incubated with primary antibodies at 4°C. Secondary antibody binding was performed at RT for 1 hour. After TBS-T washing, immunoreactive bands were incubated with enhanced chemiluminescent reagent (EuroClone) and detected via ChemiDoc™ XRS+ System (Bio-Rad). Densitometry analysis was accomplished through ImageJ software using H2B (nuclear), VDAC1 (mitochondrial), and β-actin (total) as protein normalizers. The results are representative of at least three independent experiments. The antibodies used are listed in Table 2.

2.8. Gene Expression Analysis. Total RNA was extracted from GA muscles. RNA purification was performed using the E.Z.N.A.® Total RNA Kit I (Omega Bio-tek) according to the manufacturer's instructions, and contaminant DNA was digested with DNase I enzyme (Ambion). cDNA was synthesized using the Maxima Reverse Transcriptase kit (Thermo Fisher Scientific). Real-time PCR amplifications were conducted using SensiFAST SYBR Green (Bioline) according to the manufacturer's instructions, with 300 nM primers and two μL of cDNA (20 μL final reaction volume). Specific primers used are listed in Table 3.

Thermocycling was conducted using LightCycler 480 (Roche) initiated by a 2 min incubation at 95°C, followed

TABLE 3: Summary of used primers for Beclin, Atg12, Bnip3l, Atrogin, and GAPDH.

Target	Primer sequence_forward	Primer sequence_reverse
Beclin	5'-TGAATGAGGATGACAGTGAGCA-3'	5'-CACCTGGTTCTCCACACTCTTG-3'
Atg12	5'-TCCGTGCCATCACATACACA-3'	5'-TAAGACTGCTGTGGGGCTGA-3'
Bnip3l	5'-TTGGGGCATTTTACTAACCTTG-3'	5'-TGCAGGTGACTGGTGGTACTAA-3'
Atrogin	5'-GCAAACACTGCCACATTCTCTC-3'	5'-CTTGAGGGGAAAGTGAGACG-3'
GAPDH	5'-TCAACGGCACAGTCAAGG-3'	5'-ACTCCACGACATACTCAGC-3'

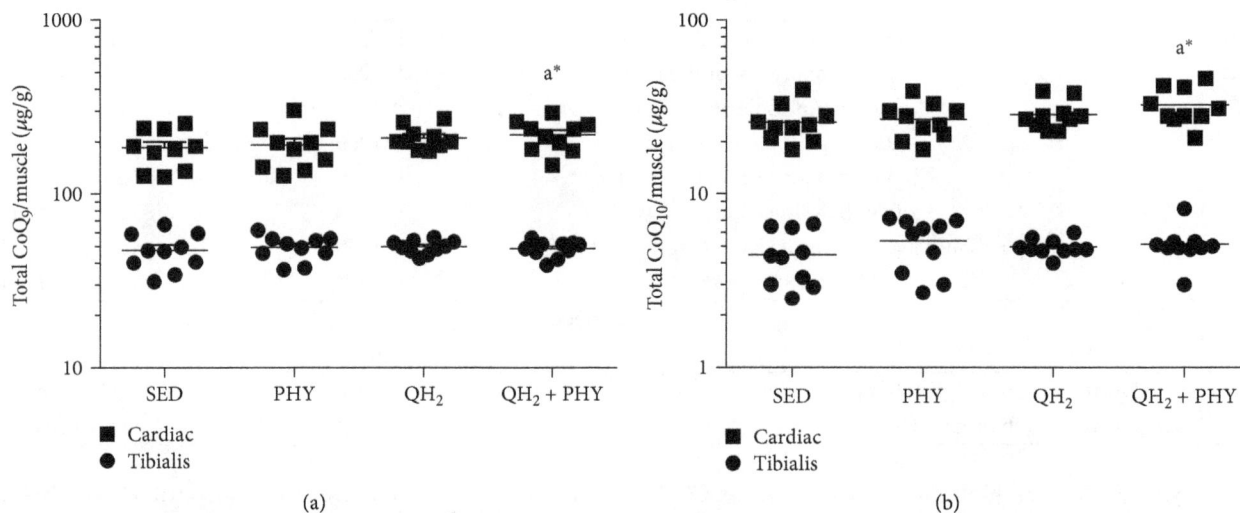

(a)

(b)

FIGURE 2: Total coenzyme Q_9 (a) and Q_{10} (b) levels in cardiac and *tibialis anterior* muscles, expressed as μg coenzyme/g of muscle in sedentary (SED), physical exercise (PHY), ubiquinol (QH$_2$), and ubiquinol associated with physical exercise (QH$_2$ + PHY) mouse groups ($n = 10$). *$p < 0.05$; a = *vs.* SED.

by 40 cycles (95°C for 5 sec, 60°C for 5 sec, and 72°C for 10 sec) with a single fluorescent reading taken at the end of each cycle. Each reaction was conducted in triplicate and completed with a melting curve analysis to confirm the specificity of amplification and lack of primer dimers. Quantification was performed according to the ΔCq method, and the expression levels of GAPDH and S16 were used as a reference [67].

3. Statistical Analysis

Data are presented as mean ± SEM. All statistical analyses were performed using GraphPad Prism® 6.0 software. Unpaired two-tailed t-test was employed when 2 groups were compared and ANOVA for comparison between three or more groups. Two-way ANOVA with Bonferroni correction for multiple comparisons was used when 3 or more groups were compared over time. The GraphPad Prism routine for outlier identification was used to identify any out-of-range values to be excluded from the statistical analysis.

4. Results

4.1. Combination of Physical Activity and Ubiquinol Supplementation Increases Q_9 and Q_{10} Content in Cardiac Muscles and Lowers the Oxidation of Endogenous Coenzyme Q_9. Total coenzyme Q_9 and Q_{10} (CoQ$_9$ and CoQ$_{10}$) levels

and oxidative status of coenzyme Q_9 were quantified by an HPLC-ECD instrument on skeletal and cardiac muscles. The results were normalized on muscle weight and expressed as $\mu g/g$ of muscle. Coenzyme Q levels were very different between skeletal and cardiac muscles, the latter showing remarkably higher levels of both coenzymes (Figure 2). After ubiquinol and physical exercise (QH$_2$ + PHY) treatment, both coenzymes were significantly increased in the cardiac tissue, in particular +23% CoQ$_9$ ($p = 0.05$, Figure 2(a)) and +27% CoQ$_{10}$ ($p = 0.03$, Figure 2(b)) with respect to the sedentary group.

To evaluate the effect of exogenous CoQ supplementation on the oxidative status of endogenous coenzyme Q_9, its oxidized form was measured as well. As shown in Figure 3, skeletal muscle is characterized by a higher extent of oxidation (on average 95% of Q_9 is oxidized) compared to cardiac muscle (35% of oxidized Q_9). Ubiquinol supplementation alone was not able to lower the oxidation of endogenous muscular CoQ. On the contrary, a significant decrease of oxidized coenzyme Q_9 was observed in skeletal muscle after regular physical exercise alone or in combination with ubiquinol supplementation (Figure 3, −4.7%, $p = 0.009$, and −3.6%, $p = 0.03$, respectively).

4.2. Physical Exercise Alone or in Combination with Ubiquinol Administration Stimulates Muscle Hypertrophy in SAMP8 Mice. To evaluate the impact of the different

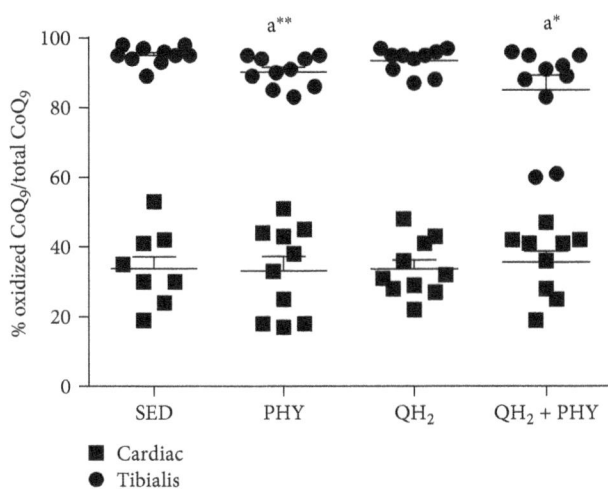

FIGURE 3: Oxidized coenzyme Q_9 level in cardiac and *tibialis anterior* muscles, expressed as percentage of oxidized of coenzyme Q_9 in sedentary (SED), physical exercise (PHY), ubiquinol (QH_2), and ubiquinol associated with physical exercise ($QH_2 + PHY$) mouse groups ($n = 10$). $^*p < 0.05$ and $^{**}p < 0.01$; (A) $= vs.$ SED.

treatments on muscle fiber atrophy/hypertrophy, fiber diameter was measured for each experimental condition. Morphometrical analyses of fiber diameter revealed a gradual increase in the ubiquinol (QH_2), ubiquinol and exercise ($QH_2 + PHY$), and exercise (PHY) groups, with the PHY fibers having the largest average diameter (+33% compared to the SED group, $p = 0.0009$, Figures 4(a) and 4(b)). Ubiquinol treatment alone did not produce any significant variation in fiber size, nor was it able to outweigh the effect of physical exercise alone (+23%; $p = 0.02$). These data suggest that physical exercise alone or in combination with ubiquinol is able to induce muscle fiber hypertrophy.

4.3. Ubiquinol Supplementation Is Able to Improve Mitochondrial Structure and Morphology Counteracting Physical Activity-Induced Mitochondrial Depolarization.
Mitochondrial ultrastructure was evaluated in skeletal muscle by transmission electron microscopy (TEM), and at functional level, mitochondrial membrane potential was evaluated in dissociated skeletal muscle cells by flow cytometry using a Nernstian fluorescent probe. As shown in Figure 5(a), in the SED experimental group, mitochondria appeared rounded or elongated, strongly damaged with rather dilated and disorganized cristae. Strikingly, muscle mitochondria of the PHY group appeared even more compromised presenting typical matrix swelling and poorly organized or absent cristae. On the contrary, mitochondria from mice supplemented with 500 mg/kg BW/day of ubiquinol alone (QH_2) or in association with physical exercise ($QH_2 + PHY$) appear slightly smaller but with well-preserved cristae. Mitochondrial membrane potential analysis (Figures 5(b) and 5(c)) confirmed that the altered mitochondrial ultrastructure observed in the PHY group was associated with significantly increased mitochondrial depolarization (+20% cells with depolarized mitochondria $vs.$ SED group, $p = 0.03$, Figure 5(c)), suggesting that exercise might account for a

bioenergetics impairment in aged muscles of 7-month-old SAMP8 mice. Notably, this increase was significantly counteracted following ubiquinol supplementation in association with regular physical exercise ($QH_2 + PHY$) (-12.7%, $p = 0.01$), while QH_2 alone was not able to decrease the basal level of depolarized cells which was similar to sedentary mice. These data suggest that ubiquinol supplementation in combination with regular physical exercise prevents exercise-dependent mitochondrial dysfunctions.

4.4. Combination of Physical Exercise and Ubiquinol Promotes Mitochondrial Biogenesis in the Muscles of the $QH_2 + PHY$ Group.
Mitochondrial DNA content and PGC-1α, Tfam, and SIRT5 protein levels of TA muscles were analyzed to evaluate the mitochondrial biogenesis. Notably, $QH_2 + PHY$ treatment was not only able to preserve mitochondrial morphology and functionality (Figure 5) but also capable of modulating mitochondrial biogenesis. In particular, a significantly higher mtDNA copy number was detected in the $QH_2 + PHY$ group compared to the two treatments alone ($QH_2 + PHY$ $vs.$ PHY, 1.35-fold change, $p = 0.03$, and $QH_2 + PHY$ $vs.$ QH_2, 1.41-fold change, $p = 0.01$, Figure 6). Moreover, the combined treatment promoted a highly significant increase in the expression of proteins involved in mitochondrial biogenesis, such as PGC-1α (+284.9%, $p < 0.0001$) and SIRT5 (+39.5%, $p = 0.02$), compared to sedentary mice (Figure 7). Regular physical exercise in association with ubiquinol supplementation was also able to increase the expression levels of TFAM although not in a significant manner. On the contrary, individual treatments, both physical exercise and ubiquinol supplementation, did not induce any changes in these markers, with the exception of a significant downregulation of SIRT5 in the trained mice.

4.5. Combination of Ubiquinol and Physical Exercise Thwarts Activation of Autophagy/Mitophagy Signals and Lowers Caspase 3-Dependent Apoptosis in the Muscles of $QH_2 + PHY$ Mice.
To assess whether the different treatments impacted muscular autophagy/mitophagy, we analyzed the mRNA expression (Figure 8) of Beclin-1 (a), Atrogin-1 (b), Atg12 (c), and Bnip3l (d) genes encoding key players involved in both these degradation processes. The association of ubiquinol supplementation and physical exercise produced a significant decrease in the mRNA expression of Beclin-1 (-1.96-fold, $p = 0.005$), Atg12 (-3.34-fold, $p = 0.003$), and Bnip3l (-4.1-fold, $p = 0.004$) if compared to the PHY group. Atrogin-1 expression decreased significantly only compared to sedentary mice ($p = 0.04$). Ubiquinol supplementation alone was able to induce a significant decrease only for Bnip3l mRNA expression to a similar extent to the combined treatment of ubiquinol and physical exercise (-3.7-fold, $p = 0.009$). To determine whether apoptosis was also modulated, cleaved caspase 3 level was also examined via Western blot assay (Figure 9). Notably, despite that all the treatments were able to significantly decrease caspase 3-dependent apoptosis with respect to SED controls, $QH_2 + PHY$ combination triggered the most pronounced antiapoptotic effect in PHY (-76.9%), QH_2 (-82.6%), and $QH_2 + PHY$ (-96.9%) mouse groups, respectively, compared

(a)

(b)

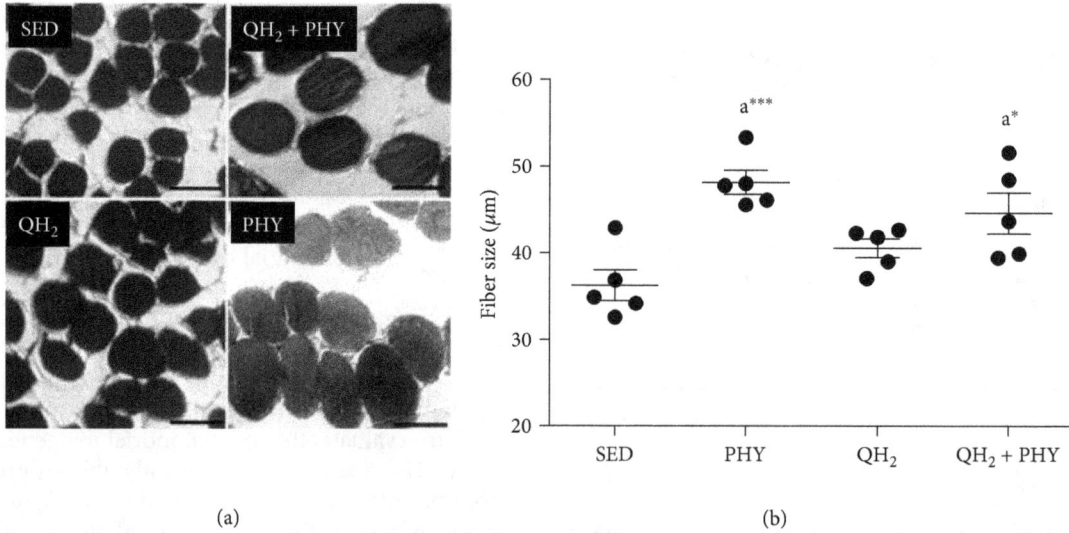

FIGURE 4: (a) Representative microphotographs of fibers (SED, bar = 25 μm; PHY, bar = 65 μm; QH$_2$, bar = 35 μm; and QH$_2$ + PHY, bar = 55 μm). (b) Fiber size quantification of *soleus* muscle, expressed in μm, in sedentary (SED), physical exercise (PHY), ubiquinol (QH$_2$), and ubiquinol associated with physical exercise (QH$_2$ + PHY) mouse groups ($n = 5$). $^*p < 0.05$ and $^{***}p < 0.001$; (A) = *vs.* SED.

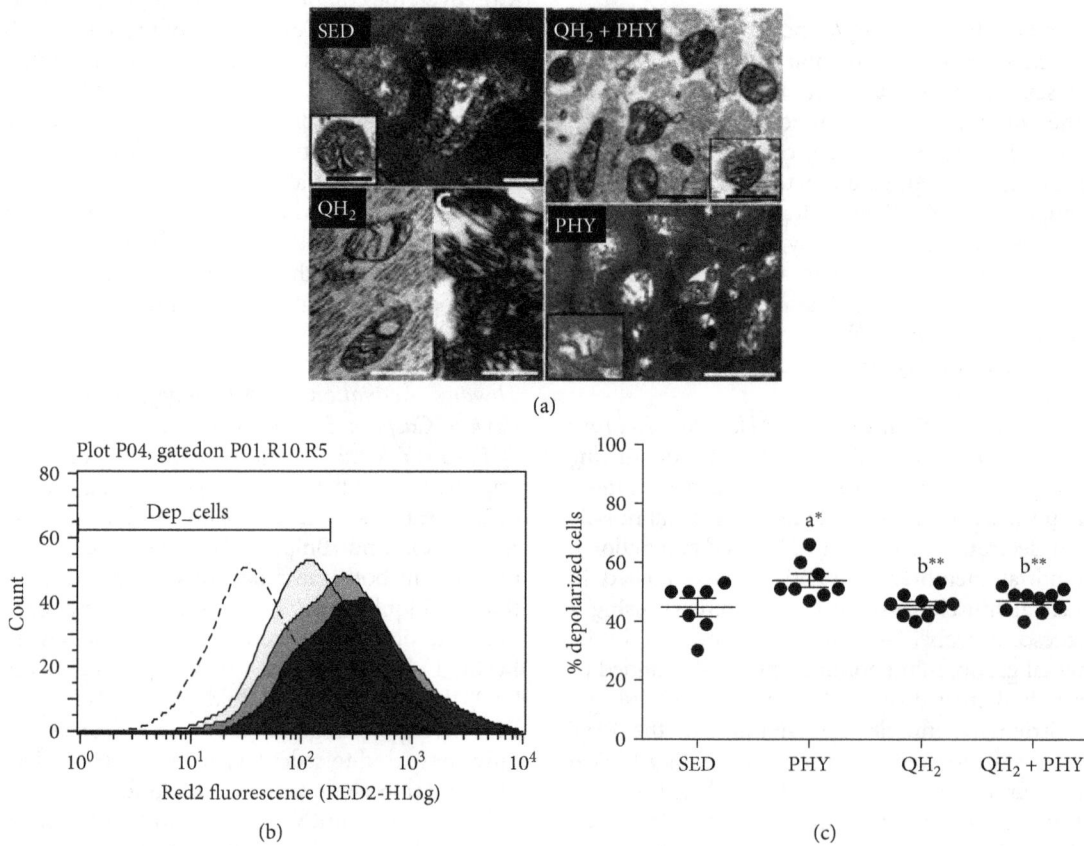

(a)

(b)

(c)

FIGURE 5: (a) TEM analysis of mitochondrial ultrastructure of *soleus* muscle (SED, bar = 200 nm; inset SED, bar = 500 nm; PHY, bar = 1 μm; QH$_2$, bar = 500 nm; and QH$_2$ + PHY, inset, and QH$_2$ + PHY, bar = 500 nm). (b) Mitochondrial membrane depolarization expressed as Red2 Fluorescent (RED2-HLog). (c) Percentage of depolarized cells of *gastrocnemius* muscle, respectively, in sedentary (black histogram; SED), physical exercise (light grey histogram; PHY), ubiquinol (dark grey histogram; QH$_2$), and ubiquinol associated with physical exercise (dark grey histogram; QH$_2$ + PHY) mouse groups ($n = 10$). Dashed histogram (b) represents sample control treated with CCCP. $^*p < 0.05$ and $^{**}p < 0.01$; (A) = *vs.* SED and (B) = *vs.* PHY.

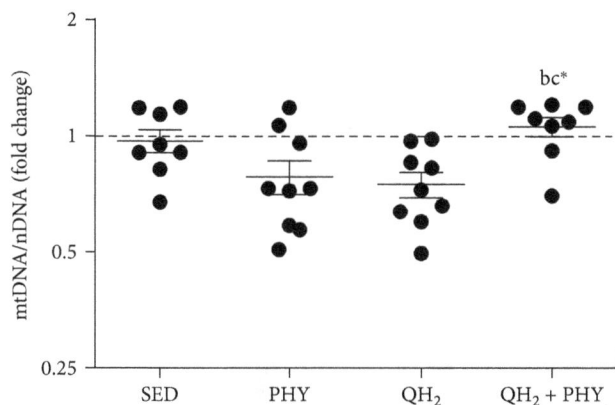

FIGURE 6: Fold change of copy number of mitochondrial DNA/nuclear DNA (mtDNA/nDNA) measured on *gastrocnemius* muscle in sedentary (SED), physical exercise (PHY), ubiquinol (QH_2), and ubiquinol associated with physical exercise (QH_2 + PHY) mouse groups ($n = 10$). $^*p < 0.05$; (b) = *vs.* PHY and c = *vs.* QH_2.

to SED ($p < 0.0001$, Figures 9(a) and 9(b)). Overall, these data suggest that QH_2 + PHY combination successfully lowers the expression of autophagy/mitophagy-associated genes and prevents apoptotic cell death inside the aging muscles.

5. Discussion

In the present study, senescence-accelerated prone 8 (SAMP8) mice, characterized by premature aging and high degree of oxidative stress [68], were used to investigate if a combined approach of mild physical exercise and ubiquinol (CoQH$_2$) supplementation was able to improve mitochondrial function and preserve skeletal muscle health during aging. In our experimental settings, SAMP8 mice were treated with ubiquinol, physical exercise, and a combination of both for two months starting in the presarcopenia phase (5 months) until sarcopenia onset (7 months) [53]. As expected, the skeletal muscle of 7-month-old SED mice (used as control) presented high oxidative stress, damaged mitochondria, high extent of apoptosis, and mitophagy. While ubiquinol or physical exercise alone was able only to partially rescue these impairments, the combination of ubiquinol and physical exercise significantly improved the overall structural and functional status of the skeletal muscle. Skeletal muscle senescence is associated with decreased muscle mass and mitochondrial dysfunction, and the excessive production of mitochondrial ROS seems to strongly associate with the disruption of mitochondrial energy metabolism [19]. In this context, physical exercise has been proposed as a strategy to stimulate mitochondrial respiration and biogenesis counteracting muscle decline in older subjects [27, 28]. Nonetheless, some studies have shown that ROS production could indeed exacerbate the oxidative stress in senescent muscle, which is characterized by a severely impaired antioxidant response [32–34, 69]. For these reasons, the association of mild regular physical activity and antioxidant therapies could be a powerful strategy to minimize the adverse effects of exercise during aging. In particular, coenzyme Q in its reduced and active form (ubiquinol), being a key player both in the mitochondrial electron transport chain and in the antioxidant response in biological membranes [48], may represent an ideal candidate in improving oxidative status and functionality of the senescent muscle.

CoQ$_{10}$ level correlates to high rates of metabolism, and for this reason, it is highest in organs such as the heart, kidney, and liver (114, 66.5, and 54.9 g/g tissue, respectively) [70], probably due to the large amounts of mitochondria where it is acting as an energy transfer molecule. In fact, coenzyme Q was first isolated from beef heart mitochondria, in 1957 [71].

Accordingly, at 7 months of age, skeletal muscle content of endogenous CoQ$_9$ was significantly lower and more oxidized in comparison to cardiac muscle. Oral ubiquinol supplementation (500 mg/kg body weight/day) alone was unable to increase skeletal and cardiac muscle CoQ content and only the association of ubiquinol supplementation and mild treadmill running significantly increased the amount of both coenzymes in the cardiac muscle but not in the skeletal muscle. Increase of both coenzymes (endogenous CoQ$_9$ and dietary absorbed CoQ$_{10}$) in the heart suggests a higher biosynthesis rate that could be related to different mitochondrial requirements triggering both biosynthesis and incorporation. In the skeletal muscle, these changes that could be required for efficient tissue incorporation seem to occur at a much lower extent or might be less evident due to a lower mitochondrial content. Accordingly, Ernster and Dallner have previously shown that feeding rats with a comparable dosage of oxidized CoQ$_{10}$ significantly increased its plasma content, while tissue CoQ$_{10}$ accumulation was very moderate and variable in different tissues/organs [47]. In particular, skeletal muscle seems to have a very low ability to incorporate CoQ. However, Sohal and Forster showed that CoQ$_{10}$ dietary supplementation in rodents was able to change the subcellular localization of CoQ, increasing the mitochondrial content of both coenzymes in various mitochondria-rich tissues, such as liver, heart, and skeletal muscle [72]. In another study, the same authors confirmed that skeletal muscle increase in CoQ$_{10}$ following supplementation was the lowest in all analyzed tissues [73]. In the present study, we verified that the use of orally administered reduced CoQ$_{10}$ did not provide any significant improvement in tissue uptake, showing results in line with previous reports where ubiquinone was used as active substance. This is a relevant observation since ubiquinol has been proposed as a more bioavailable form of Coenzyme Q$_{10}$; nonetheless, in the proposed experimental condition, the oxidative state of ubiquinol does not seem to provide any significant improvement in terms of tissue uptake.

Taken together, these data suggest that ubiquinol dietary supplementation alone might not be enough to produce its cellular accumulation, but additional stimuli, such as physical activity and mitochondrial biogenesis, could improve ubiquinol incorporation [74]. Indeed, we reported that physical exercise could therefore act as a trigger for CoQ accumulation or rearrangement at the subcellular level. This effect was particularly evident in mitochondria-rich cardiac muscle, resulting in a significant increase in the overall cellular

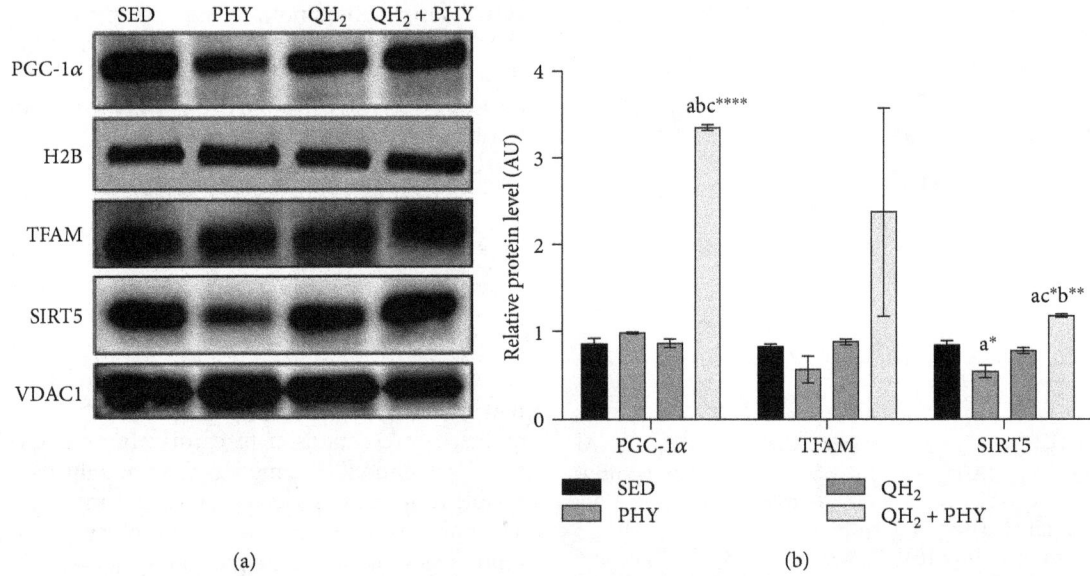

FIGURE 7: Western blot analysis (a) and relative protein quantification (b) of PGC-1α, TFAM, and SIRT5 expressed in tibialis anterior (TA) muscle, in sedentary (SED), physical exercise (PHY), ubiquinol (QH$_2$), and ubiquinol associated with physical exercise (QH$_2$ + PHY) mouse groups ($n = 5$). PGC-1α protein levels were normalized to H2B levels. TFAM and SIRT5 were normalized to VDAC1 levels. AU: arbitrary units. $^*p < 0.05$, $^{**}p < 0.01$, and $^{****}p < 0.0001$; (a) = $vs.$ SED, (b) = $vs.$ PHY, and (c) = $vs.$ QH$_2$.

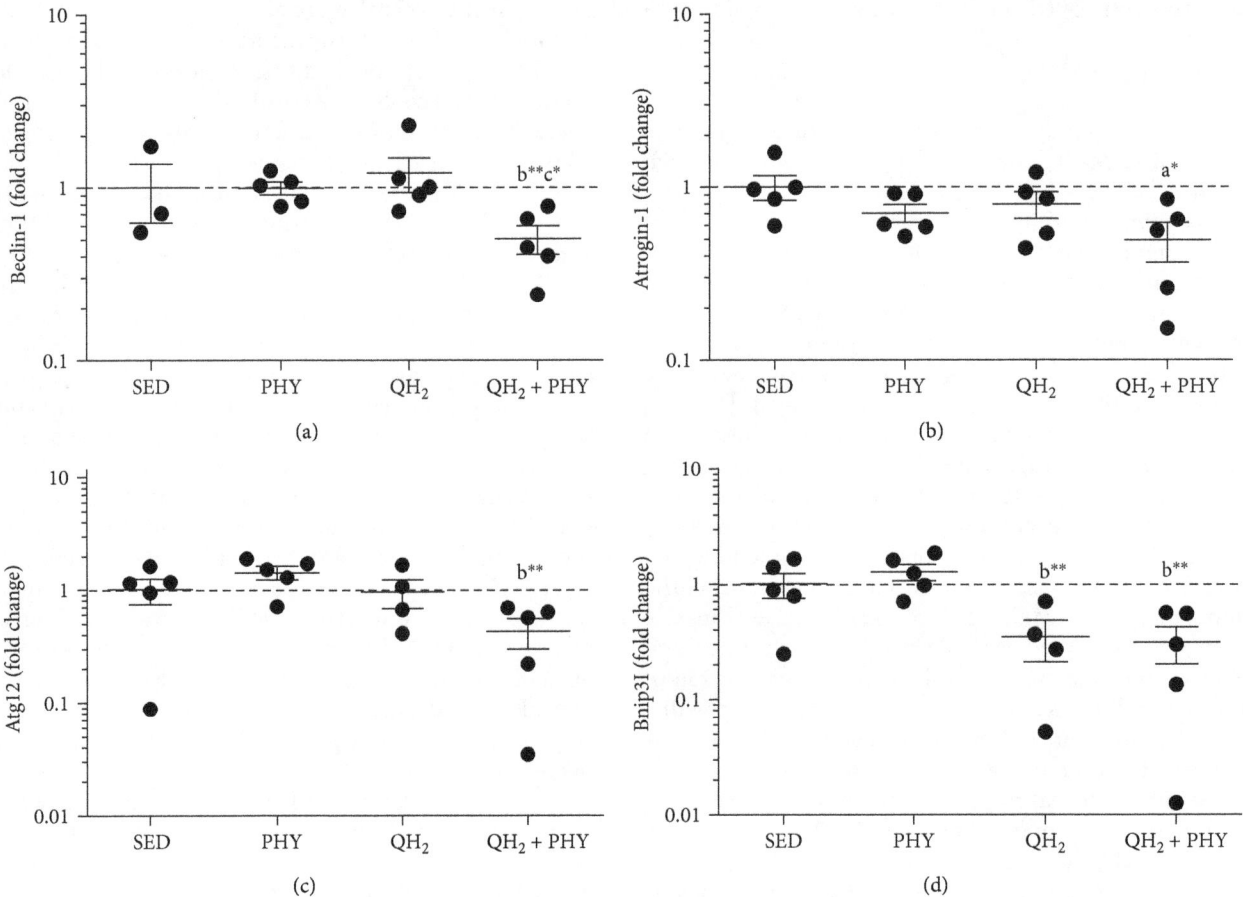

FIGURE 8: Gene expression (mRNA) expressed as fold change of genes Beclin (a), Atrogin (b), Atg12, (c) and Bnip3l (d) measured on *gastrocnemius* muscle in sedentary (SED), physical exercise (PHY), ubiquinol (QH$_2$), and ubiquinol associated with physical exercise (QH$_2$ + PHY) mouse groups ($n = 5$). $^*p < 0.05$ and $^{**}p < 0.01$; (a) = $vs.$ SED, (b) = $vs.$ PHY, and (c) = $vs.$ QH$_2$.

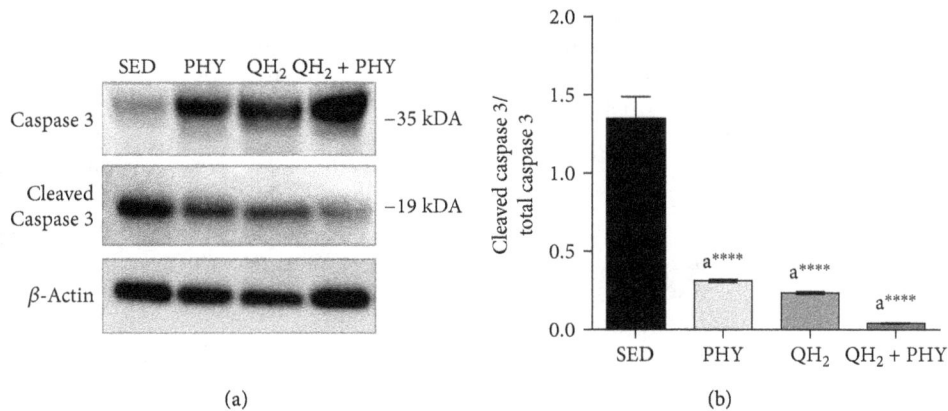

FIGURE 9: Immunoblot image (a) and relative protein quantification normalized to β-actin (b) of caspase 3 and cleaved caspase 3, measured on *tibialis anterior* muscle in sedentary (SED), physical exercise (PHY), ubiquinol (QH_2), and ubiquinol associated with physical exercise ($QH_2 + PHY$) mouse groups ($n = 5$). ****$p < 0.0001$; (a) = *vs.* SED.

content. Moreover, even if we did not observe a significant CoQ accumulation in the skeletal muscle, we observed functional modifications at mitochondrial and cellular levels suggesting CoQ activity without accumulation in this tissue.

We focused our investigation on skeletal muscle considering its primary involvement in physical exercise. In the SAMP8 model, physical exercise alone produces heterogeneous responses at the cellular level. On the one hand, it had a clear ergogenic effect being able to promote an increase in skeletal muscle fiber size and to improve the oxidative status of endogenous coenzyme Q_9. Accordingly, observational and intervention studies have demonstrated that physical exercise has a positive effect on muscle mass, muscle strength, and physical function in the older population [1, 2, 75, 76]. However, physical exercise also induced mitochondrial disturbances in terms of membrane depolarization. This result could be due to a reduced antioxidant activity [68] and to an intrinsic impairment of the electron transport chain [77]. Both conditions characterizing the presenescent SAMP8 mice might be further exacerbated by physical exercise in our experimental settings.

Notably, the combined treatment was able to counteract the mitochondrial impairment induced by physical exercise alone and also increased the mitochondrial number assessed as mtDNA/nDNA ratio. These data are confirmed by the analysis of PGC-1α muscle protein level, a key protein involved in the control of mitochondrial biogenesis, oxidative metabolism, and autophagy [23, 78, 79] which was significantly increased after 2 months of regular physical exercise associated with ubiquinol supplementation. Several studies reported that induction of PGC-1α, NRF-1, and Tfam expression [80–82] during physical exercise is triggered by oxidative stimuli [83]. On the contrary, aging-derived oxidative stress does not produce similar effects altering PGC-1α expression through different mechanisms [63].

Moreover, in our experimental model, increased fiber diameter in trained animals was not associated with a parallel increase in mtDNA copy number after 2 months of physical exercise, confirming that muscle hypertrophy was not linked with enhanced mitochondrial biogenesis.

Shrinkage of the mitochondrial pool is a feature typical of the senescence process, and it is characterized by decreased enzymatic activity and level of mitochondrial proteins [21, 84, 85] as well as low mtDNA content [63, 86]. In this regard, it is remarkable that PGC-1α upregulation was associated with a concomitant increase in mtDNA copy number only in skeletal muscle of $QH_2 + PHY$ mice and not in mice subjected to single interventions.

Moreover, SIRT5, which has been recently found to protect mitochondria from fragmentation and degradation, by supporting mitochondrial elongation [87], was significantly increased following 2 months of ubiquinol supplementation and regular physical exercise, further supporting a positive effect of the $QH_2 + PHY$ combined treatment that could suggest improvement in mitochondria biogenesis.

Intriguingly, despite the improvements in the mitochondrial pool and the functionality observed in the $QH_2 + PHY$ group, an increase in muscle fiber size was produced by physical exercise alone and to a lower extent by the combination treatment. Indeed, muscle mass depends on different factors other than mitochondrial biogenesis, such as the balance between protein synthesis and degradation. van Wessel et al. described how high oxidative fibers are small in size, despite their high capacity for protein synthesis if compared to low oxidative fibers [88]. The authors suggest that cellular energy status may be crucial in mediating either a low oxidative phenotype and a large size or a high oxidative phenotype but a small size. They also suggest that oxidative fibers have a higher rate of muscle protein degradation in the presence of low cellular energy or high oxidative stress status, a condition similar to our experimental model.

During aging, senescent cells respond to a wide range of damaging stimuli produced by the accumulation of dysfunctional proteins and organelles, among which mitochondria play a pivotal role due to their bivalent role as source, target of ROS, and master regulator of programmed cell death processes. Throughout evolution, cells developed strategies like autophagy, mitophagy, and apoptosis to manage these constraints. These tightly regulated and interconnected processes are of pivotal importance also in the maintenance muscle homeostasis, which is dysregulated during aging and sarcopenia [89, 90]. In this context, ROS originating from mitochondria have been reported to activate both autophagy machinery [91] and caspase-dependent apoptosis [92].

In this regard, the combined treatment with ubiquinol and physical exercise not only ameliorated muscle oxidative stress and bioenergetics but also associated with a decreased expression of autophagy/mitophagy-associated genes, such as Bnip3l, Atg12, and Beclin-1 known to promote mitochondrial fragmentation and mitophagy and autophagosome formation [93, 94].

Finally, the combined treatment was also able to prevent caspase 3-dependent apoptosis. Since caspase cleavage cascade is a readout of mitochondria-associated apoptotic cell death [95–97], these data strengthen the positive impact of $QH_2 + PHY$ combination on mitochondria. Furthermore, previous studies have shown that cytochrome c release from mitochondria activates caspase 3 that in turn cleaves respiratory complex proteins exacerbating mitochondrial dysfunction increasing ROS production [92]. The loss of muscle mass, caused by an imbalance between muscle protein synthesis (MPS) and muscle protein breakdown (MPB) [98] and consequently decline in strength, can also be due to increased activity of the ubiquitin proteasome pathway (UPP), which is also responsible for mitochondrial protein quality control. Our data, showing a decrease in Atrogin-1 expression and myogenin (MyoG) protein level (supplementary material (available here)) and highlighting a potential effect of the combined treatment, suggest also a possible downregulation of UPP proteolytic pathway, which might concur to muscle health preservation [99].

Taking into consideration the limitations of this study, associated to the fact that we did not take into account muscle fiber type composition and we did not measure the actual intramuscular ROS levels, overall in this context, our data demonstrate that ubiquinol might directly prevent cell death by acting both as mitochondrial nutrient and as ROS scavenger.

6. Conclusion

In conclusion, the present study shows that ubiquinol supplementation and physical exercise synergize at improving mitochondrial functionality, counteracting the deleterious effects of physical exercise-induced ROS in the muscles of a SAMP8 mouse model. These results suggest that ubiquinol could be a powerful dietary supplement in sports nutrition and in particular in the elderly. The use of antioxidants in sports practice is still a debated topic, because it was demonstrated that some of these molecules are able to turn off the hormetic signals generated by physical exercise. However, antioxidant compounds represent a very heterogeneous family of molecules with different targets and cellular tropism so that evidences reported for some of them should not be simply extended to all molecules with similar activities. Moreover, data available in the scientific literature referring to a quenching effect of antioxidants on adaptive response commonly refer to trained healthy subjects. Our study shows that ubiquinol, while reducing harmful effects generated by physical exercise, improves exercise-induced hormetic response in a model characterized by elevated oxidative stress and prone to premature aging such as SAMP8 mice.

Authors' Contributions

Andreani C. and Bartolacci C. contributed equally to this work.

Acknowledgments

This study was supported by a grant fellowship 2017 from the Fondazione Umberto Veronesi (Silvestri S. was a recipient of grant "Post-doctoral Fellowship 2017"). The authors wish to thank Kaneka for kindly providing ubiquinol.

Supplementary Materials

Immunoblot image and relative protein quantification of myogenin (MyoG) normalized to H2B (Figure 10) were measured on *tibialis anterior* muscle of all mouse groups. The results showed how ubiquinol supplementation, in association with physical exercise ($QH_2 + PHY$ mouse group), was significantly ($*p < 0.05$) able to prevent the increase in MyoG protein level induced after physical exercise alone (PHY mouse group). These data highlight a protective role of ubiquinol towards the deleterious effect of mild physical exercise in an old skeletal muscle of senescence-accelerated mice, suggesting also a possible downregulation of the UPP proteolytic pathway. Figure 10: immunoblot image and relative protein quantification of myogenin (MyoG) normalized to H2B measured on *tibialis anterior* muscle in sedentary (SED), physical exercise (PHY), ubiquinol (QH_2), and ubiquinol associated with physical exercise ($QH_2 + PHY$) mouse groups ($n = 5$), $*p < 0.05$. (*Supplementary Materials*)

References

[1] H. Kim, T. Suzuki, K. Saito et al., "Effects of exercise and tea catechins on muscle mass, strength and walking ability in community-dwelling elderly Japanese sarcopenic women: a randomized controlled trial," *Geriatrics & Gerontology International*, vol. 13, no. 2, pp. 458–465, 2013.

[2] M. Leenders, L. B. Verdijk, L. van der Hoeven, J. van Kranenburg, R. Nilwik, and L. J. C. van Loon, "Elderly men and women benefit equally from prolonged resistance-type exercise training," *The Journals of Gerontology Series A:*

Biological Sciences and Medical Sciences, vol. 68, no. 7, pp. 769–779, 2013.

[3] C.. K. Liu, X. Leng, F. -C. Hsu et al., "The impact of sarcopenia on a physical activity intervention: the Lifestyle Interventions and Independence for Elders Pilot Study (LIFE-P)," *The Journal of Nutrition, Health & Aging*, vol. 18, no. 1, pp. 59–64, 2014.

[4] K. Keller and M. Engelhardt, "Strength and muscle mass loss with aging process. Age and strength loss," *Muscles, Ligaments and Tendons Journal*, vol. 3, no. 4, p. 346, 2014.

[5] N. Montero-Fernández and J. A. Serra-Rexach, "Role of exercise on sarcopenia in the elderly," *European Journal of Physical and Rehabilitation Medicine*, vol. 49, no. 1, pp. 131–143, 2013.

[6] M. Brotto and E. L. Abreu, "Sarcopenia: pharmacology of today and tomorrow," *Journal of Pharmacology and Experimental Therapeutics*, vol. 343, no. 3, pp. 540–546, 2012.

[7] D. Scott, L. Blizzard, J. Fell, G. Giles, and G. Jones, "Associations between dietary nutrient intake and muscle mass and strength in community-dwelling older adults: the Tasmanian Older Adult Cohort Study," *Journal of the American Geriatrics Society*, vol. 58, no. 11, pp. 2129–2134, 2010.

[8] A. J. Cruz-Jentoft and F. Landi, "Sarcopenia," *Clinical Medicine*, vol. 14, no. 2, pp. 183–186, 2014.

[9] I. H. Rosenberg, "Sarcopenia: origins and clinical relevance," *Clinics in Geriatric Medicine*, vol. 27, no. 3, pp. 337–339, 2011.

[10] W. J. Evans, "Skeletal muscle loss: cachexia, sarcopenia, and inactivity," *The American Journal of Clinical Nutrition*, vol. 91, no. 4, pp. 1123S–1127S, 2010.

[11] G. A. Power, B. H. Dalton, and C. L. Rice, "Human neuromuscular structure and function in old age: a brief review," *Journal of Sport and Health Science*, vol. 2, no. 4, pp. 215–226, 2013.

[12] U. Granacher and T. Hortobágyi, "Exercise to improve mobility in healthy aging," *Sports Medicine*, vol. 45, no. 12, pp. 1625-1626, 2015.

[13] H. N. Carter, C. C. W. Chen, and D. A. Hood, "Mitochondria, muscle health, and exercise with advancing age," *Physiology*, vol. 30, no. 3, pp. 208–223, 2015.

[14] H. M. McBride, M. Neuspiel, and S. Wasiak, "Mitochondria: more than just a powerhouse," *Current Biology*, vol. 16, no. 14, pp. R551–R560, 2006.

[15] L. D. Tryon, A. Vainshtein, J. M. Memme, M. J. Crilly, and D. A. Hood, "Recent advances in mitochondrial turnover during chronic muscle disuse," *Integrative Medicine Research*, vol. 3, no. 4, pp. 161–171, 2014.

[16] M. P. Mattson, "Hormesis defined," *Ageing Research Reviews*, vol. 7, no. 1, pp. 1–7, 2008.

[17] A. R. Konopka and K. Sreekumaran Nair, "Mitochondrial and skeletal muscle health with advancing age," *Molecular and Cellular Endocrinology*, vol. 379, no. 1-2, pp. 19–29, 2013.

[18] D. Y. Seo, S. R. Lee, N. Kim, K. S. Ko, B. D. Rhee, and J. Han, "Age-related changes in skeletal muscle mitochondria: the role of exercise," *Integrative Medicine Research*, vol. 5, no. 3, pp. 182–186, 2016.

[19] I. Sanchez-Roman, A. Gómez, I. Pérez et al., "Effects of aging and methionine restriction applied at old age on ROS generation and oxidative damage in rat liver mitochondria," *Biogerontology*, vol. 13, no. 4, pp. 399–411, 2012.

[20] H. P. Indo, M. Davidson, H. C. Yen et al., "Evidence of ROS generation by mitochondria in cells with impaired electron transport chain and mitochondrial DNA damage," *Mitochondrion*, vol. 7, no. 1-2, pp. 106–118, 2007.

[21] K. R. Short, M. L. Bigelow, J. Kahl et al., "Decline in skeletal muscle mitochondrial function with aging in humans," *Proceedings of the National Academy of Sciences of the United States of America*, vol. 102, no. 15, pp. 5618–5623, 2005.

[22] O. E. Rooyackers, D. B. Adey, P. A. Ades, and K. S. Nair, "Effect of age on in vivo rates of mitochondrial protein synthesis in human skeletal muscle," *Proceedings of the National Academy of Sciences of the United States of America*, vol. 93, no. 26, pp. 15364–15369, 1996.

[23] Z. Wu, P. Puigserver, U. Andersson et al., "Mechanisms controlling mitochondrial biogenesis and respiration through the thermogenic coactivator PGC-1," *Cell*, vol. 98, no. 1, pp. 115–124, 1999.

[24] A. Vainshtein, E. M. A. Desjardins, A. Armani, M. Sandri, and D. A. Hood, "PGC-1α modulates denervation-induced mitophagy in skeletal muscle," *Skeletal Muscle*, vol. 5, no. 1, p. 9, 2015.

[25] N. Mizushima and B. Levine, "Autophagy in mammalian development and differentiation," *Nature Cell Biology*, vol. 12, no. 9, pp. 823–830, 2010.

[26] J. J. Wu, C. Quijano, E. Chen et al., "Mitochondrial dysfunction and oxidative stress mediate the physiological impairment induced by the disruption of autophagy," *Aging*, vol. 1, no. 4, pp. 425–437, 2009.

[27] L. DiPietro, "Physical activity in aging: changes in patterns and their relationship to health and function," *The Journals of Gerontology Series A: Biological Sciences and Medical Sciences*, vol. 56, no. 2, pp. 13–22, 2001.

[28] J. Dziura, C. Mendes de Leon, S. Kasl, and L. DiPietro, "Can physical activity attenuate aging-related weight loss in older people? The Yale Health and Aging Study, 1982–1994," *American Journal of Epidemiology*, vol. 159, no. 8, pp. 759–767, 2004.

[29] R. N. Baumgartner, S. J. Wayne, D. L. Waters, I. Janssen, D. Gallagher, and J. E. Morley, "Sarcopenic obesity predicts instrumental activities of daily living disability in the elderly," *Obesity Research*, vol. 12, no. 12, pp. 1995–2004, 2004.

[30] A. P. Russell, V. C. Foletta, R. J. Snow, and G. D. Wadley, "Skeletal muscle mitochondria: a major player in exercise, health and disease," *Biochimica et Biophysica Acta (BBA) - General Subjects*, vol. 1840, no. 4, pp. 1276–1284, 2014.

[31] S. Ketkar, A. Rathore, A. Kandhare et al., "Alleviating exercise-induced muscular stress using neat and processed bee pollen: oxidative markers, mitochondrial enzymes, and myostatin expression in rats," *Integrative Medicine Research*, vol. 4, no. 3, pp. 147–160, 2015.

[32] P. V. Komi, "Stretch-shortening cycle: a powerful model to study normal and fatigued muscle," *Journal of Biomechanics*, vol. 33, no. 10, pp. 1197–1206, 2000.

[33] G. S. Lynch, J. A. Faulkner, and S. V. Brooks, "Force deficits and breakage rates after single lengthening contractions of single fast fibers from unconditioned and conditioned muscles of young and old rats," *American Journal of Physiology-Cell Physiology*, vol. 295, no. 1, pp. C249–C256, 2008.

[34] I. M. Conboy, M. J. Conboy, G. M. Smythe, and T. A. Rando, "Notch-mediated restoration of regenerative potential to aged muscle," *Science*, vol. 302, no. 5650, pp. 1575–1577, 2003.

[35] Y. Shimomura, M. Suzuki, S. Sugiyama, Y. Hanaki, and T. Ozawa, "Protective effect of coenzyme Q10 on exercise-

induced muscular injury," *Biochemical and Biophysical Research Communications*, vol. 176, no. 1, pp. 349–355, 1991.

[36] M. Kon, F. Kimura, T. Akimoto et al., "Effect of Coenzyme Q10 supplementation on exercise-induced muscular injury of rats," *Exerc Immunol Rev*, vol. 13, pp. 76–88, 2007.

[37] M. Kon, K. Tanabe, T. Akimoto et al., "Reducing exercise-induced muscular injury in kendo athletes with supplementation of coenzyme Q10," *British Journal of Nutrition*, vol. 100, no. 4, pp. 903–909, 2008.

[38] A. Abadi, J. D. Crane, D. Ogborn et al., "Supplementation with α-lipoic acid, CoQ_{10}, and vitamin E augments running performance and mitochondrial function in female mice," *PLoS One*, vol. 8, no. 4, article e60722, 2013.

[39] G. Tian, J. Sawashita, H. Kubo et al., "Ubiquinol-10 supplementation activates mitochondria functions to decelerate senescence in senescence-accelerated mice," *Antioxidants & Redox Signaling*, vol. 20, no. 16, pp. 2606–2620, 2014.

[40] A. Lass, S. Agarwal, and R. S. Sohal, "Mitochondrial ubiquinone homologues, superoxide radical generation, and longevity in different mammalian species," *Journal of Biological Chemistry*, vol. 272, no. 31, pp. 19199–19204, 1997.

[41] S. Kamzalov, N. Sumien, M. J. Forster, and R. S. Sohal, "Coenzyme Q intake elevates the mitochondrial and tissue levels of Coenzyme Q and alpha-tocopherol in young mice," *The Journal of Nutrition*, vol. 133, no. 10, pp. 3175–3180, 2003.

[42] C. Gómez-Díaz, M. I. Burón, F. J. Alcaín et al., "Effect of dietary coenzyme Q and fatty acids on the antioxidant status of rat tissues," *Protoplasma*, vol. 221, no. 1-2, pp. 11–17, 2003.

[43] L. K. Kwong, S. Kamzalov, I. Rebrin et al., "Effects of coenzyme Q_{10} administration on its tissue concentrations, mitochondrial oxidant generation and oxidative stress in the rat," *Free Radical Biology & Medicine*, vol. 33, no. 5, pp. 627–638, 2002.

[44] H. Maruoka, K. Fujii, K. Inoue, and S. Kido, "Long-term effect of ubiquinol on exercise capacity and the oxidative stress regulation system in SAMP1 mice," *Journal of Physical Therapy Science*, vol. 26, no. 3, pp. 367–371, 2014.

[45] C. Schmelzer, J. G. Okun, D. Haas et al., "The reduced form of coenzyme Q_{10} mediates distinct effects on cholesterol metabolism at the transcriptional and metabolite level in SAMP1 mice," *IUBMB Life*, vol. 62, no. 11, pp. 812–818, 2010.

[46] M. Kitano, D. Watanabe, S. Oda et al., "Subchronic oral toxicity of ubiquinol in rats and dogs," *International Journal of Toxicology*, vol. 27, no. 2, pp. 189–215, 2008.

[47] L. Ernster and G. Dallner, "Biochemical, physiological and medical aspects of ubiquinone function," *Biochimica et Biophysica Acta (BBA) - Molecular Basis of Disease*, vol. 1271, no. 1, pp. 195–204, 1995.

[48] G. P. Littarru and L. Tiano, "Clinical aspects of coenzyme Q10: an update," *Nutrition*, vol. 26, no. 3, pp. 250–254, 2010.

[49] G. Dallner and P. J. Sindelar, "Regulation of ubiquinone metabolism," *Free Radical Biology & Medicine*, vol. 29, no. 3-4, pp. 285–294, 2000.

[50] G. P. Littarru, M. Battino, and K. Folkers, "Clinical aspects of coenzyme Q: improvement of cellular bioenergetics or antioxidant perfection?," in *Handbook of Antioxidants*, E. Cadenas and L. Packer, Eds., pp. 203–239, Marcel Decker, New York, NY, USA, 1996.

[51] A. Rötig, E. L. Appelkvist, V. Geromel et al., "Quinone-responsive multiple respiratory-chain dysfunction due to widespread coenzyme Q_{10} deficiency," *Lancet*, vol. 356, no. 9227, pp. 391–395, 2000.

[52] D. Alf, M. E. Schmidt, and S. C. Siebrecht, "Ubiquinol supplementation enhances peak power production in trained athletes: a double-blind, placebo controlled study," *Journal of the International Society of Sports Nutrition*, vol. 10, no. 1, p. 24, 2013.

[53] A. Y. Guo, K. S. Leung, P. M. Siu et al., "Muscle mass, structural and functional investigations of senescence-accelerated mouse P8 (SAMP8)," *Experimental Animals*, vol. 64, no. 4, pp. 425–433, 2015.

[54] T. Takeda, "Senescence-accelerated mouse (SAM): a biogerontological resource in aging research," *Neurobiology of Aging*, vol. 20, no. 2, pp. 105–110, 1999.

[55] J. E. Morley, H. J. Armbrecht, S. A. Farr, and V. B. Kumar, "The senescence accelerated mouse (SAMP8) as a model for oxidative stress and Alzheimer's disease," *Biochimica et Biophysica Acta (BBA) - Molecular Basis of Disease*, vol. 1822, no. 5, pp. 650–656, 2012.

[56] Y. Chiba, A. Shimada, N. Kumagai et al., "The senescence-accelerated mouse (SAM): a higher oxidative stress and age-dependent degenerative diseases model," *Neurochemical Research*, vol. 34, no. 4, pp. 679–687, 2009.

[57] F. Derbré, A. Gratas-Delamarche, M. C. Gómez-Cabrera, and J. Viña, "Inactivity-induced oxidative stress: a central role in age-related sarcopenia?," *European Journal of Sport Science*, vol. 14, Supplement 1, pp. S98–S108, 2014.

[58] W. Derave, B. O. Eijnde, M. Ramaekers, and P. Hespel, "Soleus muscles of SAMP8 mice provide an accelerated model of skeletal muscle senescence," *Experimental Gerontology*, vol. 40, no. 7, pp. 562–572, 2005.

[59] T. Nishikawa, J. A. Takahashi, T. Matsushita et al., "Tubular aggregates in the skeletal muscle of the senescence-accelerated mouse SAM," *Mechanisms of Ageing and Development*, vol. 114, no. 2, pp. 89–99, 2000.

[60] C. Moorwood, M. Liu, Z. Tian, and E. R. Barton, "Isometric and eccentric force generation assessment of skeletal muscles isolated from murine models of muscular dystrophies," *Journal of Visualized Experiments*, vol. 8, no. 71, article e50036, 2013.

[61] M. Romanick, L. D. V. Thompson, and H. M. Brown-Borg, "Murine models of atrophy, cachexia, and sarcopenia in skeletal muscle," *Biochimica et Biophysica Acta (BBA) - Molecular Basis of Disease*, vol. 1832, no. 9, pp. 1410–1420, 2013.

[62] T. Takeda, M. Hosokawa, S. Takeshita et al., "A new murine model of accelerated senescence," *Mechanisms of Ageing and Development*, vol. 17, no. 2, pp. 183–194, 1981.

[63] C. Kang, E. Chung, G. Diffee, and L. L. Ji, "Exercise training attenuates aging-associated mitochondrial dysfunction in rat skeletal muscle: role of PGC-1α," *Experimental Gerontology*, vol. 48, no. 11, pp. 1343–1350, 2013.

[64] N. Okudan, S. Revan, S. S. Balci, M. Belviranli, H. Pepe, and H. Gökbel, "Effects of CoQ_{10} supplementation and swimming training on exhaustive exercise-induced oxidative stress in rat heart," *Bratislava Medical Journal*, vol. 113, no. 07, pp. 393–399, 2012.

[65] S. Salucci, S. Burattini, F. Buontempo, A. M. Martelli, E. Falcieri, and M. Battistelli, "Protective effect of different antioxidant agents in UVB-irradiated keratinocytes," *European Journal of Histochemistry*, vol. 61, no. 3, p. 2784, 2017.

[66] M. Battistelli, S. Salucci, E. Olivotto et al., "Cell death in human articular chondrocyte: a morpho-functional study in micromass model," *Apoptosis*, vol. 19, no. 10, pp. 1471–1483, 2014.

[67] M. W. Pfaffl, "A new mathematical model for relative quantification in real-time RT–PCR," *Nucleic Acids Research*, vol. 29, no. 9, article e45, pp. 45e–445, 2001.

[68] S. Taniguchi, M. Hanafusa, H. Tsubone et al., "Age-dependency of the serum oxidative level in the senescence-accelerated mouse prone 8," *Journal of Veterinary Medical Science*, vol. 78, no. 8, pp. 1369–1371, 2016.

[69] M. J. Jackson and A. McArdle, "Age-related changes in skeletal muscle reactive oxygen species generation and adaptive responses to reactive oxygen species," *The Journal of Physiology*, vol. 589, no. 9, pp. 2139–2145, 2011.

[70] R. Saini, "Coenzyme Q10: the essential nutrient," *Journal of Pharmacy and Bioallied Sciences*, vol. 3, no. 3, pp. 466-467, 2011.

[71] F. L. Crane, Y. Hatefi, R. L. Lester, and C. Widmer, "Isolation of a quinone from beef heart mitochondria," *Biochimica et Biophysica Acta*, vol. 25, no. 1, pp. 220-221, 1957.

[72] R. S. Sohal and M. J. Forster, "Coenzyme Q, oxidative stress and aging," *Mitochondrion*, vol. 7, pp. S103–S111, 2007.

[73] R. S. Sohal, S. Kamzalov, N. Sumien et al., "Effect of coenzyme Q$_{10}$ intake on endogenous coenzyme Q content, mitochondrial electron transport chain, antioxidative defenses, and life span of mice," *Free Radical Biology & Medicine*, vol. 40, no. 3, pp. 480–487, 2006.

[74] M. Guescini, L. Tiano, M. L. Genova et al., "The combination of physical exercise with muscle-directed antioxidants to counteract sarcopenia: a biomedical rationale for pleiotropic treatment with creatine and coenzyme Q10," *Oxidative Medicine and Cellular Longevity*, vol. 2017, Article ID 7083049, 19 pages, 2017.

[75] J. D. Crane, L. G. MacNeil, and M. A. Tarnopolsky, "Long-term aerobic exercise is associated with greater muscle strength throughout the life span," *The Journals of Gerontology Series A: Biological Sciences and Medical Sciences*, vol. 68, no. 6, pp. 631–638, 2013.

[76] S. Zampieri, L. Pietrangelo, S. Loefler et al., "Lifelong physical exercise delays age-associated skeletal muscle decline," *The Journals of Gerontology Series A: Biological Sciences and Medical Sciences*, vol. 70, no. 2, pp. 163–173, 2015.

[77] H. Nakahara, T. Kanno, Y. Inai et al., "Mitochondrial dysfunction in the senescence accelerated mouse (SAM)," *Free Radical Biology & Medicine*, vol. 24, no. 1, pp. 85–92, 1998.

[78] M. Sandri, J. Lin, C. Handschin et al., "PGC-1α protects skeletal muscle from atrophy by suppressing FoxO3 action and atrophy-specific gene transcription," *Proceedings of the National Academy of Sciences of the United States of America*, vol. 103, no. 44, pp. 16260–16265, 2006.

[79] J. Lin, C. Handschin, and B. M. Spiegelman, "Metabolic control through the PGC-1 family of transcription coactivators," *Cell Metabolism*, vol. 1, no. 6, pp. 361–370, 2005.

[80] K. Baar, A. Wende, T. Jones et al., "Adaptations of skeletal muscle to exercise: rapid increase in the transcriptional coactivator PGC-1," *The FASEB Journal*, vol. 16, no. 14, pp. 1879–1886, 2002.

[81] J. W. Gordon, A. A. Rungi, H. Inagaki, and D. A. Hood, "Selected Contribution: Effects of contractile activity on mitochondrial transcription factor A expression in skeletal muscle," *Journal of Applied Physiology*, vol. 90, no. 1, pp. 389–396, 2001.

[82] I. Irrcher, P. J. Adhihetty, T. Sheehan, A. M. Joseph, and D. A. Hood, "PPARγ coactivator-1α expression during thyroid hormone- and contractile activity-induced mitochondrial adaptations," *American Journal of Physiology-Cell Physiology*, vol. 284, no. 6, pp. C1669–C1677, 2003.

[83] C. Kang, K. M. O'Moore, J. R. Dickman, and L. L. Ji, "Exercise activation of muscle peroxisome proliferator-activated receptor-γ coactivator-1α signaling is redox sensitive," *Free Radical Biology & Medicine*, vol. 47, no. 10, pp. 1394–1400, 2009.

[84] B. Chabi, V. Ljubicic, K. J. Menzies, J. H. Huang, A. Saleem, and D. A. Hood, "Mitochondrial function and apoptotic susceptibility in aging skeletal muscle," *Aging Cell*, vol. 7, no. 1, pp. 2–12, 2008.

[85] V. Ljubicic, A. M. Joseph, P. J. Adhihetty et al., "Molecular basis for an attenuated mitochondrial adaptive plasticity in aged skeletal muscle," *Aging*, vol. 1, no. 9, pp. 818–830, 2009.

[86] S. Welle, K. Bhatt, B. Shah, N. Needler, J. M. Delehanty, and C. A. Thornton, "Reduced amount of mitochondrial DNA in aged human muscle," *Journal of Applied Physiology*, vol. 94, no. 4, pp. 1479–1484, 2003.

[87] H. Guedouari, T. Daigle, L. Scorrano, and E. Hebert-Chatelain, "Sirtuin 5 protects mitochondria from fragmentation and degradation during starvation," *Biochimica et Biophysica Acta (BBA) - Molecular Cell Research*, vol. 1864, no. 1, pp. 169–176, 2017.

[88] T. van Wessel, A. de Haan, W. J. van der Laarse, and R. T. Jaspers, "The muscle fiber type-fiber size paradox: hypertrophy or oxidative metabolism?," *European Journal of Applied Physiology*, vol. 110, no. 4, pp. 665–694, 2010.

[89] A. Dirks and C. Leeuwenburgh, "Apoptosis in skeletal muscle with aging," *American Journal of Physiology-Regulatory, Integrative and Comparative Physiology*, vol. 282, no. 2, pp. R519–R527, 2002.

[90] R. A. Gottlieb and R. S. Carreira, "Autophagy in health and disease. 5. Mitophagy as a way of life," *American Journal of Physiology-Cell Physiology*, vol. 299, no. 2, pp. C203–C210, 2010.

[91] Y. Chen, M. B. Azad, and S. B. Gibson, "Superoxide is the major reactive oxygen species regulating autophagy," *Cell Death & Differentiation*, vol. 16, no. 7, pp. 1040–1052, 2009.

[92] J. E. Ricci, R. A. Gottlieb, and D. R. Green, "Caspase-mediated loss of mitochondrial function and generation of reactive oxygen species during apoptosis," *The Journal of Cell Biology*, vol. 160, no. 1, pp. 65–75, 2003.

[93] E. Masiero, L. Agatea, C. Mammucari et al., "Autophagy is required to maintain muscle mass," *Cell Metabolism*, vol. 10, no. 6, pp. 507–515, 2009.

[94] E. Wirawan, S. Lippens, T. vanden Berghe et al., "Beclin1: a role in membrane dynamics and beyond," *Autophagy*, vol. 8, no. 1, pp. 6–17, 2012.

[95] M. Enari, H. Sakahira, H. Yokoyama, A. Okawa, A. Iwamatsu, and S. Nagata, "A caspase-activated DNase that degrades DNA during apoptosis, and its inhibitor ICAD," *Nature*, vol. 391, no. 6662, pp. 43–50, 1998.

[96] S. Sahara, M. Aoto, Y. Eguchi, N. Imamoto, Y. Yoneda, and Y. Tsujimoto, "Acinus is a caspase-3-activated protein required for apoptotic chromatin condensation," *Nature*, vol. 401, no. 6749, pp. 168–173, 1999.

[97] M. L. Coleman, E. A. Sahai, M. Yeo, M. Bosch, A. Dewar, and M. F. Olson, "Membrane blebbing during apoptosis results from caspase-mediated activation of ROCK I," *Nature Cell Biology*, vol. 3, no. 4, pp. 339–345, 2001.

[98] R. J. Stefanetti, E. Zacharewicz, P. Della Gatta, A. Garnham, A. P. Russell, and S. Lamon, "Ageing has no effect on the regulation of the ubiquitin proteasome-related genes and proteins following resistance exercise," *Frontiers in Physiology*, vol. 5, no. 30, 2014.

[99] V. Moresi, A. H. Williams, E. Meadows et al., "Myogenin and class II HDACs control neurogenic muscle atrophy by inducing E3 ubiquitin ligases," *Cell*, vol. 143, no. 1, pp. 35–45, 2010.

6

Intravenous Anesthetic Protects Hepatocyte from Reactive Oxygen Species-Induced Cellular Apoptosis during Liver Transplantation *In Vivo*

Weifeng Yao [ID],[1] Xue Han,[2] Yihan Zhang [ID],[1] Jianqiang Guan,[1] Mian Ge,[1] Chaojin Chen,[1] Shan Wu,[1] Jiaxin Chen,[1] Gangjian Luo,[1] Pinjie Huang [ID],[1] and Ziqing Hei [ID][1]

[1]*Department of Anesthesiology, Third Affiliated Hospital, Sun Yat-sen University, Guangzhou, Guangdong 510630, China*
[2]*Department of Anesthesiology, Sun Yat-sen Memorial Hospital, Sun Yat-sen University, Guangzhou 510000, China*

Correspondence should be addressed to Pinjie Huang; hpjie@126.com and Ziqing Hei; heiziqing@sina.com

Academic Editor: Aldrin V. Gomes

Background. Liver transplantation leads to liver ischemia/reperfusion (I/R) injury, resulting in early graft dysfunction and failure. Exacerbations of oxidative stress and inflammatory response are key processes in the development of liver I/R injury. Intravenous anesthetic propofol potent effects on free radical scavenging and protects livers against I/R injury. However, the role and mechanism of propofol-mediated hepatic protection in liver transplantation is poorly understood. The aim of this study was to evaluate the role of propofol postconditioning in the liver I/R injury after liver transplantation. *Methods.* Forty-eight rats were randomly divided into six groups: rats receiving either sham operation or orthotopic autologous liver transplantation (OALT) in the absence or presence of propofol (high dose and low dose) postconditioning or intralipid control or VAS2870 (Nox2 special inhibitor). Eight hours after OALT or sham operation, parameters of organ injury, oxidative stress, inflammation, and NADPH-associated proteins were assessed. *Results.* After OALT, severe liver pathological injury was observed that was associated with increases of serum AST and ALT, which were attenuated by propofol postconditioning. In addition, especially high dose of propofol postconditioning reduced TNF-α, IL-1β, IL-6, TLR4, and NF-κB inflammatory pathway, accompanied with decrease of neutrophil elastase activity, MPO activity, 8-isoprotane, p47^{phox} and gp91^{phox} protein expressions, and increase of SOD activity. Inhibition of Nox2 by VAS2870 conferred similar protective effects in liver transplantation. *Conclusion.* Liver transplantation leads to severe inflammation and oxidative stress with NADPH oxidase activation. Propofol postconditioning reduces liver I/R injury after liver transplantation partly via inhibiting NADPH oxidase Nox2 and the subsequent inflammation and oxidative stress.

1. Introduction

Liver transplantation has become the effective surgical treatment for patients with end-stage liver disease [1]. Liver ischemia reperfusion (I/R) injury is a severe postoperative complication during the early period after transplantation. It leads to early graft dysfunction and failure, which further results in acute and chronic rejection and irreversible death [2]. Characterized by uncontrolled inflammatory response, liver I/R injury promotes hypoxic hepatocyte reoxygenation and reactive oxygen species (ROS) formation, which result in neutrophil infiltration, robust ROS generation, and ultimately programmed death of hepatocytes [3]. To date, the mechanisms accounted for liver injury, especially I/R injury during liver transplantation, are complicated and remained unclear; strategies for preventing I/R injury are still lacking. Hence, seeking protective intervention of I/R injury during perioperative period is regarded urgent and profound scientific significance and important clinical applications.

Propofol (2,6-diisopropylphenol) is widely used for anesthesia induction and maintenance during perioperation and sedation in intensive care unit (ICU) patients [4]. In addition to its clinical usages, propofol exerts anti-inflammatory and antioxidative effectiveness basing on the chemical group phenol [5]. In our previous study, we found that propofol pretreatment could attenuate pulmonary oxidative stress induced by liver transplantation through activating Nrf2 nuclear translocation and upregulating its downstream of HO-1 antioxidant enzyme formation [6, 7]. However, in most clinical situations, propofol pretreatment is not feasible while treatment at the onset or after induction of reperfusion, termed as postconditioning, is more applicable [8], which has been proven as a promising therapeutic strategy against ischemia/reperfusion damage. Whether propofol postconditioning is crucial in reducing oxidative stress in liver I/R injury and the underline mechanism remains unknown.

Nicotinamide adenine dinucleotide phosphate (NADPH) oxidase (Noxs) is one of the major sources of cellular ROS, which has been identified to play an important role in liver I/R injury [9]. Nox2 and Nox4 are two predominant Nox isoforms existing in hepatocytes in liver parenchyma [10]. Nox2-deficient mice showed lower mortality rate than wild type group when subjected to hepatic I/R injury. Whether Nox2 is correlated to liver transplantation-induced hepatic oxidative stress and contributed to the antioxidant property of propofol need to be verified.

Therefore, the current study observed the effects of propofol postconditioning on liver I/R injury induced by liver transplantation and further explored the potential mechanism whether the protective effects provided by propofol postconditioning are associated with Nox2-related oxidative stress pathway.

2. Materials and Methods

2.1. Experimental Protocols. Male Sprague-Dawley rats (220–250 g, 8 weeks) obtained from Medical Experimental Animal Center of Guangdong Province (Guangzhou, China) were housed in the animal room of Zhongshan Medical School (Guangzhou, China). Rats were fasted for 8 hours prior to the study but were allowed to access tap water ad libitum. All the animal care and research protocols were approved by the Institutional Animal Care and Use Committee of Sun Yat-sen University (Guangzhou, China) and performed in accordance with National Institutes of Health guidelines for the use of experimental animals.

The orthotopic autologous liver transplantation (OALT) model was carried out according to our previous study [11, 12]. Rats were randomly divided into six groups ($n = 8$) as follows: sham-operated control (sham) and OALT, OALT treated with intralipid (OALT + INT), OALT treated with high dose of propofol (OALT + HPro), OALT treated with low dose of propofol (OALT + LPro), and OALT treated with VAS2870 (OALT + VAS). High dose (40 mg/kg/h) or low dose (20 mg/kg/h) of propofol [13] or the same volume of intralipid was administrated continuous via tail vein for 30 min at the onset of reperfusion. Some of the rats were treated with specific Nox2 inhibitor VAS2870 (2 mg/kg, Sigma, USA) [14] intravenously after reperfusion.

2.2. Sample Harvest. Blood and liver samples were harvested eight hours after reperfusion. Under general anesthesia, animals were euthanized by a lethal injection of sodium pentobarbital. The blood was collected from carotid artery into heparinized tubes and then centrifuged for 15 min at 2000g (4°C). The supernatants were collected and stored at −80°C until measurement. Median hepatic lobes were immediately and promptly taken out (about 0.5 cm^3), washed in cold saline, fixed in 10% formalin solution, dehydrated in ascending grades of alcohol, and then embedded in paraffin. The residual parts of liver tissue were harvested and stored at −80°C until further measurement.

2.3. Serum Aspartate Aminotransferase (AST) and Alanine Aminotransferase (ALT) Levels. The activity of AST and ALT in serum, indicators of liver cellular damage, was measured by a clinical chemistry analyzer system.

2.4. Histological Examination of Liver Sections. Median hepatic lobes were fixed in 4% buffered formalin. After embedding and cutting of 4 μm slices, all samples were stained with hematoxylin/eosin. The staining sections were visualized and images were acquired using a microscope with 10x and 40x objectives. Histological evaluation was performed in a blinded manner. The severity of liver injury was graded with modified Suzuki criteria [15].

2.5. Assay of Inflammatory Cytokines and Oxidative Stress Markers. Part of the liver was homogenized with a Potter liver homogenizer at 500 g and centrifuged at 800 g for 10 min. The supernatant was pipetted into a fresh Eppendorf cup for the detection of cytokines. Inflammatory cytokines including TNF-α, IL-1β, and IL-6 in the liver were quantified with commercial ELISA kits (KeyGen BioTech, China). And the neutrophil elastase and 8-isoprostane were detected using ELISA kits (Cayman Chemical). Superoxide dismutase (SOD) and myeloperoxidase (MPO) activities were measured according to our previous methods [16].

2.6. Immunohistochemical Staining of p47^{phox}. Immunohistochemical staining was performed in a previous study [16]. Liver tissue sections were deparaffinized, hydrated, and incubated at 4°C overnight with a p47^{phox} primary antibody (Cell Signaling Technology, Danvers, USA, diluted 1 : 500), followed by incubation with a horseradish peroxidase-coupled anti-rabbit IgG secondary antibody at room temperature for 2 hours and then colored with diaminobenzidine (DAB) for 3 minutes. Phosphate-buffered saline (PBS) was used to replace primary antibody in the negative control. DAB staining intensity was observed under light microscope (Leica Microsystems Digital Imaging, Cambridge, UK) and assessed with a microscopic image analysis system (ImageJ, National Institutes of Health, USA).

2.7. TUNEL for DNA Fragmentation. The nuclear DNA fragmentation, a specific biochemical hallmark of apoptosis, was labeled by TUNEL staining with a Dead End Fluorometric TUNEL system kit (Promega Corp., Madison, Wisconsin, USA) according to the manufacturer's protocol and our previous study [17]. Liver sections were incubated with proteinase K solution (20 μg/ml in PBS) at room temperature for 10 minutes after deparaffinization and hydration. TUNEL labeling was conducted with a 100 μl mix of equilibration buffer, nucleotide mix, and recombinant terminal

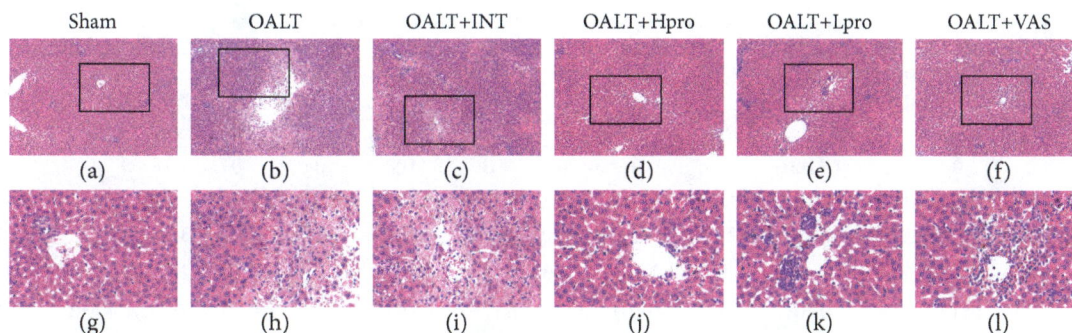

FIGURE 1: Representative photomicrographs of the livers after 8 hours of OALT. The liver tissue sections were stained with hematoxylin and eosin (H&E staining, 100x and 400x). $n = 8$ per group. $^{\#}P < 0.01$ vs. the sham group; $^{*}P < 0.05$ and $^{**}P < 0.01$ vs. the OALT group. HPro = high dose of propofol; LPro = low dose of propofol; INT = intralipid; VAS = VAS2870; OALT = orthotopic autologous liver transplantation.

deoxynucleotidyl transferase (rTdT) enzyme (the volume ratio was 45:5:1) in a humidified, lucifugal chamber for 1 hour at 37°C, from which step to the end of experiment, the slides were protected from direct light. The reaction was terminated by immersing the slides in a 2 × SSC buffer for 15 minutes at room temperature and then were rinsed with PBS. Nuclear was visualized by DAPI staining. The liver tissues were covered by an antifade solution and mounted by glass coverslips with clear nail polish sealing the edges. The slides were immediately analyzed by a fluorescence microscope and then stored at −20°C in dark if necessary.

2.8. Immunoblotting.

Western blot analysis was performed in our previous studies [18]. In brief, the hepatic tissues were homogenized and nuclear proteins were extracted with a Nuclear-Cytosol Extraction kit (Applygen Technology Inc., Beijing, China) according to the manufacturer's instructions. The protein concentration had been determined by the BCA protein assay (Bio-Rad, Hemel Hempstead, Herts, UK). Sixty micrograms of each protein sample was subjected to Western blot analysis using the following primary antibodies incubated overnight at 4°C: anti-gp91^{phox} at 1:8000 dilution (Cell Signaling Technology Inc.), anti-p47^{phox} at 1:1000 dilution (Cell Signaling Technology Inc.), anti-Na/K-ATPase at 1:1000 dilution (Cell Signaling Technology Inc.), anti-cleaved caspase-3 at 1:1000 dilution (Cell Signaling Technology Inc.), anti-procaspase-3 at 1:1000 dilution (Cell Signaling Technology Inc.), anti-nuclear factor kappa B (NF-κB) p65 at 1:1000 dilution (Cell Signaling Technology Inc.), anti-Toll-like receptor 4 (TLR4) at 1:1000 dilution (Santa Cruz Biotechnology Inc.), and anti-β-actin at 1:1500 dilution (Merck Millipore, Germany). The secondary antibodies were goat anti-mouse or anti-rabbit IgG antibodies at 1:2000 dilution (Thermo Fisher Scientific, Fremont, CA, USA). The enhanced chemiluminescence system was used to detect the protein-antibody complex (KGP1125, Nanjing KeyGEN Biotech. Co. Ltd.). The AlphaView software (Cell Biosciences, Santa Clara, CA) was used to measure the optical density of the interesting protein band signals which were correlated to the protein levels and normalized to those of β-actin.

2.9. Analysis of Data.

Data were expressed as means ± SD. Statistical significance among groups was determined by one-way ANOVA followed by Newman-Keuls post hoc analysis using the GraphPad Prism 6 software (San Diego, CA, USA). Statistical significance was accepted at $P < 0.05$.

3. Results

3.1. Propofol Postconditioning Reduced Liver Injury after OALT.

As shown in Figure 1, compared with the sham group, there was a massive cellular necrosis (Table 1) in the centrilobular regions of the livers at 8 hours after OALT, accompanied with severe cell ballooning and infiltration of inflammatory cell, which was assessed and scaled according to the modified Suzuki criteria ($P < 0.01$ vs. the sham group). Propofol postconditioning, especially administrated at high dose (40 mg/kg/h), significantly reduced the extent of necrosis, cell ballooning, and inflammatory cell infiltration ($P < 0.01$ vs. the OALT group or intralipid group). Similarly, the Nox2 inhibitor VAS2870 exerted the same protective effects in the livers against I/R injury following OALT, evidenced by ameliorated cell necrosis, cell ballooning, and inflammatory cell infiltration ($P < 0.05$ vs. the OALT group). Consisted with the pathological results, as shown in Figures 2(a) and 2(b), high dose of propofol dramatically attenuated AST and ALT levels compared with the OALT group or intralipid group. These results indicated that propofol postconditioning and Nox2 inhibition could both provide liver protection in the early stage of OALT.

3.2. Nox2 Inhibition Was Involved in the Protective Effects Conferred by Propofol Postconditioning.

In order to test whether the antioxidative effect of propofol postconditioning was linked to Nox2, the Nox2 subunits p47^{phox} on cell membrane and gp91^{phox} in cytoplasm were detected. As shown in Figures 3(a)–3(d), OALT leads to upregulation of p47^{phox} and gp91^{phox} protein expressions, while propofol postconditioning significantly decreased these two Nox2 subunit protein expressions in the liver following OALT. Moreover, Nox2 specific inhibitor VAS2870 was used as a positive control showing dramatically inhibition of p47^{phox} and gp91^{phox} protein expressions after VAS2870 treatment.

TABLE 1: Histological score of liver injury by OALT.

Groups	Centrilobular cell death Grade				Average	Ballooning Grade				Average	Inflammation Grade				Average
	+3	+2	+1	0		+3	+2	+1	0		+3	+2	+1	0	
Sham	0	0	0	8 (100)	0	0	0	0	8 (100)	0	0	0	0	8 (100)	0
OALT	2 (25)	3 (38)	3 (38)	0 (0)	$1.9^{\#}$	3 (38)	3 (38)	2 (25)	0 (0)	$2.1^{\#}$	5 (63)	2 (25)	1 (13)	0 (0)	$2.5^{\#}$
OALT + INT	2 (25)	4 (50)	2 (25)	0 (0)	$2.0^{\#}$	2 (25)	4 (50)	2 (25)	0 (0)	$2.0^{\#}$	4 (50)	3 (38)	1 (13)	0 (0)	$2.4^{\#}$
OALT + HPro	0 (0)	1 (13)	6 (75)	1 (13)	1.0^{**}	0 (0)	1 (13)	7 (88)	0 (0)	1.1^{**}	0 (0)	2 (25)	5 (63)	1 (13)	1.1^{**}
OALT + LPro	0 (0)	1 (13)	7 (88)	0 (0)	1.1^{**}	0 (0)	2 (25)	6 (75)	0 (0)	1.3^{*}	0 (0)	4 (50)	4 (50)	0 (0)	1.5^{*}
OALT + VAS	0 (0)	2 (25)	6 (75)	0 (0)	1.3^{*}	0 (0)	2 (25)	5 (63)	1 (13)	1.1^{**}	0 (0)	3 (38)	4 (50)	1 (13)	1.3^{*}

Numbers of rats are shown, with percentages enclosed within parenthesis. Grade indication: no change (0), mild (1), moderate (2), and severe (3). $^{\#}P < 0.01$ vs. the sham group, $^{*}P < 0.05$ vs. the OALT group, and $^{**}P < 0.01$ vs. the OALT group.

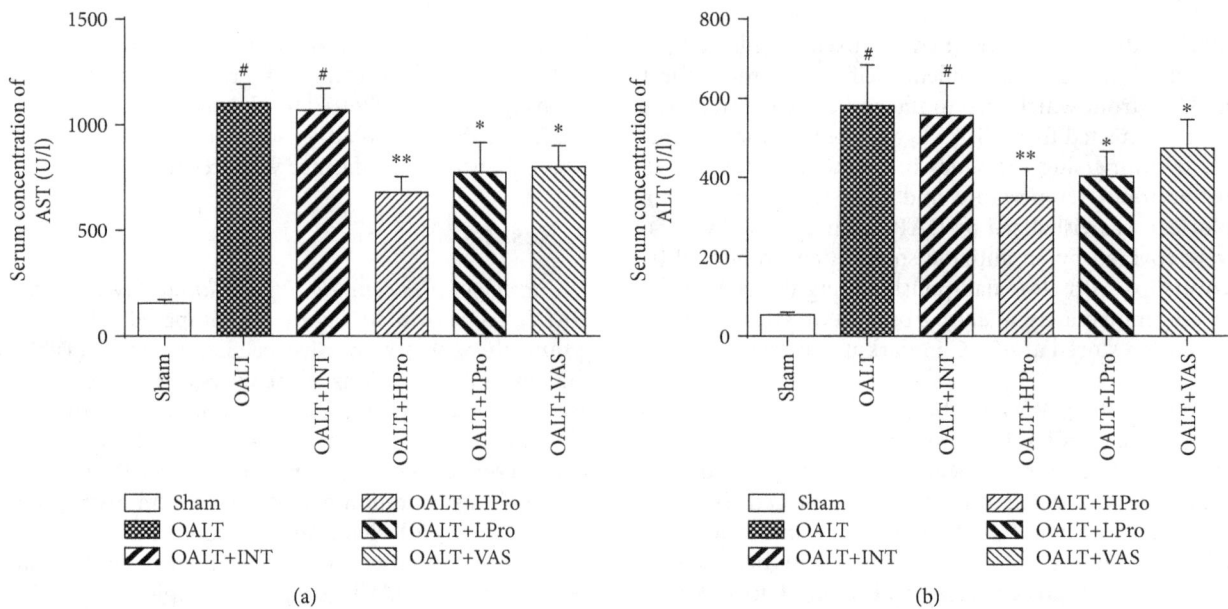

FIGURE 2: Serum alanine aminotransferase (ALT) (a) and aspartate aminotransferase (AST) (b) levels of experimental rats 8 hours after OALT. The results are expressed as the mean ± SD. $n = 8$ per group. $^{\#}P < 0.01$ vs. the sham group; $^{*}P < 0.05$ and $^{**}P < 0.01$ vs. the OALT group. HPro = high dose of propofol; LPro = low dose of propofol; INT = intralipid; VAS = VAS2870; OALT = orthotopic autologous liver transplantation.

Taken together, these results revealed that propofol postconditioning may reduce hepatic oxidative stress via inhibiting NADPH oxidase Nox2 activity and the subsequent ROS generation.

3.3. Propofol Postconditioning Attenuated Liver Inflammatory Response following OALT.

According to the pathological results, we found inflammatory infiltration during liver injury in the early stage of OALT; we then tested the inflammatory cytokines and inflammation-related TLR4/NF-κB pathway. As shown in Figures 4(a)–4(c), hepatic proinflammatory cytokines TNF-α, IL-1β, and IL-6 were all increased in the OALT group. Propofol postconditioning of both doses but not intralipid treatment significantly reduced the releases of proinflammatory cytokines compared to the OALT group. Treatment with Nox2 inhibitor

VAS2870 presented similar anti-inflammation effects with decrease of levels of cytokines TNF-α, IL-1β, and IL-6. Both propofol postconditioning and Nox2 inhibition could inhibit the TLR4/NF-κB inflammatory pathway, evidenced by reduced nuclear protein expressions of NF-κB p65 protein and downregulated total TLR4 expression (Figures 4(d)–4(f)) ($P < 0.05$ vs. OALT).

3.4. Propofol Postconditioning Mitigated Neutrophil Infiltration and Hepatic Oxidative Stress.

ROS scavenging is one of the characteristics of propofol. In order to detect the antioxidative effects of propofol postconditioning on liver I/R injury after OALT, neutrophil infiltration and hepatic oxidative stress were measured. As shown in Figures 5(a) and 5(b), hepatic neutrophil elastase (NE) activity and MPO activity, both of which were associated with

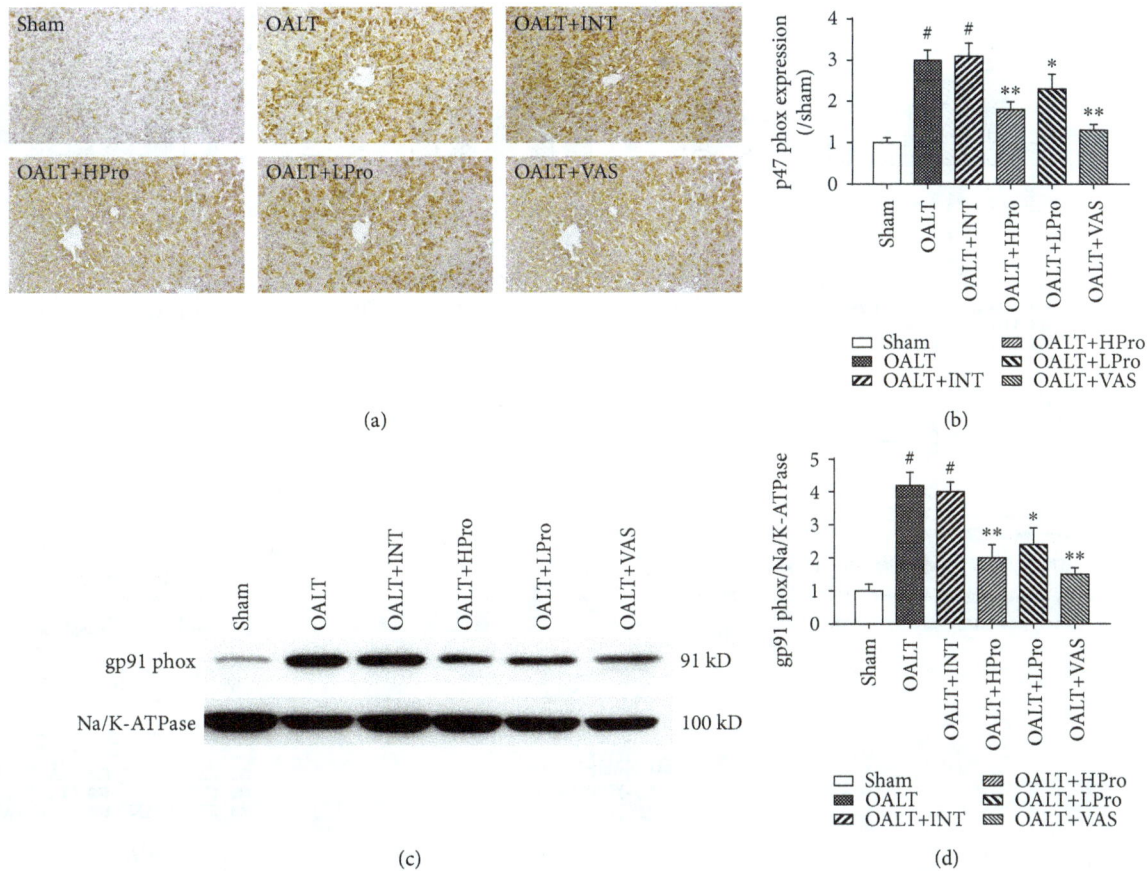

(a)

(b)

(c)

(d)

FIGURE 3: Hepatic NADPH oxidase expression changed due to OALT. Protein p47^{phox} expression was detected by immunohistochemistry method (a). The amount of protein p47^{phox} was calculated by gray scanning and was analyzed (b). Protein gp91^{phox} expression was detected by Western blot method (c). The amount of protein gp91^{phox} was calculated by gray scanning and was analyzed (d). The results are expressed as the mean ± SD. $n = 8$ per group. $^{\#}P < 0.01$ vs. the sham group; $^{*}P < 0.05$ and $^{**}P < 0.01$ vs. the OALT group. HPro = high dose of propofol; LPro = low dose of propofol; INT = intralipid; VAS = VAS2870; OALT = orthotopic autologous liver transplantation.

neutrophil infiltration, were significantly elevated in rats subjected to OALT. Both propofol postconditioning and VAS2870 treatment inhibited neutrophil infiltration caused by OALT and reduced lipid peroxidation product 8-isoprostane generation and increased SOD activity (Figures 5(c) and 5(d)) in the livers ($P < 0.05$ vs. OALT). These results indicated that propofol postconditioning and Nox2 inhibition protected the liver from oxidative stress via reduced neutrophil infiltration and ROS generation.

3.5. Propofol Postconditioning Protected Hepatocytes from Apoptosis. Oxidative stress and inflammation can finally lead to hepatocyte apoptosis or necrosis and cause liver I/R injury. As shown in Figures 6(a)–6(c), we identified a significant amount of cell apoptosis occurred in the liver following OALT compared to the sham group ($P < 0.01$ vs. the sham group). High dose of propofol postconditioning significantly reduced the number of apoptotic cells, which was consistent with the decrease of cleaved caspase-3/procaspase-3 ratio. Similarly, Nox2 inhibition by VAS2870 reduced hepatocyte apoptosis compared to the OALT group. These results indicated that propofol postconditioning reduced hepatocyte ROS generation and finally protected hepatocyte from apoptosis.

4. Discussion

In the current study, we demonstrated that propofol postconditioning reduced hepatocellular apoptosis after liver transplantation and its antioxidative property was related to inhibition of NADPH oxidase. We established an OALT model to mimic clinical liver transplantation and then detected the hepatic pathology, oxidative mediators, and inflammation response including TLR4/NF-κB signaling pathway. To further clarify the protective effects of propofol, VAS2870, a specific inhibitor of NADPH oxidase Nox2, was used as a positive control. Our results suggested that propofol postconditioning exerted protective effects against liver injury following OALT. And inhibition of Nox2 maybe a possible mechanism for liver protection conferred by propofol postconditioning (Figure 7).

Liver I/R injury has been identified as one of the most important factors to the etiology after liver transplantation, which contributes to early graft dysfunction and failure [19]. I/R processed is triggered when a donor liver is transiently deprived of oxygen and reoxygenation, leading to uncontrolled inflammatory response and reactive oxygen species release in the early stages of reperfusion [20]. In the present study, we found dramatically increased hepatic inflammatory

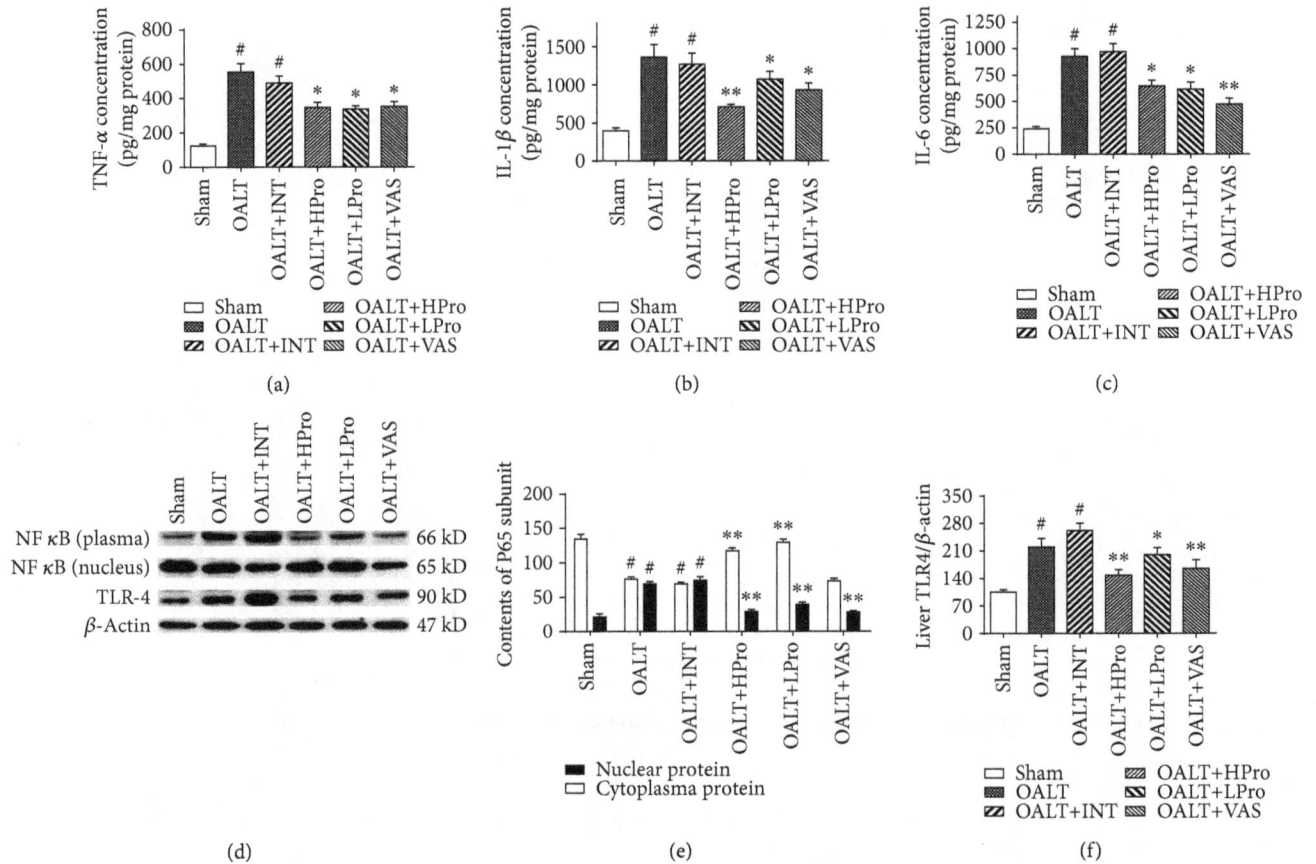

FIGURE 4: Hepatic inflammatory response after OALT. Proinflammatory cytokines TNF-α (a), IL-1β (b), and IL-6 (c) levels were measured by ELISA assay. Cytoplasm and nuclear NF-κB p65 and TLR4 proteins were detected by Western blot (d). The amount of target proteins NF-κB p65 (e) and TLR4 (f) was calculated by gray scanning and was analyzed. $n = 8$ per group. $^\#P < 0.01$ vs. the sham group; $^*P < 0.05$ and $^{**}P < 0.01$ vs. the OALT group. HPro = high dose of propofol; LPro = low dose of propofol; INT = intralipid; VAS = VAS2870; OALT = orthotopic autologous liver transplantation.

cytokines including TNF-α, IL-1β, and IL-6 as well as activated TLR4/NF-κB signaling pathway after OALT. These cytokines were proved to be vital to the initiation and propagation of liver I/R injury, whose main role was to recruit circulating neutrophils to the injured liver tissue during reperfusion [21]. In our study, hepatic MPO and neutrophil elastase were increased, which indicated that neutrophil extensively infiltrates the liver in the early stage of OALT. Along with neutrophil infiltration was excessive ROS generation and subsequent oxygen-derived product formation [22].

Strong evidences have illustrated the importance of ROS in pathogenesis of liver I/R injury [23, 24]. One of the currently promising intervention strategies is ischemic preconditioning (IPC), which is an intrinsic process whereby repeated short episode of ischemia to protect the liver against subsequent ischemia [25]. However, IPC may lead to potential vascular injury and thermogenesis [26]. We previously used propofol pretreatment during liver transplantation and found that propofol protected the lung from oxidative stress via enhancing antioxidant enzyme HO-1 expression. However, it takes several days to pretreat with propofol but most liver transplantations are emergency operations [6, 7]. Thus, we preferred propofol postconditioning and

demonstrated its protective function in reducing early liver damage after transplantation. In the model of rats' middle cerebral artery occlusion, it has proved that propofol postconditioning (20 mg/kg/h for 2 hours at the onset of reperfusion) led to long-term recovery of brain functions and upregulating the activity of the PKMζ/KCC2 pathway [27]. Li et al. found that propofol postconditioning enhanced cell viability and alleviated apoptosis to protect cardiomyocytes against hypoxia/reoxygenation injury through ERK signaling pathway [28]. Of interest, Li et al. found that alternative use of isoflurane and propofol conferred superior cardioprotection against postischemic myocardial injury and dysfunction, and this function was probably mediated through attenuating cardiac oxidative damage [29], which indicated that anesthesia may play an important role in organ protection during I/R injury.

NADPH oxidase activation and subsequent ROS formation are important upstream events which can activate hepatocytes and amplify the production of multiple proinflammatory cytokines, such as TNF-α or interlukin-1β [30]. Hepatic NADPH oxidase activation and the ROS production have been implicated as critical regulators of liver I/R injury [23]. Although propofol has been shown to reduce oxidative stress

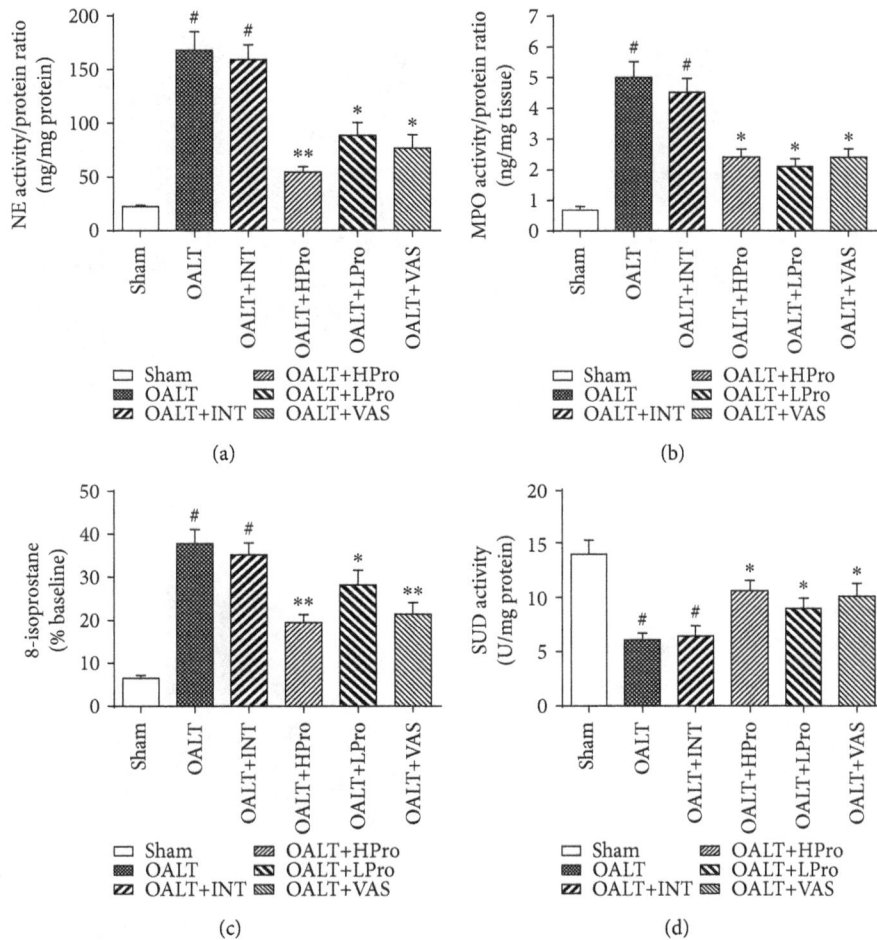

FIGURE 5: Neutrophil infiltration and oxidative stress in the liver. Neutrophil elastase (NE) (a) and myeloperoxidase (MPO) (b) activities reflected neutrophil infiltration. 8-Isoprostane (c) and superoxide dismutase (SOD) (d) were detected to reflect hepatic oxidative stress level. $n = 8$ per group. $^\#P < 0.01$ vs. the sham group; $^*P < 0.05$ and $^{**}P < 0.01$ vs. the OALT group. HPro = high dose of propofol; LPro = low dose of propofol; INT = intralipid; VAS = VAS2870; OALT = orthotopic autologous liver transplantation.

as an ROS scavenger, the current study shows that propofol can also suppress Nox2 to reduce the consequent production of ROS. Notably, propofol downregulated the hepatic expression of the NADPH oxidase membrane components $p47^{phox}$ and glycosylated subunit $gp91^{phox}$ after OALT. We speculated that this may be an important mechanism of propofol actions. Luo et al. showed that siRNA silencing of $p22^{phox}$ significantly attenuated the protective effects of propofol [31]. Recent studies have also identified other receptors as potential molecular targets of propofol including nicotinic and M1 muscarinic receptors [32, 33]. Whether these receptors act as upstream regulators, NADPH oxidase remains to be determined.

Of note, in the current study, the OALT model is superior in mimicking the pathophysiological variation during liver ischemia/reperfusion in liver transplantation and ischemia/reperfusion-mediated liver injury without interference of immunoactivities between grafts and hosts. However, as the cold ischemia time in this model is about 20 minutes, so it is not able to represent the long (6 to 8 hours) cold preservation time that occurs in the liver graft before being transplanted. Propofol postconditioning was performed at the onset of

reperfusion with continuous infusion for 30 min and proved to be protective against liver I/R injury. However, whether the dose and the duration we chose was the best intervention required further investigation. Moreover, although we have confirmed that the protective effect of propofol postconditioning was related to Nox2 activity inhibition, whether it acts on the other NADPH oxidase subunit such as Nox4 also remains unknown. It is also still unclear that how propofol acts on Nox2, directly or indirectly. Those questions remain unanswered. More studies will be involved to clarify these mechanisms and make this intervention more safe and reliable.

In summary, liver transplantation leads to severe inflammation and oxidative stress accompanied with NADPH oxidase Nox2 activation. Propofol postconditioning exerted prominently protective function against the I/R injury after liver transplantation, which presented as lower levels of inflammatory mediators and oxidative products accompanied with less neutrophil filtration and weaker induction of Nox2. Collectively, propofol postconditioning had been proved to reduce liver inflammation and oxidative stress probably via inhibiting NADPH oxidase Nox2.

(a)

(b)

(c)

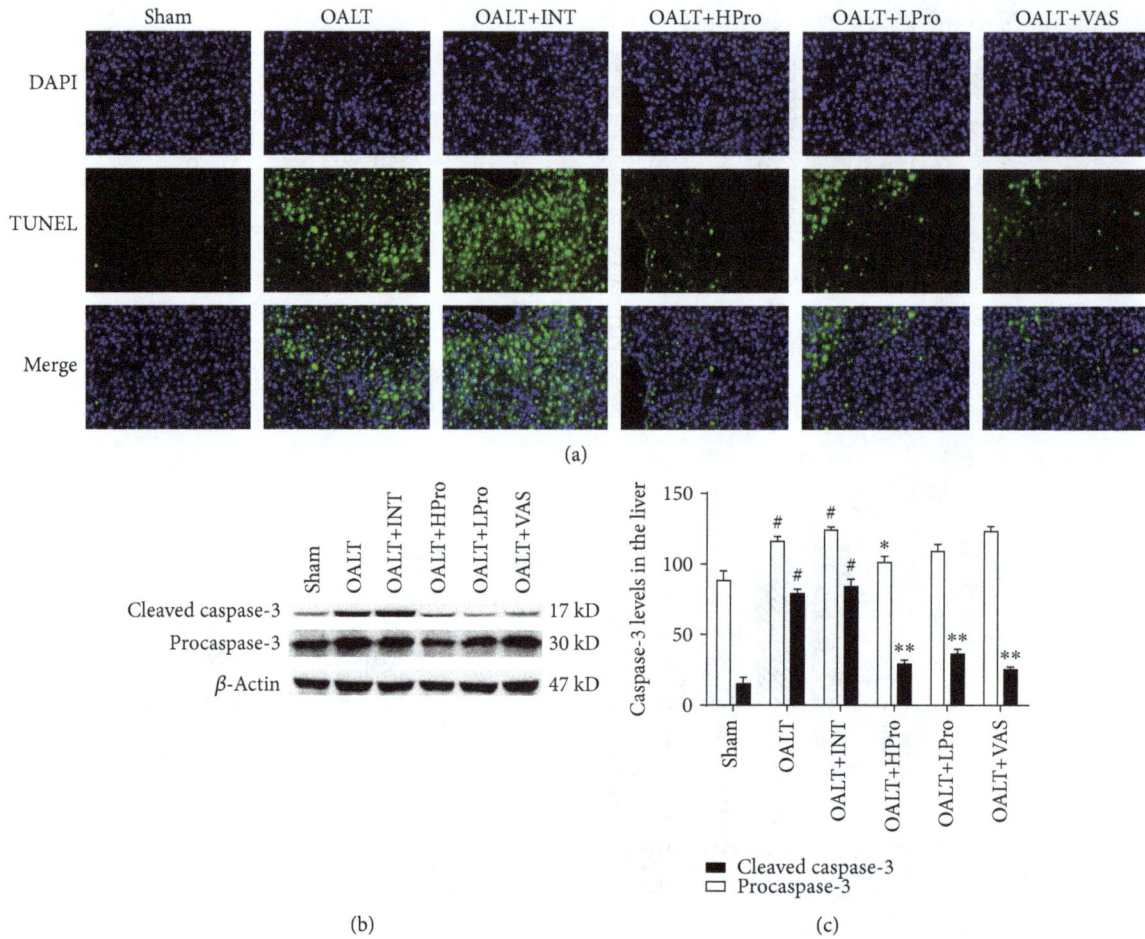

FIGURE 6: Propofol postconditioning protected hepatocyte from apoptosis. Fluorescent TUNEL staining of liver tissue (40x) (a). Cleaved caspase-3 and procaspase-3 proteins were detected by Western blot method (b). The amount of target proteins cleaved caspase-3 and procaspase-3 was calculated by gray scanning and was analyzed (c). The results are expressed as the mean ± SD. $n = 8$ per group. [#]$P < 0.01$ vs. the sham group; [*]$P < 0.05$ and [**]$P < 0.01$ vs. the OALT group. HPro = high dose of propofol; LPro = low dose of propofol; INT = intralipid; VAS = VAS2870; OALT = orthotopic autologous liver transplantation.

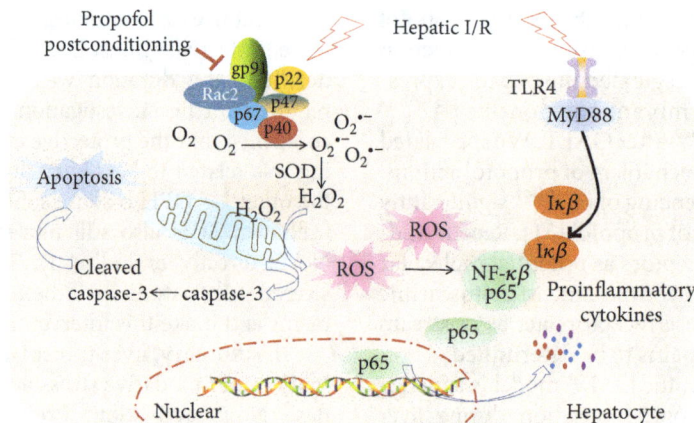

FIGURE 7: Propofol postconditioning reduces liver injury and the possible mechanisms. Under hepatic I/R condition, NADPH oxidase and TLR4/NF-κB pathway are activated. Endogenously, ROS were generated due to NADPH oxidase activation, resulting in the caspase-3-related apoptosis pathway as well as NF-κB pathway activation. Amount of proinflammatory cytokines was produced after NF-κB p65 pathway activation. Propofol postconditioning inhibited Nox2 (gp91[phox] and p47[phox]) which could lead to downregulation of ROS generation and finally reduced hepatic I/R injury.

Authors' Contributions

Weifeng Yao and Xue Han contributed equally to this study. Weifeng Yao, Ziqing Hei, and Pinjie Huang conceived and designed the experiments. Weifeng Yao, Xue Han, Yihan Zhang, Jianqiang Guan, Mian Ge, Chaojin Chen, Shan Wu, Jiaxin Chen, Gangjian Luo, and Pinjie Huang performed the experiments. Weifeng Yao analyzed the data. Xue Han contributed the reagents/materials/analysis tools. Weifeng Yao wrote the paper. All authors read and approved the manuscript.

Acknowledgments

The study was supported in part by grants from the National Natural Science Foundation of China (no. 81601724 for Weifeng Yao; no. 81501693 for Pinjie Huang and no. 81770649 for Gangjian Luo; no. 81772127 for Ziqing Hei). The study also was supported in part by grants from the Natural Science Foundation of Guangdong Province (no. 2016A030313232 for Pinjie Huang).

References

[1] F. Durand, "How to improve long-term outcome after liver transplantation?," *Liver International*, vol. 38, Supplement 1, pp. 134–138, 2018.

[2] R. F. Saidi and S. K. H. Kenari, "Liver ischemia/reperfusion injury: an overview," *Journal of Investigative Surgery*, vol. 27, no. 6, pp. 366–379, 2014.

[3] J. Li, R. J. Li, G. Y. Lv, and H. Q. Liu, "The mechanisms and strategies to protect from hepatic ischemia-reperfusion injury," *European Review for Medical and Pharmacological Sciences*, vol. 19, no. 11, pp. 2036–2047, 2015.

[4] P. Tang and R. Eckenhoff, "Recent progress on the molecular pharmacology of propofol," *F1000Res*, vol. 7, p. 123, 2018.

[5] I. Vasileiou, T. Xanthos, E. Koudouna et al., "Propofol: a review of its non-anaesthetic effects," *European Journal of Pharmacology*, vol. 605, no. 1-3, pp. 1–8, 2009.

[6] M. Ge, W. Yao, Y. Wang et al., "Propofol alleviates liver oxidative stress via activating Nrf2 pathway," *The Journal of Surgical Research*, vol. 196, no. 2, pp. 373–381, 2015.

[7] W. Yao, G. Luo, G. Zhu et al., "Propofol activation of the Nrf2 pathway is associated with amelioration of acute lung injury in a rat liver transplantation model," *Oxidative Medicine and Cellular Longevity*, vol. 2014, Article ID 258567, 9 pages, 2014.

[8] D. Bracco, "Post-conditioning: promising answers and more questions," *Critical Care*, vol. 16, no. 6, p. 180, 2012.

[9] H. Harada, I. N. Hines, S. Flores et al., "Role of NADPH oxidase-derived superoxide in reduced size liver ischemia and reperfusion injury," *Archives of Biochemistry and Biophysics*, vol. 423, no. 1, pp. 103–108, 2004.

[10] S. H. Ellmark, G. J. Dusting, M. N. T. Fui, N. Guzzo-Pernell, and G. R. Drummond, "The contribution of Nox4 to NADPH oxidase activity in mouse vascular smooth muscle," *Cardiovascular Research*, vol. 65, no. 2, pp. 495–504, 2005.

[11] W. Yao, H. Li, G. Luo et al., "SERPINB1 ameliorates acute lung injury in liver transplantation through ERK1/2-mediated STAT3-dependent HO-1 induction," *Free Radical Biology & Medicine*, vol. 108, pp. 542–553, 2017.

[12] C. Luo, D. Yuan, X. Li et al., "Propofol attenuated acute kidney injury after orthotopic liver transplantation via inhibiting gap junction composed of connexin 32," *Anesthesiology*, vol. 122, no. 1, pp. 72–86, 2015.

[13] A. G. Hudetz, X. Liu, S. Pillay, M. Boly, and G. Tononi, "Propofol anesthesia reduces Lempel-Ziv complexity of spontaneous brain activity in rats," *Neuroscience Letters*, vol. 628, pp. 132–135, 2016.

[14] Y. H. Tuo, Z. Liu, J. W. Chen et al., "NADPH oxidase inhibitor improves outcome of mechanical reperfusion by suppressing hemorrhagic transformation," *Journal of NeuroInterventional Surgery*, vol. 9, no. 5, pp. 492–498, 2017.

[15] A. Naiki-Ito, M. Asamoto, T. Naiki et al., "Gap junction dysfunction reduces acetaminophen hepatotoxicity with impact on apoptotic signaling and connexin 43 protein induction in rat," *Toxicologic Pathology*, vol. 38, no. 2, pp. 280–286, 2010.

[16] X. Huang, W. Zhao, D. Hu et al., "Resveratrol efficiently improves pulmonary function via stabilizing mast cells in a rat intestinal injury model," *Life Sciences*, vol. 185, pp. 30–37, 2017.

[17] W. Yao, H. Li, X. Han et al., "MG53 anchored by dysferlin to cell membrane reduces hepatocyte apoptosis which induced by ischaemia/reperfusion injury in vivo and in vitro," *Journal of Cellular and Molecular Medicine*, vol. 21, no. 10, pp. 2503–2513, 2017.

[18] M. Ge, W. Yao, D. Yuan et al., "Brg1-mediated Nrf2/HO-1 pathway activation alleviates hepatic ischemia-reperfusion injury," *Cell Death & Disease*, vol. 8, no. 6, article e2841, 2017.

[19] M. Mendes-Braz, M. Elias-Miro, M. B. Jimenez-Castro, A. Casillas-Ramirez, F. S. Ramalho, and C. Peralta, "The current state of knowledge of hepatic ischemia-reperfusion injury based on its study in experimental models," *Journal of Biomedicine & Biotechnology*, vol. 2012, Article ID 298657, 20 pages, 2012.

[20] M. Abu-Amara, S. Y. Yang, N. Tapuria, B. Fuller, B. Davidson, and A. Seifalian, "Liver ischemia/reperfusion injury: processes in inflammatory networks-a review," *Liver Transplantation*, vol. 16, no. 9, pp. 1016–1032, 2010.

[21] K. M. Quesnelle, P. V. Bystrom, and L. H. Toledo-Pereyra, "Molecular responses to ischemia and reperfusion in the liver," *Archives of Toxicology*, vol. 89, no. 5, pp. 651–657, 2015.

[22] H. Jaeschke, "Reactive oxygen and mechanisms of inflammatory liver injury: present concepts," *Journal of Gastroenterology and Hepatology*, vol. 26, Suppl 1, pp. 173–179, 2011.

[23] H. Jaeschke and B. L. Woolbright, "Current strategies to minimize hepatic ischemia-reperfusion injury by targeting reactive oxygen species," *Transplantation Reviews*, vol. 26, no. 2, pp. 103–114, 2012.

[24] H. Jaeschke, "Mechanisms of liver injury. II. Mechanisms of neutrophil-induced liver cell injury during hepatic ischemia-reperfusion and other acute inflammatory conditions," *American Journal of Physiology-Gastrointestinal and Liver Physiology*, vol. 290, no. 6, pp. G1083–G1088, 2006.

[25] S. Yan, L. M. Jin, Y. X. Liu, L. Zhou, H. Y. Xie, and S. S. Zheng, "Outcomes and mechanisms of ischemic preconditioning in liver transplantation," *Hepatobiliary & Pancreatic Diseases International*, vol. 9, no. 4, pp. 346–354, 2010.

[26] R. S. Koti, A. M. Seifalian, and B. R. Davidson, "Protection of the liver by ischemic preconditioning: a review of mechanisms and clinical applications," *Digestive Surgery*, vol. 20, no. 5, pp. 383–396, 2003.

[27] C. Y. Yang, S. Y. Liu, H. Y. Wang et al., "Neuroprotection by propofol post-conditioning: focus on PKMζ/KCC2 pathway activity," *Cellular and Molecular Neurobiology*, vol. 38, no. 3, pp. 691–701, 2018.

[28] H. Li, J. Tan, Z. Zou, C. G. Huang, and X. Y. Shi, "Propofol post-conditioning protects against cardiomyocyte apoptosis in hypoxia/reoxygenation injury by suppressing nuclear factor-kappa B translocation via extracellular signal-regulated kinase mitogen-activated protein kinase pathway," *European Journal of Anaesthesiology*, vol. 28, no. 7, pp. 525–534, 2011.

[29] T. Li, W. Wu, Z. You et al., "Alternative use of isoflurane and propofol confers superior cardioprotection than using one of them alone in a dog model of cardiopulmonary bypass," *European Journal of Pharmacology*, vol. 677, no. 1-3, pp. 138–146, 2012.

[30] K. Kimura, K. Shirabe, T. Yoshizumi et al., "Ischemia-reperfusion injury in fatty liver is mediated by activated NADPH oxidase 2 in rats," *Transplantation*, vol. 100, no. 4, pp. 791–800, 2016.

[31] T. Luo, J. Wu, S. V. Kabadi et al., "Propofol limits microglial activation after experimental brain trauma through inhibition of nicotinamide adenine dinucleotide phosphate oxidase," *Anesthesiology*, vol. 119, no. 6, pp. 1370–1388, 2013.

[32] S. S. Jayakar, W. P. Dailey, R. G. Eckenhoff, and J. B. Cohen, "Identification of propofol binding sites in a nicotinic acetylcholine receptor with a photoreactive propofol analog," *The Journal of Biological Chemistry*, vol. 288, no. 9, pp. 6178–6189, 2013.

[33] O. Murasaki, M. Kaibara, Y. Nagase et al., "Site of action of the general anesthetic propofol in muscarinic M1 receptor-mediated signal transduction," *The Journal of Pharmacology and Experimental Therapeutics*, vol. 307, no. 3, pp. 995–1000, 2003.

7

5-Aminolevulinic Acid-Based Photodynamic Therapy Pretreatment Mitigates Ultraviolet A-Induced Oxidative Photodamage

Hui Hua,[1] Jiawei Cheng(iD),[1] Wenbo Bu,[2] Juan Liu,[1] Weiwei Ma,[1] Chenchen Si,[1] Jie Wang,[1] Bingrong Zhou(iD),[1] and Dan Luo(iD)[1]

[1]Department of Dermatology, The First Affiliated Hospital of Nanjing Medical University, Nanjing 210029, China
[2]Institute of Dermatology, Chinese Academy of Medical Sciences (CAMS) & Peking Union Medical College (PUMC), Nanjing, Jiangsu, China

Correspondence should be addressed to Bingrong Zhou; bingrong.2002@163.com and Dan Luo; daniluo2005@163.com

Academic Editor: Demetrios Kouretas

Aim. To determine whether 5-aminolevulinic acid-based photodynamic therapy (ALA-PDT) is effective in combating ultraviolet A- (UVA-) induced oxidative photodamage of hairless mice skin *in vivo* and human epidermal keratinocytes *in vitro*. *Methods.* In *in vitro* experiments, the human keratinocyte cell line (HaCaT cells) was divided into two groups: the experimental group was treated with ALA-PDT and the control group was left untreated. Then, the experimental group and the control group of cells were exposed to $10 \, J/m^2$ of UVA radiation. ROS, O_2^- species, and MMP were determined by fluorescence microscopy; p53, OGG1, and XPC were determined by Western blot analysis; apoptosis was determined by flow cytometry; and 8-oxo-dG was determined by immunofluorescence. Moreover, HaCaT cells were also treated with ALA-PDT. Then, SOD1 and SOD2 were examined by Western blot analysis. In *in vivo* experiments, the dorsal skin of hairless mice was treated with ALA-PDT or saline-PDT, and then, they were exposed to $20 \, J/m^2$ UVA light. The compound 8-oxo-dG was detected by immunofluorescence. *Conclusion.* In human epidermal keratinocytes and hairless mice skin, UVA-induced oxidative damage can be prevented effectively with ALA-PDT pretreatment.

1. Introduction

Skin photodamage has become a major public health issue given the tremendous increase in the number of patients suffering from it. Skin photodamage is caused by excessive exposure to ultraviolet (UV) radiation of the sun [1–4]. Ultraviolet radiation can cause acute reactions, such as erythema and edema; moreover, constant exposure to UV radiation can also lead to chronic skin reactions, such as photoaging and carcinoma [5, 6].

The major source of UV radiation is sunlight. There are two types of UV radiation that can reach the earth's atmosphere: UV radiation A (UVA) and UV radiation B (UVB), of which UVA constitutes 95%. Compared to UVB, the wavelength of UVA is longer; therefore, UVA penetrates deeper into the skin than UVB. Recent studies have reported that UVA is probably more mutagenic than UVB [7]. The UVA-induced skin damage may be indirect; it can trigger excessive production of ROS, which causes oxidative damage to proteins, lipids, and DNA. This leads to the generation of several types of oxidative products, such as 7,8-dihydro-8-oxo-guanosine (8-oxoG) and 8-oxo-7,8-dihydro-2'-deoxyguanosine (8-oxo-dG) [8, 9]. If the human body fails to remove UV mutagenic photoproducts within a definite period of time, the DNA cannot be repaired completely. These adverse products finally lead to the development of skin cancer.

Skin photodamage can be prevented by adopting effective measures of UV protection. Currently, sunscreen lotions and protective clothing are the most effective photoprotective measures [10, 11]; however, many people find it difficult to use them on a regular basis. Previous studies have shown that these strategies have only caused a modest reduction in actinic keratosis (AKs) and squamous cell carcinomas (SCCs) of the skin; however, there has been no reduction in basal cell carcinomas (BCCs) of the skin [12, 13]. Some ingredients in sunscreens, such as benzophenone-3 (BP-3), can cause skin irritation and phototoxicity in susceptible populations; BP-3 is extensively used in organic sunscreens [14]. Currently, there is no worldwide consensus on the testing and labeling of sunscreens that offer UVA protection [15]. In fact, sunscreen alone may not be able to provide adequate protection from ultraviolet A. Therefore, it is very important to develop targeted chemoprevention strategies.

5-Aminolevulinic acid-based photodynamic therapy (ALA-PDT) is a noninvasive therapy; photosensitizer, oxygen, and light are the key components of ALA-PDT. Moreover, ALA is a precursor of protoporphyrin IX (PpIX). A topical formulation of ALA is used to target skin tissues; light of appropriate wavelength is used to activate the photosensitizer, which produces reactive oxygen species (ROS). Ultimately, this leads to cell necrosis and apoptosis [16, 17]. Previous studies have shown that ALA-PDT has a therapeutic effect on a variety of photodamage diseases, such as skin tumors and photoaging [18, 19]; moreover, it also prevents the onset of photodamage diseases, such as nonmelanoma skin cancers (NMSCs) and actinic keratoses (AKs). Goldberg et al. conducted a study on patients with a history of NMSCs and multiple AKs; they found that the onset of NMSCs can be prevented and delayed in these patients [20]. Togsverd-Bo et al. conducted a study on high-risk renal transplant recipients; they found that the onset of AK was significantly delayed when patients' normal skin was treated with repeated PDT for a long period of time [21]. The results indicate that ALA-PDT can prevent the occurrence of photodamage diseases, but we still do not know the exact mechanism through which ALA-PDT exerts inhibitory effect on UV-induced damages. In this study, hairless mice skin and HaCaT cells were pretreated with ALA-PDT. Then, they were exposed to UVA radiation to determine whether UVA-induced photodamage can be prevented with ALA-PDT pretreatment. We also determined the potential mechanisms through which ALA-PDT inhibits UVA-induced photodamage. The results indicate that UVA-induced DNA damage can be significantly reduced by ALA-PDT pretreatment, which upregulates p53-dependent DNA repair and activates the antioxidant enzymes. This indicates that UVA-induced oxidative damage can be inhibited with ALA-PDT pretreatment.

2. Material and Methods

2.1. Cell Culture, ALA-PDT Treatment, and UVA Irradiation. The immortalized human keratinocyte cell line (HaCaT) was grown at 37°C in a humidified atmosphere of 5% CO_2; the cell culture medium was Dulbecco's modified Eagle's medium (DMEM), which was supplemented with 10% fetal bovine serum (FBS) and 1% penicillin-streptomycin. Thereafter, HaCaT cells were subcultured by trypsinization, and they were used in subsequent passages. Under standard conditions, HaCaT cells were grown to >70% confluency.

Then, subsequent experiments were performed. The cells were divided into three groups, namely, control group, UVA group, and ALA-PDT + UVA group. No treatment was provided to cells in the control group. In the UVA group, cells were irradiated with 10 J/cm^2 of UVA light. In the ALA-PDT + UVA group, cells were incubated with 0.5 mmol/L of ALA for 4 h. Then, the cells were exposed to red laser light of 3 J/cm^2 intensity (50 mW/cm^2 for 60 s). Finally, these cells were irradiated with 10 J/cm^2 of UVA light (3.7 mW/cm^2 for 45 min). The UVA radiation was delivered using a UVA fluorescent lamp (340–400 nm wavelength, a peak at 305 nm, Sigma SS-04P, Shanghai, China). The intensity of UVA radiation was measured with a UV radiometer (Philips, Amsterdam, Netherlands). Before irradiating the cells with UVA light, the medium was removed and the cells were covered with a thin layer of phosphate-buffered saline (PBS).

2.2. Cell Viability Measurement. Cell viability was measured using a CCK-8 Kit (Beyotime Biotechnology, Shanghai, China). In brief, HaCaT cells (2000/100 μL) were seeded into 96-well plates. Then, they were treated with ALA-PDT and UVA alone or in combinations. Thereafter, cells of each well were incubated with 10 μL of CCK-8 solution for 2 h. To determine cell density, we measured the absorbance of cell culture at 450 nm with a Thermo Scientific Microplate Reader.

2.3. Measurement of Intracellular ROS and O_2^-. A fluorescent probe was used to measure the intracellular ROS and O_2^- species produced by HaCaT cells. Cells were plated in 6-well plates or 96-well plates. Then, they were incubated in the dark with 10 μmmol/L DCFH-DA or 5 μmmol/L Dihydroethidium for 20 min at 37°C (Beyotime Biotechnology, Shanghai, China). The fluorescence intensity was measured with a SpectraMax 190 microplate reader (Molecular Devices, Sunnyvale, USA). Cells were observed under a fluorescence microscope, and they were also photographed randomly by a Nikon camera with constant time, exposure, and gain (Nikon, Tokyo, Japan).

2.4. Flow Cytometry Analysis of Apoptosis. HaCaT cells had been treated with ALA-PDT by the abovementioned process. Then, these cells were harvested and washed with PBS. Finally, these cells were double-stained with an Annexin-V-FITC apoptosis detection kit (Beyotime Biotechnology, Shanghai, China). The cells were incubated with PI (10 μL) and Annexin-V-FITC (5 μL) at room temperature for 15 min in the dark. Then, they were quantitatively analyzed with a FACScan flow cytometer (BD, Franklin Lakes, NJ, USA). Cells stained with Annexin-V(+)/PI(−) were apoptotic in nature.

2.5. Evaluation of Mitochondrial Membrane Potential (MMP). The fluorescent probe JC-1 (Beyotime Biotechnology, Shanghai, China) was used to determine the mitochondrial membrane potential (MMP) of HaCaT cells. Cells were cultured in 96-well plates and 6-well plates; these cells were incubated with JC-1 staining solution (5 μg/mL) for 20 min at 37°C and rinsed twice with JC-1 staining buffer. A fluorescence microscope (Nikon, Tokyo, Japan) was used to determine the relative amounts of dual emissions from mitochondrial JC-1 monomers (490 nm excitation and 530 nm emission) or aggregates (525 nm excitation and 590 nm emission). The fluorescence intensity of mitochondrial JC-1 monomers and aggregates was determined with a Spectra-Max 190 microplate reader (Molecular Devices, Sunnyvale, USA). An increase in the green/red fluorescence intensity ratio indicates mitochondrial depolarization.

2.6. Immunofluorescence Analysis for Detection of 8-Oxo-dG. HaCaT cells were cultured on coverslips and fixed in 4% paraformaldehyde for 15 min. Then, they were permeabilized with 0.5% Triton X-100 for 10 min. This blocked the nonspecific binding with PBS, which contained 1% bovine serum albumin (BSA) for 30 min. Then, they were incubated overnight with anti-8-oxo-dG monoclonal antibody at 4°C (1:800; Trevigen, Gaithersburg, USA). Subsequently, cells were washed again and incubated with Cy3-conjugated secondary antibody (1:1000, Beyotime Biotechnology, Shanghai, China) for 2 h. After washing stained cells with PBS, photomicrographs were taken with a fluorescence microscope (Nikon, Tokyo, Japan). The 8-oxo-dG-positive nuclei appeared red in color.

2.7. Western Blotting for Detection of SOD1, SOD2, p53, XPC, and OGG1. After treating HaCaT cells with ALA-PDT mentioned above, Western blot analysis was performed on these cells. Cells were lysed in a RIPA buffer (Beyotime Biotechnology, Shanghai, China). Protein concentrations were quantified with a bicinchoninic acid protein assay kit (BCA, Beyotime Biotechnology, Shanghai, China). Then, equal amounts of 20 μg protein/sample were separated with sodium dodecyl sulfate polyacrylamide gel electrophoresis (SDS-PAGE). After transferring the samples into PVDF membranes, the samples were allowed to react with specific primary antibodies: SOD1 (1:1000; CST, Boston, MA, USA), SOD2 (1:500; CST), p53 (1:1000; Sigma, St. Louis, MO, USA), XPC (1:1000; CST), and OGG1 (1:500; Sigma). Subsequently, the cells were incubated with HRP-conjugated anti-mouse or anti-rabbit IgG for 2 h. Protein expression levels were determined with an enhanced chemiluminescence (ECL) detection system. β-Actin was used as an internal control.

2.8. Animal. All animal experiments were performed after receiving approval from the Animal Use Committee of Nanjing Medical University in China. We included 28 female BALB/c athymic nude mice, 4–6 weeks old, and the weight of each mouse was between 19 and 22 g. We purchased these mice from Model Animal Research Center of Nanjing University in China. After acclimatizing the mice to experimental conditions, they were randomly divided to three groups (10 animals in each group): the control group (no treatment), the ALA-PDT + UVA group (10% ALA + 12 J/cm^2 PDT + 20 J/cm^2 UVA), and the UVA group (saline + 20 J/cm^2 UVA).

2.9. ALA-PDT Treatment and UVA Irradiation. A piece of medical cotton was soaked with a specific concentration of

ALA solution (10%; Fudan-Zhangjiang Bio-Pharmaceutical Co., Shanghai, China). Then, the cotton soaked with ALA solution was applied on approximately 4.0 cm^2 of dorsal skin. In the UVA group, physiological saline was used as a negative control. The treated areas were covered with layers of plastic wrap and black plastic sheeting, and they were secured with a medical tape. We removed these dressings after 2 h. The treated tissues were irradiated for 10 min with a PDT laser (XD-635AB; Fudan-Zhangjiang Bio-Pharmaceutical Co., Shanghai, China) of wavelength 635 nm; the energy density of the PDT laser was 12 J/cm^2 (50 m W/cm^2 for 4 min). The mice were treated with ALA-PDT or physiological saline for two days. After these mice were anesthetized with 0.4% chloral hydrate (0.1 mL/10 g), they were irradiated with 20 J/cm^2 of UVA light (3.7 mW/cm^2 for 90 min).

2.10. Immunofluorescence Analysis of 8-Oxo-dG. After fixing the specimens in 4% paraformaldehyde, they were embedded in a paraffin bath. After blocking endogenous proteins, sections were incubated overnight at 4°C with anti-8-oxo-dG monoclonal antibody (1:1000; Trevigen, Gaithersburg, USA). After washing the sections with PBS, they were incubated with Cy3-labeled secondary antibodies (1:2000; Beyotime Biotechnology, Shanghai, China) at 37°C for 1 h. Then, the slides were observed and pictures were captured under a fluorescence microscope.

2.11. Statistical Analysis. Statistical analysis was performed using the SPSS software for Windows, version 16.0 (SPSS, Chicago, IL, USA). Statistical analysis was carried out by one-way analysis of variance (ANOVA) and Student-Newman-Keuls (SNK-q) test. Data are expressed as the mean ± SD for each group. The values of $^*p < 0.05$ were considered to be statistically significant, and they are indicated in the figures.

3. Results

3.1. Sublethal Dose of ALA-PDT Induced Intracellular ROS. We determined whether sublethal doses of ALA-PDT affected intracellular ROS levels. We incubated HaCaT cells with 0.5 mmol/L of ALA for 4 h. Cells were exposed to 3 J/cm^2 intensity of red laser light. The results of the CCK-8 assay indicated that there was no significant difference between the cell viability of the ALA-PDT group and the control group ($p > 0.05$) (Figure 1(a)). The ROS levels were determined by the fluorescent probe DCFH-DA. The HaCaT cells were treated with sublethal doses of ALA-PDT. Compared to the control group, these cells showed stronger green fluorescence and increased fluorescence intensity ($p < 0.05$; Figure 1(c)).

3.2. Sublethal Dose of ALA-PDT Increased the Levels of SOD1 and SOD2 Proteins. The expression of SOD1 and SOD2 proteins was tested by Western blot analysis to evaluate the level of antioxidant enzymes in HaCaT cells treated with a sublethal dose of ALA-PDT. Compared to the control group, the levels of SOD1 protein increased by 117.56%, 151.15%, and 123.66% in HaCaT cells treated with ALA-PDT at 24 h, 36 h, and 48 h, respectively. The levels of SOD2 protein in the ALA-PDT group increased by 64.94%, 86.36%, and

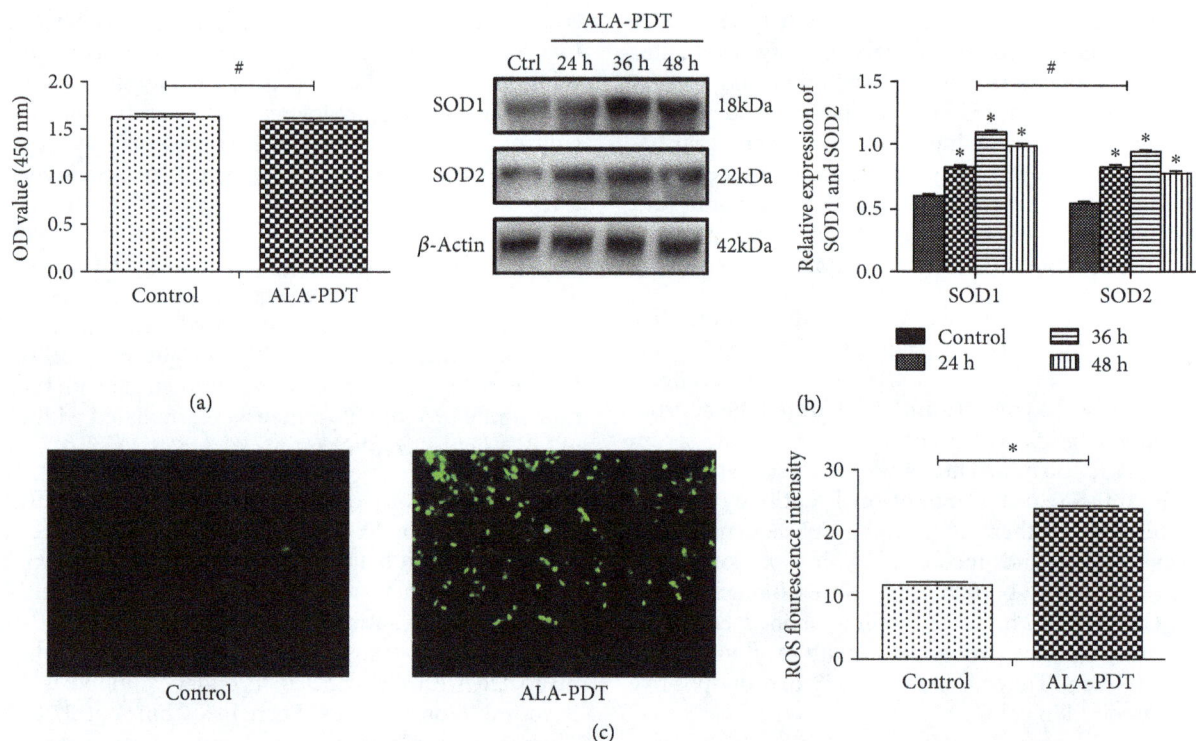

(a)

(b)

(c)

FIGURE 1: Sublethal doses of ALA-PDT induced intracellular ROS, and the expression levels of SOD1 and SOD2 were determined in HaCaT cells. The ALA-PDT group was treated with the following components: 0.5 mmol/L of ALA and 3 J/cm^2 of red laser light. (a) Cell viability was detected by the CCK-8 assay at 450 nm after being treated with a sublethal dose of ALA-PDT. (b) The expression levels of SOD1 and SOD2 proteins were determined 24 h, 36 h, and 48 h after receiving a sublethal dose of ALA-PDT. Protein expression levels were quantified by using β-actin as a control. (c) Cells in the ALA-PDT group were treated with a sublethal dose of ALA-PDT. The intracellular ROS showed green fluorescence under a fluorescence microscope, and the fluorescence intensity was determined by a fluorescence microplate reader. Data were expressed as mean $\pm$ SD, $n = 3$ for each group, $^*p < 0.05$, $^\#p > 0.05$.

58.44% at 24 h, 36 h, and 48 h, respectively, compared to those of the control group ($p < 0.05$; Figure 1(b)).

3.3. ALA-PDT Pretreatment Reduces UVA-Induced Oxidative Damage.
After irradiating HaCaT cells with UVA light, we assessed the extent of oxidative damage by measuring the amount of ROS and O_2^- species generated in this process. The number of ROS and O_2^- species increased tremendously in HaCaT cells when they were irradiated with UVA light. However, the UVA-induced oxidative damage was reduced significantly when HaCaT cells were subjected to ALA-PDT pretreatment: the number of ROS and O_2^- species declined tremendously in HaCaT cells subjected to ALA-PDT pretreatment, and the fluorescence intensities were reduced by 34.54% and 35.44%, respectively ($p < 0.05$ and $p < 0.05$, respectively; Figure 2).

3.4. ALA-PDT Pretreatment Inhibits UVA-Irradiated Cytotoxicity.
The cytotoxic effects of UVA and ALA-PDT were determined by performing the CCK-8 assay. The results indicated that cell viability decreased by 36.14% at 24 h after the samples were irradiated with UVA light. However, ALA-PDT pretreatment reduced by 15.07% UVA-induced cytotoxicity in those UVA-irradiated HaCaT cells ($p < 0.05$; Figure 3(a)).

3.5. ALA-PDT Pretreatment Suppressed UVA-Induced Apoptosis.
In this study, HaCaT cells were doubly stained with Annexin-V/PI. Then, the apoptosis rate of these cells was determined by flow cytometry. Annexin-V(−)/PI(−) cells are live cells and Annexin-V(+)/PI(−) cells are early-stage apoptotic cells. Annexin-V(+)/PI(+) cells are late-stage apoptotic or necrotic cells. The apoptosis rate was expressed as a percentage of apoptotic cells in total cells. As shown in Figure 3(b), the early and late-stage apoptosis was significantly increased with UVA light. Compared to the UVA group, apoptosis significantly decreased by 31.60% in HaCaT cells subjected to ALA-PDT pretreatment ($p < 0.05$).

3.6. ALA-PDT Pretreatment Alleviates the UVA-Induced Mitochondrial Dysfunction.
In order to determine the effect of ALA-PDT and UVA on mitochondria, we performed an assay to determine the changes in MMP by performing flow cytometry with the lipophilic fluorochrome JC-1. The accumulation of JC-1 in mitochondria led to the formation of JC-1 aggregates detected in the red channel. When the MMP was depolarized, JC-1 remained in the cytoplasm as monomers; these monomers were detected in the green channel. As shown in Figure 3(c), control cells exhibited bright red fluorescence. This indicated that control cells had a strong MMP. After being exposed to UVA, cells

(a)

(b)

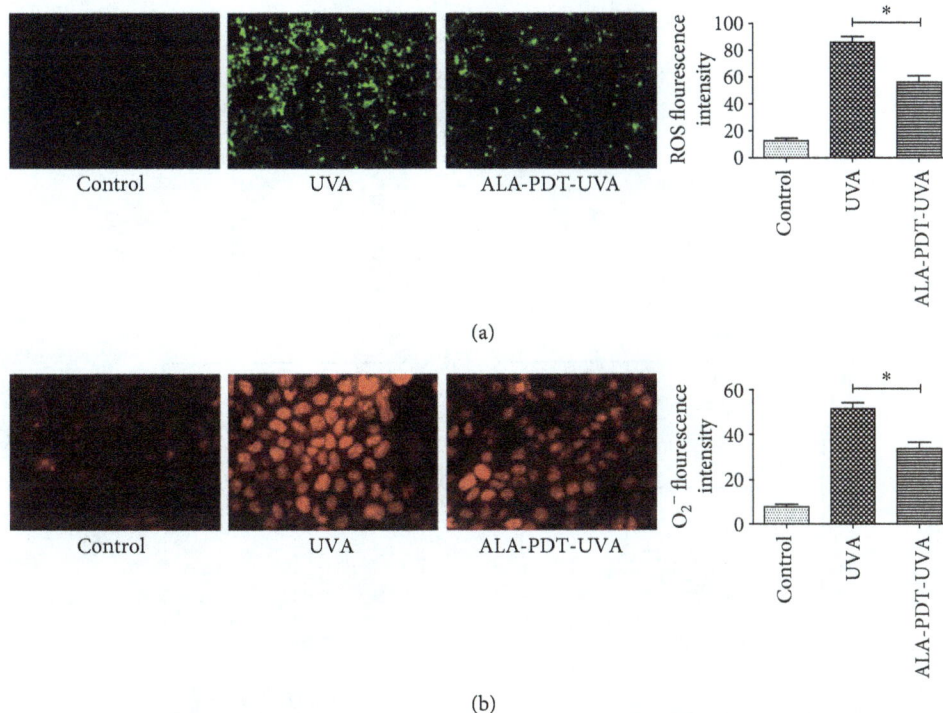

Figure 2: UVA-induced oxidative damage was reduced with ALA-PDT pretreatment. (a, b) Cells were treated with a sublethal dose of ALA-PDT, then these cells were irradiated with $10 J/cm^2$ of UVA light. Cells were incubated with $10 \mu mmol/L$ DCFH-DA or $5 \mu mmol/L$ Dihydroethidium for 20 min, after which ROS and O_2^- production was visualized by fluorescence microscopy. Intracellular ROS and O_2^- species exhibited green and red fluorescence under a fluorescence microscope; the fluorescence intensity was determined by a fluorescence microplate reader. Data were expressed as mean ± SD, $n = 3$ for each group, $^*p < 0.05$.

typically lost their MMP. Mitochondrial fluorescence intensity was undetected in these cells. The UVA-induced reduction of MMP can be significantly prevented by subjecting HaCaT cells to ALA-PDT pretreatment.

3.7. ALA-PDT Pretreatment Inhibited the Level of 8-Oxo-dG.
Immunofluorescence detected 8-oxo-dG, which is the characteristic product of UVA-induced oxidative damage on DNA. When HaCaT cells were exposed to UVA, there was a significant increase in 8-oxo-dG generation. However, ALA-PDT pretreatment could significantly reduce the elevated levels of 8-oxo-dG in HaCaT cells subjected to UVA light ($p < 0.05$; Figure 4(a)). In vivo, we also observed that UVA light induced the production of 8-oxo-dG in the skin of hairless mice; however, ALA-PDT can inhibit the excessive generation of 8-oxo-dG in the skin of hairless mice, which was exposed to UVA radiation ($p < 0.05$; Figure 4(b)).

3.8. ALA-PDT Pretreatment Increased the Levels of p53, XPC, and OGG1 Proteins.
To determine whether ALA-PDT pretreatment can increase the expression level of proteins involved in DNA damage repair, we determined the expression of p53, XPC, and OGG1 proteins in HaCaT cells by Western blot analysis. The results indicated that compared to the unirradiated group, the expression of p53, XPC, and OGG1 proteins significantly increased by 36.48%, 48.97%, and 136.45% in the UVA-irradiated group ($p < 0.05$). In the ALA-PDT pretreatment group, the levels of p53, XPC, and

OGG1 significantly increased by 25.38%, 33.80%, and 29.64%, respectively, than those in the UVA group ($p < 0.05$; Figure 5).

4. Discussion

When human epidermal keratinocytes and the skin of hairless mice were pretreated with ALA-PDT, the UVA-induced oxidative damage was reduced significantly. ROS plays a significant role in the mechanism of ALA-PDT [22]. High-level ROS can disrupt cellular processes, while low-level ROS can mediate cellular signaling [23]. Moreover, ROS can elicit oxidative damage and apoptosis in photoaged fibroblasts, which may be the basis for the rejuvenating effects on photoaged skin [24]. The mechanism of acne treatment is as follows: ROS suppresses the expression of IL-1α on keratinocyte hyperkeratosis via the FGFR2b pathway [25]. In our previous study, low concentration of ALA (0.5 mmol/L) and low intensity of red light ($3 J/cm^2$) did not have a significant effect on cell viability; however, the p53-dependent pathway was activated sufficiently with excessive production of ROS. Therefore, a sublethal dose of ALA-PDT was used in subsequent cell experiments.

When HaCaT cells were exposed to UVA radiation, the production of reactive oxygen species (ROS) increased tremendously; the UVA radiation interacted with endogenous chromophores to produce ROS, such as superoxide radical (O_2^-) and singlet oxygen (O_2). The reactive oxygen species

(a)

(b)

(c)

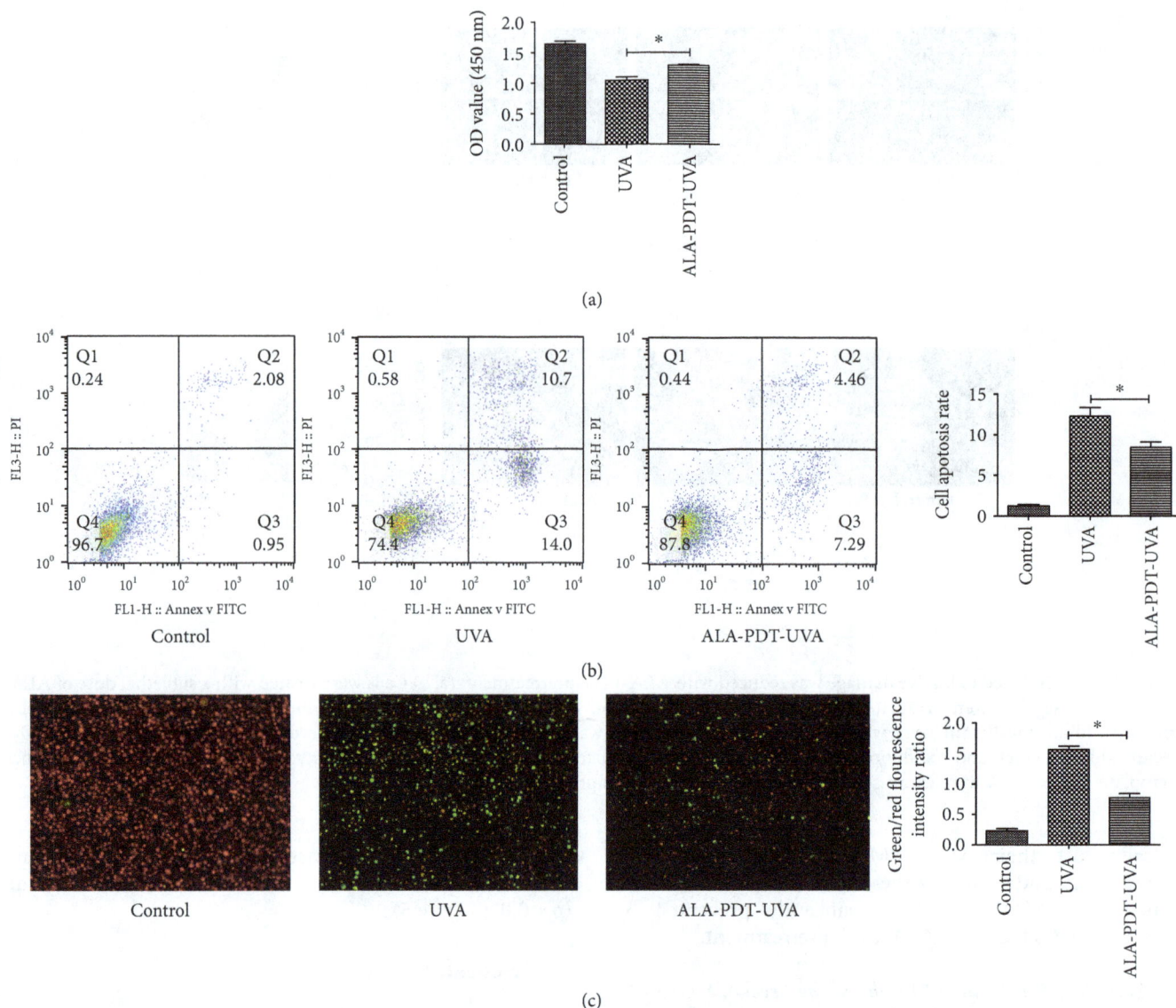

FIGURE 3: ALA-PDT pretreatment inhibits cytotoxicity and apoptosis of cells irradiated with UVA. Cells were treated with a sublethal dose of ALA-PDT, then these cells were irradiated with 10 J/cm^2 of UVA light. (a) The cell viability was detected by CCK-8 assay at 450 nm. (b) The apoptosis of HaCaT cells was measured by using Annexin-V and PI in conjunction with flow cytometry; Annexin-V(+)/PI(−) cells were early-stage apoptotic cells. (c) Early apoptosis was indicated by a decrease in mitochondrial membrane potential. When the fluorescence probe JC-1 underwent a transition from red light to green light, it indicated a decrease in cell membrane potential. This was an indicator of early apoptosis. The fluorescence intensity of the green/red ratio was determined by a fluorescence microplate reader. Data were expressed as mean ± SD, $n = 3$ for each group, $^*p < 0.05$, $^\#p > 0.05$.

can cause damage to cellular proteins, lipids, and DNA, which leads to the formation of oxidative DNA lesions [26]. Moreover, 8-oxo-dG is a characteristic biomarker of DNA oxidation because guanine bases are most susceptible to oxidation [27]. Hu et al. pretreated keratinocytes with oxyresveratrol or kuwanon O; the two phenolic compounds were extracted from the roots of *Morus australis*. They reported both of them were able to inhibit the generation of ROS in keratinocytes, which were irradiated with UVA, and enhanced the cell viability and antioxidative defense capability of keratinocytes [28]. In our study, when HaCaT cells were exposed to UVA light, it increased the generation of ROS, O_2^-, and 8-oxo-dG species. Moreover, ALA-PDT pretreatment protected HaCaT

cells from UVA-induced damage by suppressing the generation of cellular ROS, O_2^-, and 8-oxo-dG.

UVA-mediated apoptosis was partially induced indirectly by generating ROS. It has been well established that after being exposed to UVA light, keratinocytes undergo apoptosis [29–31]. When HaCaT cells were exposed to UVA, apoptosis was induced in these cells; the signs of apoptosis were as follows: cell viability decreased, the fragmentation of DNA increased, and cell morphology is alerted. A previous study reported that ellagic acid pretreatment can successfully suppress UVA-induced apoptosis [32]. In our study, we proved that ALA-PDT pretreatment could successfully suppress UVA-induced apoptosis in HaCaT cells.

(a)

(b)

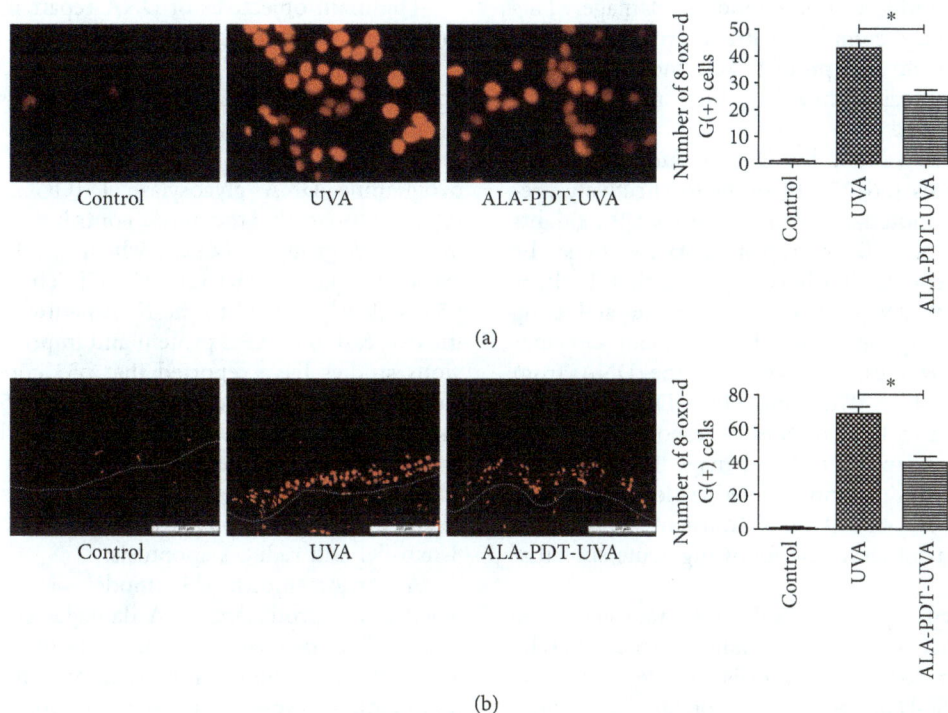

FIGURE 4: The expression level of 8-oxo-dG was inhibited with ALA-PDT pretreatment. Cells were treated with a sublethal dose of ALA-PDT, then these cells were irradiated with 10 J/cm^2 of UVA light. The expression level of 8-oxo-dG was detected by immunofluorescence. (a, b) Red fluorescence represented 8-oxo-dG-positive cells. Photographs were taken randomly under a fluorescence microscope, and the number of positive cells was counted; this represented the data for each group. Data were expressed as mean ± SD, $n = 3$ for each group, $^*p < 0.05$.

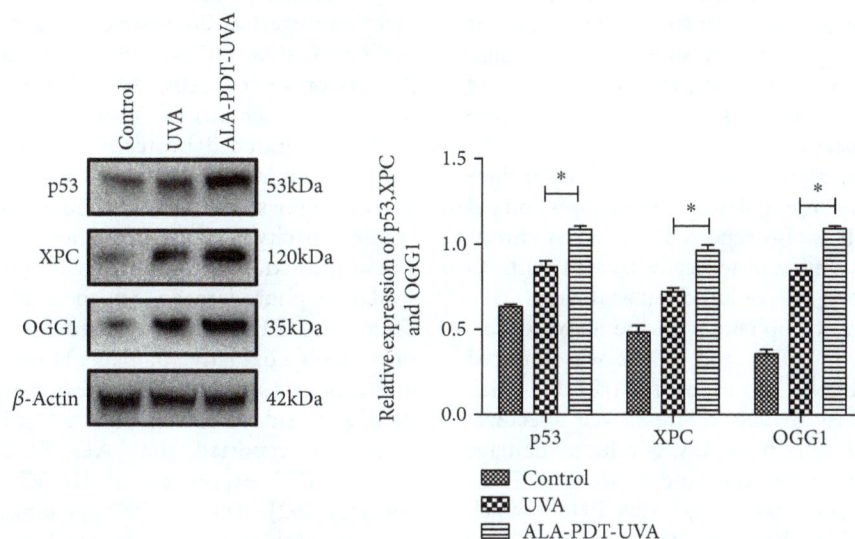

FIGURE 5: ALA-PDT pretreatment increased the levels of p53, XPC, and OGG1 proteins. Cells were treated with a sublethal dose of ALA-PDT, then these cells were irradiated with 10 J/cm^2 of UVA light. A Western blot analysis was carried out to detect the expression levels of p53, XPC, and OGG1 proteins. Protein expression levels were quantified by using β-actin as control. Data were expressed as mean ± SD, $n = 3$ for each group, $^*p < 0.05$.

Complex pathways are involved in the initiation and progression of UV-mediated apoptosis of keratinocytes. Mitochondrial-, death receptor-, ER stress-, and ROS-mediated apoptosis have been reported in these studies [33, 34]. Petruk et al. reported that *Opuntia* raw extract, which is a phenolic antioxidant, was able to protect cells against UVA-induced apoptosis by inhibiting the activation of caspase-3 and caspase-7 [35]. We confirmed that MMP of HaCaT cells was significantly affected by UVA radiation; moreover, ALA-PDT pretreatment can significantly protect HaCaT cells against UVA-induced mitochondrial damage. This observation completely complies with a previous report, which states that ellagic acid protects keratinocytes against UVA-induced apoptosis through the mitochondrial apoptotic pathway [32].

Skin diseases are caused by UVA-induced oxidative damage and apoptosis [36–38]. In order to effectively prevent UVA-induced photodamage, endogenous antioxidants must be induced and DNA repair capacity must be improved [39]. Several studies have reported that T-oligos induced a protective DNA-damage response by activating p53, leading to the upregulation of antioxidant enzymes and DNA-repair enzymes. This protects the DNA from future insults [40–42]. The inducible DNA damage response, which is also known as SOS response, was first found in bacteria. Adaptive DNA damage responses are elicited in cells by administering sublethal doses of DNA-damaging agents [43, 44]. And a transient increase in DNA repair rate was observed by following acute sublethal DNA damage [45].

Reactive oxygen species (ROS)/free radicals were scavenged from a network of antioxidant enzymes, thereby maintaining cellular redox homeostasis [36, 46]. Superoxide dismutases (SODs), especially copper and zinc-dependent superoxide dismutase (SOD1) and the mitochondrial manganese-dependent superoxide dismutase (SOD2), efficiently catalyze the conversion of super oxides into oxygen and hydrogen peroxides. It is well known to be a major antioxidant enzyme that protects cells from oxidative stress, and it prevents carcinogenesis [47–49]. Effect of UVA irradiation on antioxidant enzymes has been reported. Skin cells prepare for subsequent exposure to damaging radiation by upregulating the activities of the antioxidant enzymes SOD1 and SOD2, which also demonstrated the existence of an SOS-like adaptive response [50]. Lee et al. reported that T-oligo can induce antioxidant defenses by upregulating the expression of SOD1 and SOD2 [40]. It is also reported that when chronically irradiated mouse skin was topically treated with T-oligo, the level of 8-oxo-dG reduced substantially [51]. Our data was completely compliant with the above observation: the expression of SOD1 and SOD2 was induced and activated with sublethal doses of ALA-PDT, which offered protection against oxidative stress. We speculate that ALA-PDT protects cells from UVA-induced damage by reducing the generation of ROS and 8-oxo-dG. Thus, apoptosis of cells is suppressed by ALA-PDT, which mainly induces antioxidant defenses. SODs are important antioxidant components of antioxidant systems. However, the activation mechanisms of SODs are still unclear. It has been reported that bread crust extract could activate SOD through the receptor for advanced glycation end products (AGEs). But high doses of bread crust extract are independent of AGE receptors, indicating that additional mechanisms are involved in the activation of SOD [52]. In our experiments, sublethal doses of ALA-PDT induced an antioxidant response by activation of SOD1 and SOD2, but the specific activation mechanism of SODs remained to be further studied.

The main objectives of DNA repair mechanisms are as follows: (i) to ensure genomic stability and (ii) to eliminate DNA lesions [53, 54]. The ubiquitous DNA oxidation product 8-oxo-dG is repaired predominantly via base excision repair (BER) pathway and nucleotide excision repair (NER) pathway [55]. The BER DNA glycosylase 8-oxoguanine DNA glycosylase 1 (OGG1) dominates the repair of 8-oxo-dG; the minor contributor is xeroderma pigmentosum group C (XPC), which is related to nucleotide excision repair (NER) [26, 56, 57]. The tumor suppressor p53 is closely related to the NER pathway, which promotes the expression of XPC protein and improves NER [58]. Previous studies have reported that p53 coordinates the BER pathway to prevent genomic instability [59]. In our study, the levels of OGG1 and XPC proteins can be improved with ALA-PDT pretreatment. The above results indicate that ALA-PDT can induce NER- and BER-based DNA damage repair by activating p53, which accelerates the removal of 8-oxo-dG and reduces apoptosis.

A hairless mouse skin model was used to determine whether the protective DNA damage response was elicited *in vivo*. The *in vivo* results indicate that the expression of 8-oxo-dG was significantly reduced with ALA-PDT pretreatment. However, we failed to observe sunburn cells and TUNEL-positive cells in hairless mice skin. This observation completely complied with previous reports, stating that sunburn cells are absent or rare *in vivo* after being exposed to UVA; however, UVA can induce apoptosis in cultured cells [60, 61].

In summary, our results prove that ALA-PDT pretreatment can exert antioxidative damage by reducing the generation of ROS, O_2^-, and 8-oxo-dG, as well as diminishing the apoptosis of cells. We also elucidated the possible molecular mechanisms through which sublethal doses of ALA-PDT induced protective DNA damage responses in human keratinocytes. The inducible antioxidant responses are as follows: the p53-dependent upregulation of DNA repair capacity and the activation of antioxidant enzymes. These antioxidant responses can protect skin cells from oxidative photodamage, which is induced by UVA light. Thus, ALA-PDT might be used for the prevention of diseases due to oxidative damage. However, in addition to the inducible antioxidant responses, more detailed studies on their antioxidant mechanism are still needed. Wang and Sun have reported that ALA-PDT suppressed IFN-γ-induced K17 expression in HaCaT cells via the MAPK pathway [62]. The MAPK signaling pathway is involved in many biological processes, such as cell proliferation, differentiation, gene expression, and apoptosis [63]. Further experiments are required to determine whether the MAPK pathway participated in the process of ALA-PDT exerting antioxidant effects. Also, our present experiments have failed to fully confirm whether ALA-PDT can prevent UVA-induced photodamage *in vivo*. In subsequent studies, we will further confirm whether ALA-PDT exerts photoprotective effect by eliciting an SOS-like response *in vivo*. The possibility of using ALA-PDT for skin photoprotection or the prevention of oxidative damage in humans deserves further investigation.

Authors' Contributions

Hui Hua, Jiawei Cheng, and Wenbo Bu contributed equally to this work.

Acknowledgments

This work was supported by Grants from the China National Natural Science Foundation (81573072, 81301384, and 81703142) and the Priority Academic Program Development (PAPD) of Jiangsu Higher Education Institutions. Bingrong Zhou is funded by the Project of Key Youth Medical Talent of Jiangsu Province (QNNRC 2016583) and Outstanding Young Backbone Teachers of Nanjing Medical University (2017).

References

[1] M. K. Tripp, M. Watson, S. J. Balk, S. M. Swetter, and J. E. Gershenwald, "State of the science on prevention and screening to reduce melanoma incidence and mortality: the time is now," *CA: A Cancer Journal for Clinicians*, vol. 66, no. 6, pp. 460–480, 2016.

[2] Health, US Department of, and Human Services, "The surgeon general's call to action to prevent skin cancer," *Environmental Policy Collection*, vol. 5, Supplement 1, p. 192, 2014.

[3] R. E. B. Watson, N. K. Gibbs, C. E. M. Griffiths, and M. J. Sherratt, "Damage to skin extracellular matrix induced by UV exposure," *Antioxidants & Redox Signaling*, vol. 21, no. 7, pp. 1063–1077, 2014.

[4] J. Moan, Z. Baturaite, A. C. Porojnicu, A. Dahlback, and A. Juzeniene, "UVA, UVB and incidence of cutaneous malignant melanoma in Norway and Sweden," *Photochemical & Photobiological Sciences*, vol. 11, no. 1, pp. 191–198, 2012.

[5] L. R. Sklar, F. Almutawa, H. W. Lim, and I. Hamzavi, "Effects of ultraviolet radiation, visible light, and infrared radiation on erythema and pigmentation: a review," *Photochemical & Photobiological Sciences*, vol. 12, no. 1, pp. 54–64, 2013.

[6] B. A. Gilchrest, "Photoaging," *Journal of Investigative Dermatology*, vol. 133, no. E1, pp. E2–E6, 2013.

[7] T. M. Rünger, B. Farahvash, Z. Hatvani, and A. Rees, "Comparison of DNA damage responses following equimutagenic doses of UVA and UVB: a less effective cell cycle arrest with UVA may render UVA-induced pyrimidine dimers more mutagenic than UVB-induced ones," *Photochemical & Photobiological Sciences*, vol. 11, no. 1, pp. 207–215, 2012.

[8] H. T. Wang, B. Choi, and M. S. Tang, "Melanocytes are deficient in repair of oxidative DNA damage and UV-induced photoproducts," *Proceedings of the National Academy of Sciences of the United States of America*, vol. 107, no. 27, pp. 12180–12185, 2010.

[9] N. Maddodi, A. Jayanthy, and V. Setaluri, "Shining light on skin pigmentation: the darker and the brighter side of effects of UV radiation," *Photochemistry and Photobiology*, vol. 88, no. 5, pp. 1075–1082, 2012.

[10] S. González, M. Fernández-Lorente, and Y. Gilaberte-Calzada, "The latest on skin photoprotection," *Clinics in Dermatology*, vol. 26, no. 6, pp. 614–626, 2008.

[11] S. Q. Wang, Y. Balagula, and U. Osterwalder, "Photoprotec-

tion: a review of the current and future technologies," *Dermatologic Therapy*, vol. 23, no. 1, pp. 31–47, 2010.

[12] S. C. Thompson, D. Jolley, and R. Marks, "Reduction of solar keratoses by regular sunscreen use," *The New England Journal of Medicine*, vol. 329, no. 16, pp. 1147–1151, 1993.

[13] A. Green, G. Williams, R. Nèale et al., "Daily sunscreen application and betacarotene supplementation in prevention of basal-cell and squamous-cell carcinomas of the skin: a randomised controlled trial," *The Lancet*, vol. 354, no. 9180, pp. 723–729, 1999.

[14] H.-J. Kim, E. Lee, M. Lee et al., "Phosphodiesterase 4b plays a role in benzophenone-3-induced phototoxicity in normal human keratinocytes," *Toxicology and Applied Pharmacology*, vol. 338, pp. 174–181, 2018.

[15] S. Q. Wang, H. Xu, J. W. Stanfield, U. Osterwalder, and B. Herzog, "Comparison of ultraviolet a light protection standards in the United States and European Union through in vitro measurements of commercially available sunscreens," *Journal of the American Academy of Dermatology*, vol. 77, no. 1, pp. 42–47, 2017.

[16] C. H. Kim, C. Chung, K. H. Choi et al., "Effect of 5-aminolevulinic acid-based photodynamic therapy via reactive oxygen species in human cholangiocarcinoma cells," *International Journal of Nanomedicine*, vol. 6, pp. 1357–1363, 2011.

[17] L. W. Zhang, Y. P. Fang, and J. Y. Fang, "Enhancement techniques for improving 5-aminolevulinic acid delivery through the skin," *Dermatologica Sinica*, vol. 29, no. 1, pp. 1–7, 2011.

[18] J. Ji, L. L. Zhang, H. L. Ding et al., "Comparison of 5-aminolevulinic acid photodynamic therapy and red light for treatment of photoaging," *Photodiagnosis and Photodynamic Therapy*, vol. 11, no. 2, pp. 118–121, 2014.

[19] X. Ge, J. Liu, Z. Shi et al., "Inhibition of Mapk signaling pathways enhances cell death induced by 5-aminolevulinic acid-photodynamic therapy in skin squamous carcinoma cells," *European Journal of Dermatology*, vol. 26, no. 2, pp. 164–172, 2016.

[20] L. H. Goldberg, J. M. Landau, M. N. Moody et al., "Evaluation of the chemopreventative effects of ALA PDT in patients with multiple actinic keratoses and a history of skin cancer," *Journal of Drugs in Dermatology*, vol. 11, no. 5, pp. 593–597, 2012.

[21] K. Togsverd-Bo, S. H. Omland, H. C. Wulf, S. S. Sørensen, and M. Haedersdal, "Primary prevention of skin dysplasia in renal transplant recipients with photodynamic therapy: a randomized controlled trial," *American Journal of Transplantation*, vol. 15, no. 11, pp. 2986–2990, 2015.

[22] Z. Zhou, J. Song, L. Nie, and X. Chen, "Reactive oxygen species generating systems meeting challenges of photodynamic cancer therapy," *Chemical Society Reviews*, vol. 45, no. 23, pp. 6597–6626, 2016.

[23] P. T. Schumacker, "Reactive oxygen species in cancer: a dance with the devil," *Cancer Cell*, vol. 27, no. 2, pp. 156–157, 2015.

[24] B. R. Zhou, L. C. Zhang, F. Permatasari, J. Liu, Y. Xu, and D. Luo, "ALA-PDT elicits oxidative damage and apoptosis in UVB-induced premature senescence of human skin fibroblasts," *Photodiagnosis and Photodynamic Therapy*, vol. 14, pp. 47–56, 2016.

[25] M. V. Gozali, F. Yi, J.-a. Zhang et al., "Photodynamic therapy inhibit fibroblast growth factor-10 induced keratinocyte differentiation and proliferation through ROS in fibroblast growth factor receptor-2b pathway," *Scientific Reports*, vol. 6, no. 1, p. 27402, 2016.

[26] A. Svobodová and J. Vostálová, "Solar radiation induced skin damage: review of protective and preventive options," *International Journal of Radiation Biology*, vol. 86, no. 12, pp. 999–1030, 2010.

[27] A. Valavanidis, T. Vlachogianni, and C. Fiotakis, "8-Hydroxy-2′-deoxyguanosine (8-ohdg): a critical biomarker of oxidative stress and carcinogenesis," *Journal of Environmental Science and Health, Part C*, vol. 27, no. 2, pp. 120–139, 2009.

[28] S. Hu, F. Chen, and M. Wang, "Photo-protective effects of oxyresveratrol and kuwanon O on DNA damage induced by UVA in human epidermal keratinocytes," *Chemical Research in Toxicology*, vol. 28, no. 3, pp. 541–548, 2015.

[29] E. Maverakis, Y. Miyamura, M. P. Bowen, G. Correa, Y. Ono, and H. Goodarzi, "Light, including ultraviolet," *Journal of Autoimmunity*, vol. 34, no. 3, pp. J247–J257, 2010.

[30] M. S. Cooke, M. D. Evans, M. Dizdaroglu, and J. Lunec, "Oxidative DNA damage: mechanisms, mutation, and disease," *The FASEB Journal*, vol. 17, no. 10, pp. 1195–1214, 2003.

[31] N. Morley, A. Rapp, H. Dittmar et al., "UVA-induced apoptosis studied by the new apo/necro-Comet-assay which distinguishes viable, apoptotic and necrotic cells," *Mutagenesis*, vol. 21, no. 2, pp. 105–114, 2006.

[32] Y. C. Hseu, C. W. Chou, K. J. Senthil Kumar et al., "Ellagic acid protects human keratinocyte (HaCaT) cells against UVA-induced oxidative stress and apoptosis through the upregulation of the HO-1 and Nrf-2 antioxidant genes," *Food and Chemical Toxicology*, vol. 50, no. 5, pp. 1245–1255, 2012.

[33] M. Ichihashi, M. Ueda, A. Budiyanto et al., "UV-induced skin damage," *Toxicology*, vol. 189, no. 1-2, pp. 21–39, 2003.

[34] C. Q. Yuan, Y. N. Li, and X. F. Zhang, "Down-regulation of apoptosis-inducing factor protein by RNA interference inhibits UVA-induced cell death," *Biochemical and Biophysical Research Communications*, vol. 317, no. 4, pp. 1108–1113, 2004.

[35] G. Petruk, F. di Lorenzo, P. Imbimbo et al., "Protective effect of Opuntia ficus-indica L. cladodes against UVA-induced oxidative stress in normal human keratinocytes," *Bioorganic & Medicinal Chemistry Letters*, vol. 27, no. 24, pp. 5485–5489, 2017.

[36] L. Chen, J. Y. Hu, and S. Q. Wang, "The role of antioxidants in photoprotection: a critical review," *Journal of the American Academy of Dermatology*, vol. 67, no. 5, pp. 1013–1024, 2012.

[37] A. Svobodová, A. Zdarilová, J. Malisková, H. Mikulková, D. Walterová, and J. Vostalová, "Attenuation of UVA-induced damage to human keratinocytes by silymarin," *Journal of Dermatological Science*, vol. 46, no. 1, pp. 21–30, 2007.

[38] Y. Liu, F. Chan, H. Sun et al., "Resveratrol protects human keratinocytes HaCaT cells from UVA-induced oxidative stress damage by downregulating Keap1 expression," *European Journal of Pharmacology*, vol. 650, no. 1, pp. 130–137, 2011.

[39] L. Marrot, C. Jones, P. Perez, and J.-R. Meunier, "The significance of Nrf2 pathway in (photo)-oxidative stress response in melanocytes and keratinocytes of the human epidermis," *Pigment Cell & Melanoma Research*, vol. 21, no. 1, pp. 79–88, 2008.

[40] M. S. Lee, M. Yaar, M. S. Eller, T. M. Rünger, Y. Gao, and B. A. Gilchrest, "Telomeric DNA induces P53-dependent reactive oxygen species and protects against oxidative damage," *Journal of Dermatological Science*, vol. 56, no. 3, pp. 154–162, 2009.

[41] S. Arad, N. Konnikov, D. A. Goukassian, and B. A. Gilchrest, "T-Oligos augment UV-induced protective responses in human skin," *The FASEB Journal*, vol. 20, no. 11, pp. 1895–1897, 2006.

[42] B. A. Gilchrest, "Telomere-based protective responses to DNA damage," *Journal of Investigative Dermatology Symposium Proceedings*, vol. 17, no. 1, pp. 15-16, 2015.

[43] S. Arad, N. Konnikov, D. A. Goukassian, and B. A. Gilchrest, "Quantification of inducible SOS-like photoprotective responses in human skin," *Journal of Investigative Dermatology*, vol. 127, no. 11, pp. 2629–2636, 2007.

[44] D. M. Smith and G. P. Raaphorst, "Adaptive responses in human glioma cells assessed by clonogenic survival and DNA strand break analysis," *International Journal of Radiation Biology*, vol. 79, no. 5, pp. 333–339, 2009.

[45] M. Radman, "SOS repair hypothesis: phenomenology of an inducible DNA repair which is accompanied by mutagenesis," in *Molecular Mechanisms for Repair of DNA*, Basic Life Sciences, P. C. Hanawalt and R. B. Setlow, Eds., pp. 355–367, Springer, Boston, MA, USA, 1975.

[46] Y. C. Hseu, H. W. Lo, M. Korivi, Y. C. Tsai, M. J. Tang, and H. L. Yang, "Dermato-protective properties of ergothioneine through induction of Nrf2/ARE-mediated antioxidant genes in UVA-irradiated human keratinocytes," *Free Radical Biology & Medicine*, vol. 86, pp. 102–117, 2015.

[47] V. C. Culotta, M. Yang, and T. V. O'Halloran, "Activation of superoxide dismutases: putting the metal to the pedal," *Biochimica et Biophysica Acta (BBA) - Molecular Cell Research*, vol. 1763, no. 7, pp. 747–758, 2006.

[48] F. Johnson and C. Giulivi, "Superoxide dismutases and their impact upon human health," *Molecular Aspects of Medicine*, vol. 26, no. 4-5, pp. 340–352, 2005.

[49] I. N. Zelko, T. J. Mariani, and R. J. Folz, "Superoxide dismutase multigene family: a comparison of the CuZn-SOD (Sod1), Mn-SOD (Sod2), and EC-SOD (Sod3) gene structures, evolution, and expression," *Free Radical Biology & Medicine*, vol. 33, no. 3, pp. 337–349, 2002.

[50] M. T. Leccia, M. Yaar, N. Allen, M. Gleason, and B. A. Gilchrest, "Solar simulated irradiation modulates gene expression and activity of antioxidant enzymes in cultured human dermal fibroblasts," *Experimental Dermatology*, vol. 10, no. 4, pp. 272–279, 2001.

[51] S. Arad, E. Zattra, J. Hebert, E. H. Epstein Jr, D. A. Goukassian, and B. A. Gilchrest, "Topical thymidine dinucleotide treatment reduces development of ultraviolet-induced basal cell carcinoma in Ptch-1+/− mice," *The American Journal of Pathology*, vol. 172, no. 5, pp. 1248–1255, 2008.

[52] B. Leuner, S. Ruhs, H. J. Brömme et al., "RAGE-dependent activation of gene expression of superoxide dismutase and vanins by AGE-rich extracts in mice cardiac tissue and murine cardiac fibroblasts," *Food & Function*, vol. 3, no. 10, pp. 1091–1098, 2012.

[53] J. H. J. Hoeijmakers, "Genome maintenance mechanisms for preventing cancer," *Nature*, vol. 411, no. 6835, pp. 366–374, 2001.

[54] E. C. Friedberg, "DNA damage and repair," *Nature*, vol. 421, no. 6921, pp. 436–440, 2003.

[55] E. Parlanti, M. D'Errico, P. Degan et al., "The cross talk between pathways in the repair of 8-oxo-7,8-dihydroguanine in mouse and human cells," *Free Radical Biology & Medicine*, vol. 53, no. 11, pp. 2171–2177, 2012.

[56] M. D'Errico, E. Parlanti, M. Teson et al., "New functions of XPC in the protection of human skin cells from oxidative dam-

age," *EMBO Journal*, vol. 25, no. 18, pp. 4305–4315, 2006.

[57] K. L. Brown, M. Roginskaya, Y. Zou, A. Altamirano, A. K. Basu, and M. P. Stone, "Binding of the human nucleotide excision repair proteins XPA and XPC/HR23B to the 5R-thymine glycol lesion and structure of the cis-(5R,6S) thymine glycol epimer in the 5′-GTgG-3′ sequence: destabilization of two base pairs at the lesion site," *Nucleic Acids Research*, vol. 38, no. 2, pp. 428–440, 2010.

[58] S. Adimoolam and J. M. Ford, "P53 and DNA damage-inducible expression of the xeroderma pigmentosum group C gene," *Proceedings of the National Academy of Sciences of the United States of America*, vol. 99, no. 20, pp. 12985–12990, 2002.

[59] M. Poletto, A. J. Legrand, S. C. Fletcher, and G. L. Dianov, "P53 coordinates base excision repair to prevent genomic instability," *Nucleic Acids Research*, vol. 44, no. 7, pp. 3165–3175, 2016.

[60] S. Takeuchi, W. Zhang, K. Wakamatsu et al., "Melanin acts as a potent UVB photosensitizer to cause an atypical mode of cell death in murine skin," *Proceedings of the National Academy of Sciences of the United States of America*, vol. 101, no. 42, pp. 15076–15081, 2004.

[61] S. Jiang, X.-M. Liu, X. Dai et al., "Regulation of DHICA-mediated antioxidation by dopachrome tautomerase: implication for skin photoprotection against UVA radiation," *Free Radical Biology & Medicine*, vol. 48, no. 9, pp. 1144–1151, 2010.

[62] X. L. Wang and Q. Sun, "Photodynamic therapy with 5-aminolevulinic acid suppresses IFN-γ-induced K17 expression in HaCaT cells via MAPK pathway," *European Review for Medical and Pharmacological Sciences*, vol. 21, no. 20, pp. 4694–4702, 2017.

[63] J. M. Kyriakis and J. Avruch, "Mammalian MAPK signal transduction pathways activated by stress and inflammation: a 10-year update," *Physiological Reviews*, vol. 92, no. 2, pp. 689–737, 2012.

8

Thymoquinone Attenuates Cardiomyopathy in Streptozotocin-Treated Diabetic Rats

Mustafa S. Atta ⓘ,[1] Ali H. El-Far ⓘ,[2] Foad A. Farrag,[3] Mohamed M. Abdel-Daim ⓘ,[4] Soad K. Al Jaouni,[5] and Shaker A. Mousa ⓘ[6]

[1]*Department of Physiology, Faculty of Veterinary Medicine, Kafrelsheikh University, Kafrelsheikh 33516, Egypt*
[2]*Department of Biochemistry, Faculty of Veterinary Medicine, Damanhour University, Damanhour 22511, Egypt*
[3]*Department of Anatomy and Embryology, Faculty of Veterinary Medicine, Kafrelsheikh University, Kafrelsheikh 33516, Egypt*
[4]*Department of Pharmacology, Faculty of Veterinary Medicine, Suez Canal University, Ismailia 41522, Egypt*
[5]*Hematology/Pediatric Oncology, King Abdulaziz University Hospital and Scientific Chair of Yousef Abdullatif Jameel of Prophetic Medicine Application, Faculty of Medicine, King Abdulaziz University, Jaddah 21589, Saudi Arabia*
[6]*Pharmaceutical Research Institute, Albany College of Pharmacy and Health Sciences, Rensselaer, NY 12144, USA*

Correspondence should be addressed to Mustafa S. Atta; mostafa.ataa@vet.kfs.edu.eg
and Mohamed M. Abdel-Daim; abdeldaim.m@vet.suez.edu.eg

Guest Editor: Ayman M. Mahmoud

Diabetic cardiomyopathy is a diabetic complication due to oxidative stress injuries. This study examined the protecting influence of thymoquinone (TQ) on diabetes-caused cardiac complications. The intracellular means by which TQ works against diabetes-caused cardiac myopathy in rats is not completely understood. In this study, Wistar male rats ($n = 60$) were assigned into four groups: control, diabetic (diabetes induced by IP infusion of streptozotocin, 65 mg/kg), diabetic + TQ (diabetic rats given TQ (50 mg/kg) administered once per day by stomach gavage), and TQ (50 mg/kg) for 12 weeks. TQ supplementation appreciably recovered the cardiac parameters alongside significant declines in plasma nitric oxide concentrations and total superoxide dismutase (T.SOD) activities. Importantly, TQ downgraded expression of cardiac-inducible nitric oxide synthase in addition to significantly upregulating vascular endothelial growth factor and erythropoietin genes and nuclear factor-erythroid-2-related factor 2 (Nrf2) protein. TQ normalized plasma triacylglycerol and low-density lipoprotein-cholesterol and significantly improved the high-density lipoprotein-cholesterol levels. Additionally, TQ administration improved the antioxidant ability of cardiac tissue via significantly increased cardiac T.SOD and decreased cardiac malondialdehyde levels. Oral supplementation with TQ prevented diabetic-induced cardiomyopathy via its inhibitory effect on the E-selectin level, C-reactive protein, and interleukin-6. The TQ protecting effect on the heart tissue was shown by normalization of the plasma cardiac markers troponin I and creatine kinase. This experiment shows the aptitude of TQ to protect cardiac muscles against diabetic oxidative stress, mainly through upregulation of Nrf2, which defeated oxidative damage by improvement of the antioxidant power of cardiac muscle that consequently protected the cardiac muscles and alleviated the inflammatory process.

1. Introduction

Diabetes mellitus (DM) is a metabolic ailment that occurs due to different factors including either genetic or environmental influences. DM is distinguished by disturbances in insulin metabolism that consequently alter carbohydrates, lipids, and protein metabolisms [1]. A cascade of myocardial variations that occur in DM with fibrosis, hypertrophy, and microcirculatory imperfections characterizes diabetic cardiomyopathy. These circulatory complaints hinder the heart efficiency, then concomitantly result in cardiac failure [2]. Diabetic-induced cardiac complication is distinguished by myocardial functional alterations in which oxidative stresses are the main cause [3]. DM-generated reactive oxygen species (ROS) that led to injuries to cellular structures subsequently led to functional, structural, and metabolic impairments [4]. ROS creation triggers cardiomyocytes' necrosis besides apoptosis, which induces cardiac alterations and dysfunction. Therefore, the cellular antioxidant molecules try to abolish the harmful effect of ROS to maintain cellular integrity [5]. Oxidative stress-associated pathological processes can be attenuated by the nuclear factor-erythroid-2- (NF-E2-) related factor 2 (Nrf2) molecule that sustains cellular redox homeostasis [6].

Diabetic cardiomyopathy is influenced by vascular endothelial growth factor (VEGF) that is responsible for blood vessels' formation to counteract cellular degeneration [7]. Concomitantly, downregulation of VEGF occurs with lowering of endothelial cells' apoptosis [8]. Treatment with erythropoietin (EPO) during cardiac ischemia decreases the chance of myocardial apoptosis [9]. EPO enhanced heart efficiency by incitement of endothelial ancestor cell-interceded endothelial turnover and VEGF upregulation [10].

Nigella sativa seeds (black cumin) have various beneficial pharmacological properties [11]. Thymoquinone (TQ; 2-isopropyl-5-methyl-1,4-benzoquinone) is a potent antioxidant phytochemical constituent present in *N. sativa* seeds that acts mainly by scavenging ROS and prevents cellular damage due to different prooxidants [12]. Herein, we investigated the defensive role of TQ against cardiomyopathy due to diabetes induction in rats regarding the intracellular pathway by which TQ may relegate diabetic cardiomyopathy.

2. Materials and Methods

2.1. Chemicals. Streptozotocin (STZ, S0130), dimethyl sulfoxide (DMSO, D2650), ethylenediaminetetraacetic acid (EDS), thymoquinone (274666), glucose (D9434), 0.1 M citrate buffer, phosphate-buffered saline (PBS, P5493), and sodium chloride solution (0.9%, 07982) were obtained from Sigma-Aldrich (St. Louis, MO, USA). β-Actin and Nrf2 antibodies were purchased from Santa Cruz Biotechnology Inc. (Santa Cruz, CA, USA).

2.2. Animals. The morals advisory group of Kafrelsheikh University, Egypt, permitted this study (KVM021/2016; March 2016). Sixty male rats weighing 180–200 g each were raised in the Physiology Unit, Faculty of Veterinary Medicine, Kafrelsheikh University, Egypt. Rats were maintained and fed in the constant conditions recommended in our previous work [13].

2.3. Experimental Design. Animals were assigned into four different groups (control, diabetic, diabetic + TQ, and TQ; 15 each), and every group was allocated into three repeats (5 each). Control and TQ groups were injected intraperitoneally (IP) once with 0.5 ml citrate buffer (pH 4.5) per rat. Diabetes was induced and monitored in diabetic and diabetic + TQ groups according to Atta et al. [13]. At the end of 12 weeks, the rats were anesthetized with intravenous infusion of sodium pentobarbital (30 mg/kg) to prevent suffering for accurate sampling.

2.4. Sampling. After 12 weeks, whole blood, serum, and heart samples for Western blot and RT-PCR were taken according to Atta et al. [13].

2.5. Biochemical Analysis. Kits from Merck (India Ltd.) were used for determination of plasma total cholesterol, triacylglycerol (TAG), and high-density lipoprotein-cholesterol (HDL-C). Low-density lipoprotein-cholesterol (LDL-C) was calculated by the method of Friedewald et al. [14]. Commercial ELISA diagnostic kits from BioCheck (Foster City, CA, USA) were used for determination of plasma troponin I (BC-1105) and creatine kinase-MB (CK-MB, BC-1121).

Heart inflammatory cytokines were assayed with ELISA kits for E-selectin (MBS762069, MyBioSource, San Diego, CA, USA), high sensitive C reactive protein (CRP) (MBS268328, MyBioSource), and interleukin-6 (IL-6) (MBS726707, MyBioSource). Malondialdehyde (MDA) concentrations in plasma and tissue homogenates were assessed using a thiobarbituric acid method [15]. Total superoxide dismutase (T.SOD) was measured in the plasma and cardiac tissue supernatant using nitro blue tetrazolium following the method of Nishikimi et al. [16]. Nitric oxide (NO) quantities in tissue supernatant were quantified according to the method of Miranda et al. [17].

Protein concentrations of cardiac homogenates were assessed with the Bradford assay (5000002, Bio-Rad Laboratories, Watford, UK) for calibration of biochemical assessment [18].

2.6. Assessment of Gene Expression. Total RNA contents were extracted from heart tissue samples in 1 ml QIAzol (79306, QIAGEN Inc., Valencia, CA, USA) with chloroform. The RNA pellets were rinsed with 70% ethanol, dried, and suspended in diethylpyrocarbonate (DEPC, 129112, QIAGEN Inc.). RNA amount and purity were assessed using a spectrophotometer at 260 nm. The ratio of the 260/280 optical density of all RNA tested was 1.7–1.9. RNA in samples was transcribed to the corresponding cDNA with RevertAid Premium reverse transcriptase (EP0733, Thermo Fisher Scientific, Deutschland, Germany). EPO, VEGF, and inducible nitric oxide synthase (iNOS) gene expressions' concentration were examined with RT-PCR using a Bio-Rad MJ Mini Opticon Real-Time PCR System. The primer sequences for EPO, VEGF, iNOS, and GAPDH (housekeeping) genes are listed in Table 1. Data are presented relative to control values using three separate experiments.

2.7. Western Blotting. Heart tissue was homogenized in ice-cold lysis buffer and then centrifuged at 14,000 ×g for 20 min at 4°C. Samples' protein amount was evaluated following Bradford [18]. Samples of equivalent protein amounts were subjected to electrophoresis using SDS/PAGE and transferred to PVDF membrane (88518, Thermo Fisher Scientific) after 1 h, and then blocked using 5% nonfat dried milk in Tris-Tween. The membrane was kept with a polyclonal rabbit anti-Nrf2 antibody (1 : 200, Santa Cruz Biotechnology) and anti-β-actin (Santa Cruz Biotechnology) as internal control diluted 1 : 1000 in Tris-Tween buffer. The

TABLE 1: Primers for gene expression by RT-PCR.

Gene	Direction	Primer sequence	References
GAPDH	Sense	CAAGGTCA TCCATGACAACTTTG	[19]
	Antisense	GTCCACCACCCTG TTGCTGTAG	
EPO	Sense	TACGTAGCCTCACTTCACTGCTT	[19]
	Antisense	GCAGAAAGTATCCGCTGTGAGTGTTC	
iNOS	Sense	TCTGTGCCTTTGCTCATGAC	[20]
	Antisense	CATGGTGAACACGTTCTTGG	
VEGF	Sense	TATGTTT GACTGCTGTGGACTTGA	[19]
	Antisense	AGGGATGGG TTTGTCGTGT	

membranes were treated with the secondary antibodies (1 : 3000) (611-1302, Rockland Immunochemical, Boyertown, PA, USA) incubated with membranes for 1 h at room temperature and rinsed. Protein bands were densitometrically assessed by means of Image J software version 1.48 (National Institutes of Health, Bethesda, MD, USA). Band density was normalized to the equivalent density of β-actin.

2.8. Histological Study. Heart samples were fixed in 10% neutral buffer formaldehyde (F8775, Sigma-Aldrich) solution for a minimum of one day. Fixed tissues were handled via paraffin embedding method and dehydrated via ascending sorts of ethanol (32205, Sigma-Aldrich), clearing in xylene, and immersed in paraffin (327204, Sigma-Aldrich), then implanted in paraffin wax at 60°C. Five μm thick sections were dyed with hematoxylin and eosin [21]. Vacuolation percentages in the photomicrographs of all groups were quantified with Image J software.

2.9. Statistical Assessment. Variance analysis (one-way ANOVA) and results were subjected to Bonferroni's multiple comparisons post hoc test using GraphPad Prism 5 (GraphPad Software, San Diego, CA, USA) with $p < 0.05$ considered statistically significant. Results are shown as means ± standard error.

3. Results

3.1. Thymoquinone and Plasma Biochemical Factors Related to Cardiac Activity. Plasma TAG, LDL-C, troponin I, and creatine kinase were significantly elevated in the diabetic rats although they returned to close to control group levels in the TQ group (Figure 1), while the diabetic group showed significant decreases in HDL-C compared to other groups as presented in Figure 1(c). Plasma NO was significantly elevated in the diabetic rats and was reduced in diabetic + TQ rats (Figure 1(f)). Plasma T.SOD activities were significantly reduced in the diabetic rats matched with control and TQ groups, which might be owing to damage due to diabetes (Figure 1(g)).

3.2. Thymoquinone and the Proinflammatory Markers of Cardiac Tissues. The protecting influence of TQ on the inflammatory cytokines was evaluated. As presented in Figure 2, E-selectin, CRP, and IL-6 levels were significantly

raised ($p < 0.01$) in the diabetic group vs. control and other treated rats.

3.3. Thymoquinone and Cardiac Tissue Antioxidant Status. Diabetic rats displayed a significant increase ($p < 0.001$) in lipid peroxidation levels as monitored with levels of MDA, as well as a significant decrease ($p < 0.001$) in the activities of T.SOD as compared to control. Diabetic + TQ rats had significantly decreased levels of MDA ($p < 0.001$) and expressed a significant increase in T.SOD levels ($p < 0.01$). Conversely, the diabetic + TQ group showed significantly decreased ($p < 0.001$) T.SOD activity and significantly increased ($p < 0.001$) MDA level, significantly increased in comparison to control, as shown in Figure 3.

3.4. Thymoquinone and Cardiac EPO, VEGF, and iNOS mRNA Levels and the Nrf2 Protein Level. The mRNA expression of EPO significantly decreased ($p < 0.05$) in the diabetic group while the EPO mRNA expression increased significantly ($p < 0.05$) in the diabetic + TQ group, even more than control (Figure 4(a)). The VEGF gene significantly decreased ($p < 0.01$) in the diabetic group, whereas in the diabetic + TQ rats, the VEGF mRNA expression was significantly increased ($p < 0.001$) in comparison to the diabetic group (Figure 4(b)). Cardiac iNOS mRNA was significantly elevated ($p < 0.001$) in the diabetic group vs. control, while in the TQ group, the level of iNOS expression was similar to control (Figure 4(c)). The protein level of Nrf2 assessed with Western blot is displayed in Figure 4(d). The diabetic group showed significant downregulation ($p < 0.001$) of Nrf2 protein expression in comparison to control and other TQ-treated groups. The diabetic + TQ group displayed upregulation of Nrf2 protein expression.

3.5. Histopathology. The histopathological assay of cardiac tissue from control and TQ groups showed regular morphological appearances, normal myocardial fiber structure, and architecture with no evidence of degeneration and vacuolation (Figure 5(a) and 5(d)). The myocardial sections of the diabetic group revealed marked myolysis and degeneration in addition to the vacuolation of myocardial fibers (Figure 5(b)). The myocardial sections of the diabetic + TQ group showed small areas of slight degeneration and vacuolation (Figure 5(c)). Compared to control, the vacuolation percentages in diabetic, diabetic + TQ, and TQ groups were 9.00 ± 2.54, 2.00 ± 0.65, and 0%, respectively (Figure 5(e)).

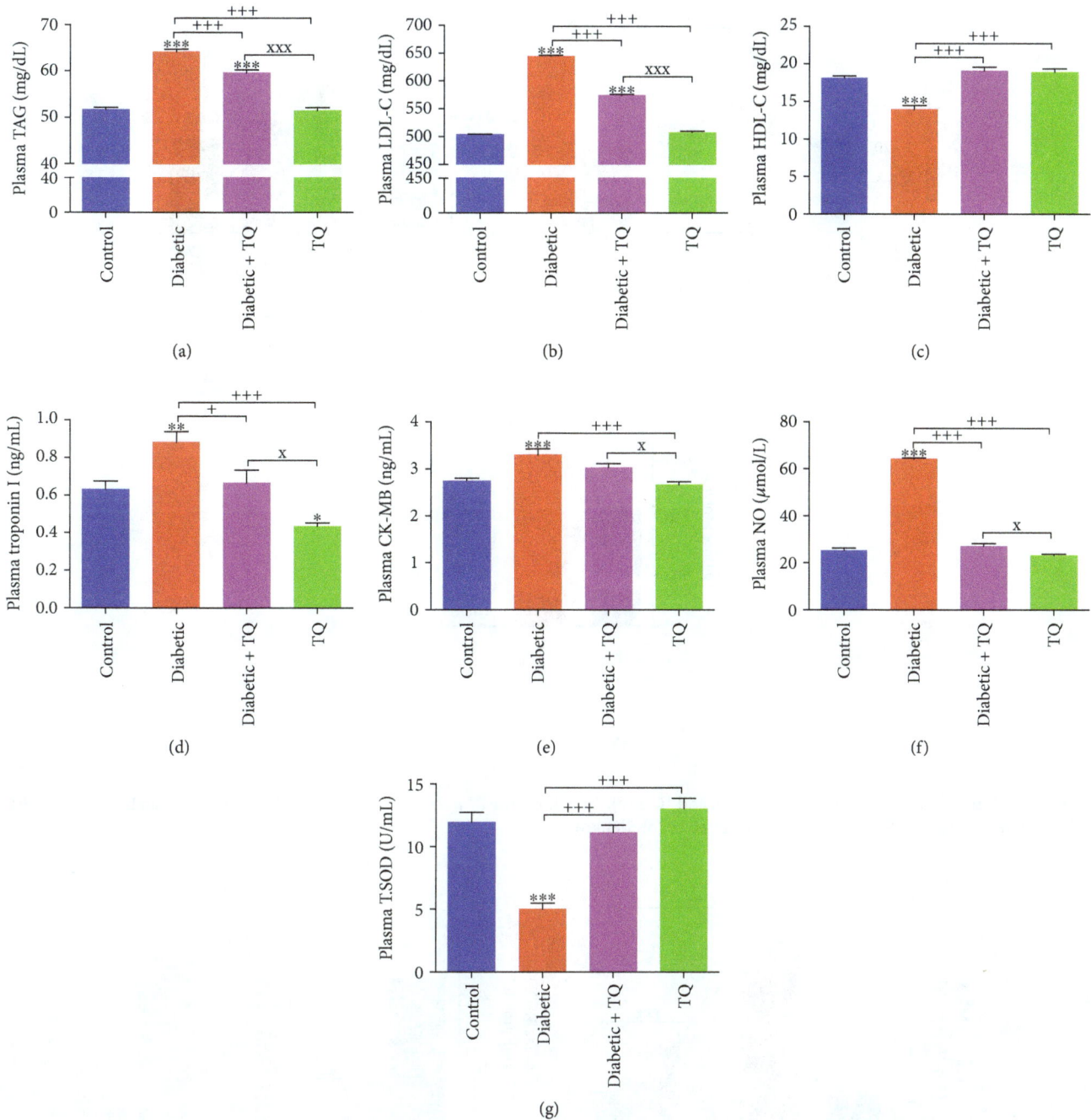

FIGURE 1: Plasma levels of TAG (a), LDL-C (b), HDL-C (c), troponin I (d), CK-MB (e), NO (f), and T.SOD (g). $^*p < 0.05$, $^{**}p < 0.01$ and $^{***}p < 0.001$ vs. control. $^+p < 0.05$ and $^{+++}p < 0.001$ vs. diabetic. $^xp < 0.05$ and $^{xxx}p < 0.001$ vs. TQ. TQ: thymoquinone; TAG: triacylglycerol; LDL-C: low-density lipoprotein cholesterol; HDL-C: high-density lipoprotein cholesterol; CK-MB: creatine kinase-MB; NO: nitric oxide; T.SOD: total superoxide dismutase.

4. Discussion

Diabetes mellitus is a disorder accompanied by an increased glucose level and hyperlipidemia along with problems in insulin and erythrocytic hemoglobin glycosylation [22]. In this study, we have similar data of body weights, serum insulin levels, and HbA1c (%) as presented in our previous study [13], whereas the body weights and insulin concentrations in the diabetic group were significantly reduced compared to the control and TQ-treated rats. TQ caused significant improvement in the body weights in addition to the insulin pattern in the diabetic + TQ group as opposed to the diabetic group. The diabetic group had a significant increase in the HbA1c (%) compared to control and other rat groups. Additionally, there were no marked changes among the TQ and control groups.

Diabetic rats had a significant elevation in plasma TAG and LDL-C levels, while HDL-C levels were significantly

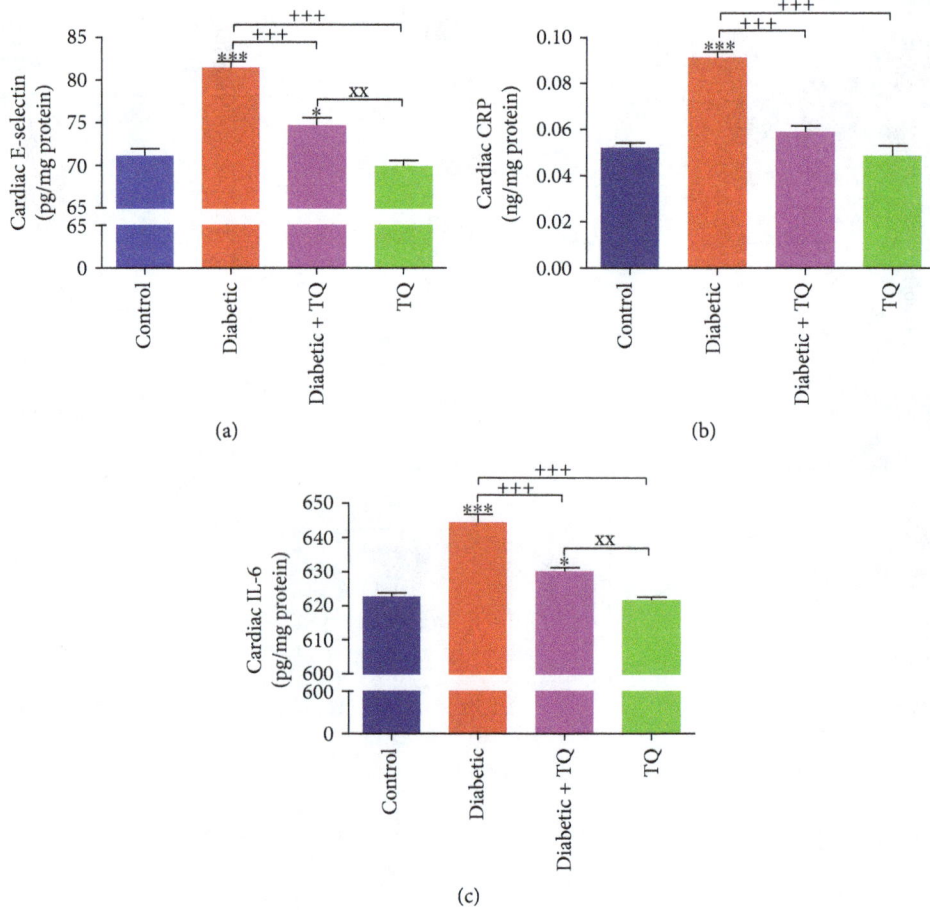

(a)

(b)

(c)

FIGURE 2: Cardiac levels of E-selectin (a), CRP (b), and IL-6 (c). $^*p < 0.05$ and $^{***}p < 0.001$ vs. control. $^{+++}p < 0.001$ vs. diabetic. $^{xx}p < 0.01$ vs. TQ. TQ: thymoquinone; CRP: C reactive protein; IL-6: interleukin-6.

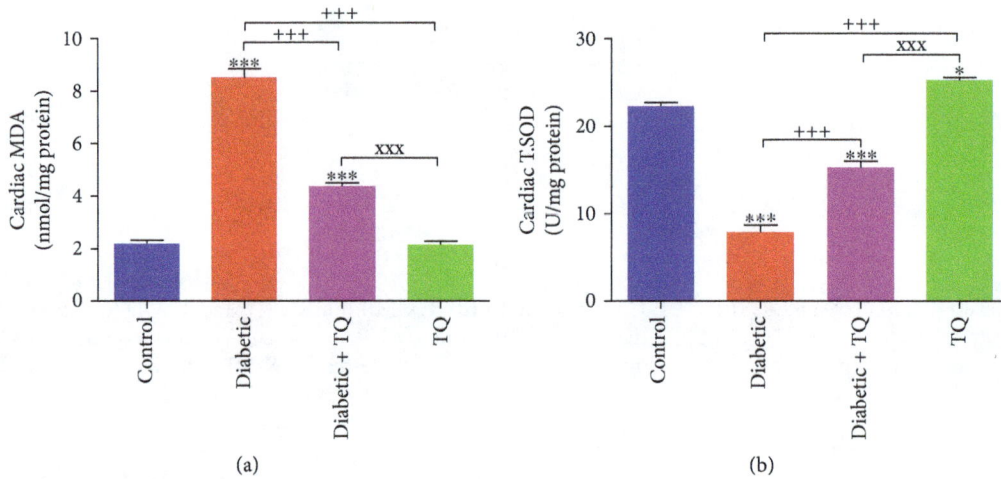

(a)

(b)

FIGURE 3: Cardiac MDA levels (a) and T.SOD activities (b). $^*p < 0.05$ and $^{***}p < 0.001$ vs. control. $^{+++}p < 0.001$ vs. diabetic. $^{xxx}p < 0.001$ vs. TQ. TQ: thymoquinone; MDA: malondialdehyde; T.SOD: total superoxide dismutase.

reduced when compared to control rats. These findings are consistent with results of Ighodaro et al. [23] and Zhang et al. [24] in which the authors reported significant elevations in total cholesterol, TAG, HDL-C, and LDL-C of STZ-treated rats, and with our previous results that the plasma concentration of insulin was significantly reduced in diabetic rats, which led to hyperglycemia with a high percentage of HbA1C [13]. Alternatively, TQ significantly improved the plasma

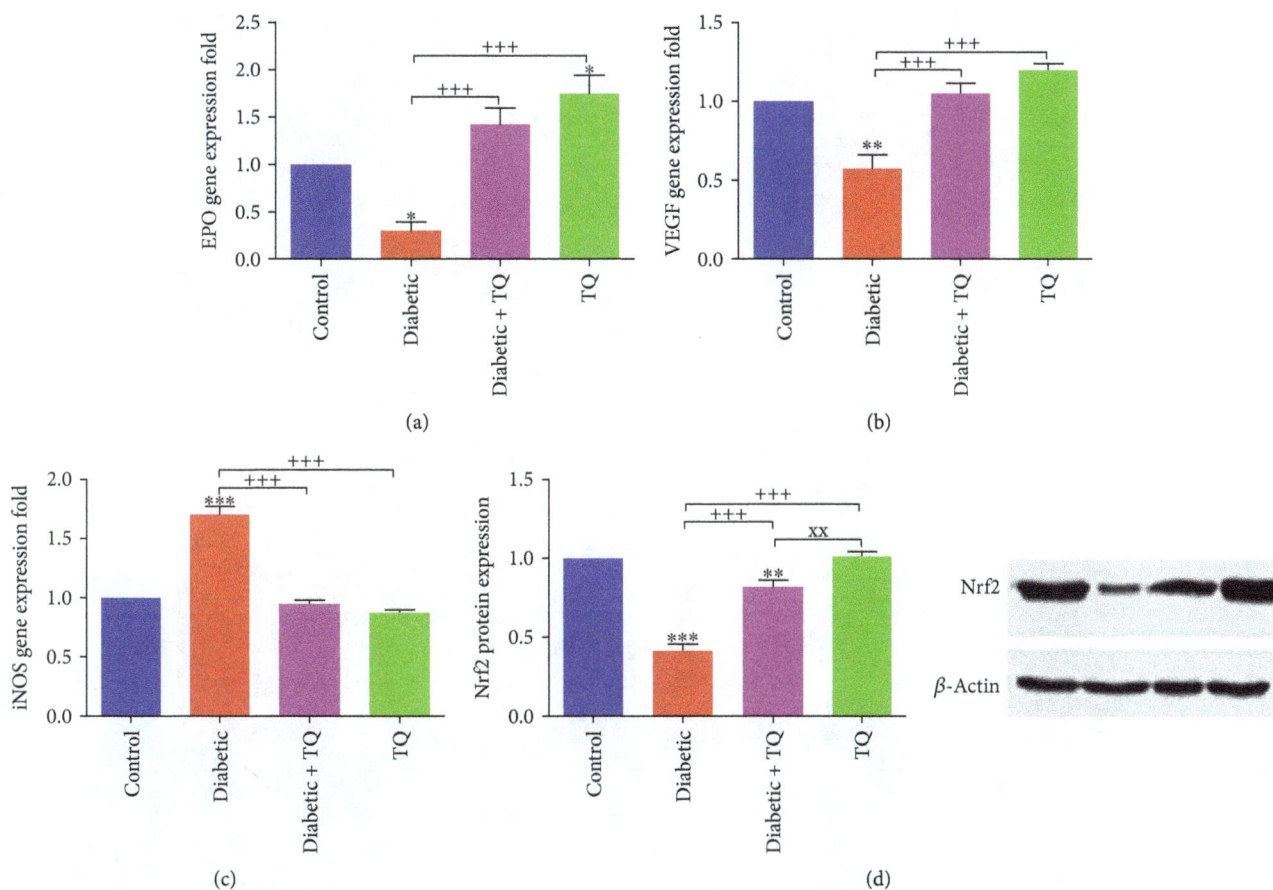

(a)

(b)

(c)

(d)

FIGURE 4: Gene expression folds of cardiac EPO (a), VEGF (b), and iNOS (c) genes and Western blot of Nrf2 (d). $^*p < 0.05$, $^{**}p < 0.01$, and $^{***}p < 0.001$ vs. control. $^{+++}p < 0.001$ vs. diabetic. $^{xx}p < 0.01$ vs. TQ. VEGF: vascular endothelial growth factor; EPO: erythropoietin; iNOS: inducible nitric oxide synthase; Nrf2: nuclear factor erythroid 2-related factor 2.

levels of TAG, LDL-C, and HDL-C in the diabetic + TQ group in relation to the diabetic group. Prabhakar et al. [25] reported the antihyperlipidemic consequence of TQ in contradiction to a high-fructose diet-induced metabolic disorder in rats. Also, TQ attenuated the significant increase in TAG and total cholesterol of cyclophosphamide-induced cardiomyopathies in rats [26]. We previously reported that TQ supplementation to diabetic rats reverted the plasma level of insulin and erythrocytic HbA1C to near their normal levels, indicating the importance of TQ in the regeneration of β-cells injured by STZ [13]. Concomitantly, TQ modulates hyperglycemia and decreases the rate of hemoglobin glycation.

Troponin I and CK-MB are plasma cardiac biomarkers that aid in the laboratory diagnosis of heart attack. STZ induced a significant increase in plasma troponin I and CK-MB, while TQ counteracted the oxidative injuries in cardiac muscles due to STZ. Giribabu et al. [27] stated that STZ-nicotinamide-induced cardiac injuries were accompanied by significant increases in troponin I and CK-MB in diabetic rats. On the contrary, TQ ameliorated the cardiac injuries that occurred in diabetic rats through hindering inflammatory progression and enhancing antioxidant status [28]. This experiment revealed that TQ potentiated the antioxidant status of plasma along with cardiac muscles of STZ-treated rats

via significant decreases in plasma NO and cardiac MDA, while significantly increasing the plasma and cardiac T.SOD. Similarly, TQ significantly decreased MDA levels and increased T.SOD activities in β-cells of the STZ-induced diabetic group [29]. In addition, TQ significantly defeated oxidative damages induced by STZ in rats via significant decreases in testicular NO and MDA levels. Likewise, TQ increased testicular reduced glutathione levels and T.SOD activities, alleviating testicular injuries of diabetic rats [13].

Diabetes accompanied by inflammation and heart disorder is correlated with increased inflammatory biomarkers and cytokines [30], and therefore, plasma E-selectin, CRP, and IL-6 can be augmented in diabetic rats. Nawale et al. [28] stated that alloxan-induced diabetic rats had a significant level of CRP. Also, CRP, IL-6, E-selectin, and TNF-α were significantly raised in diabetic rats in response to oxidative damage [5, 31, 32]. On the contrary, TQ lowered the plasma levels of E-selectin, CRP, and IL-6. This result agreed with Karaca et al. [33], who noticed a significant reduction in interleukin-1 beta (IL-1β), IL-6, tumor necrosis factor-alpha (TNF-α), and monocyte chemoattractant protein-1 (MCP-1) in rats subjected to experimental induction of esophagitis. Also, it was found that TQ has a role against inflammatory progression in the hippocampal tissues due to lipopolysaccharide-induced inflammation in rats [34].

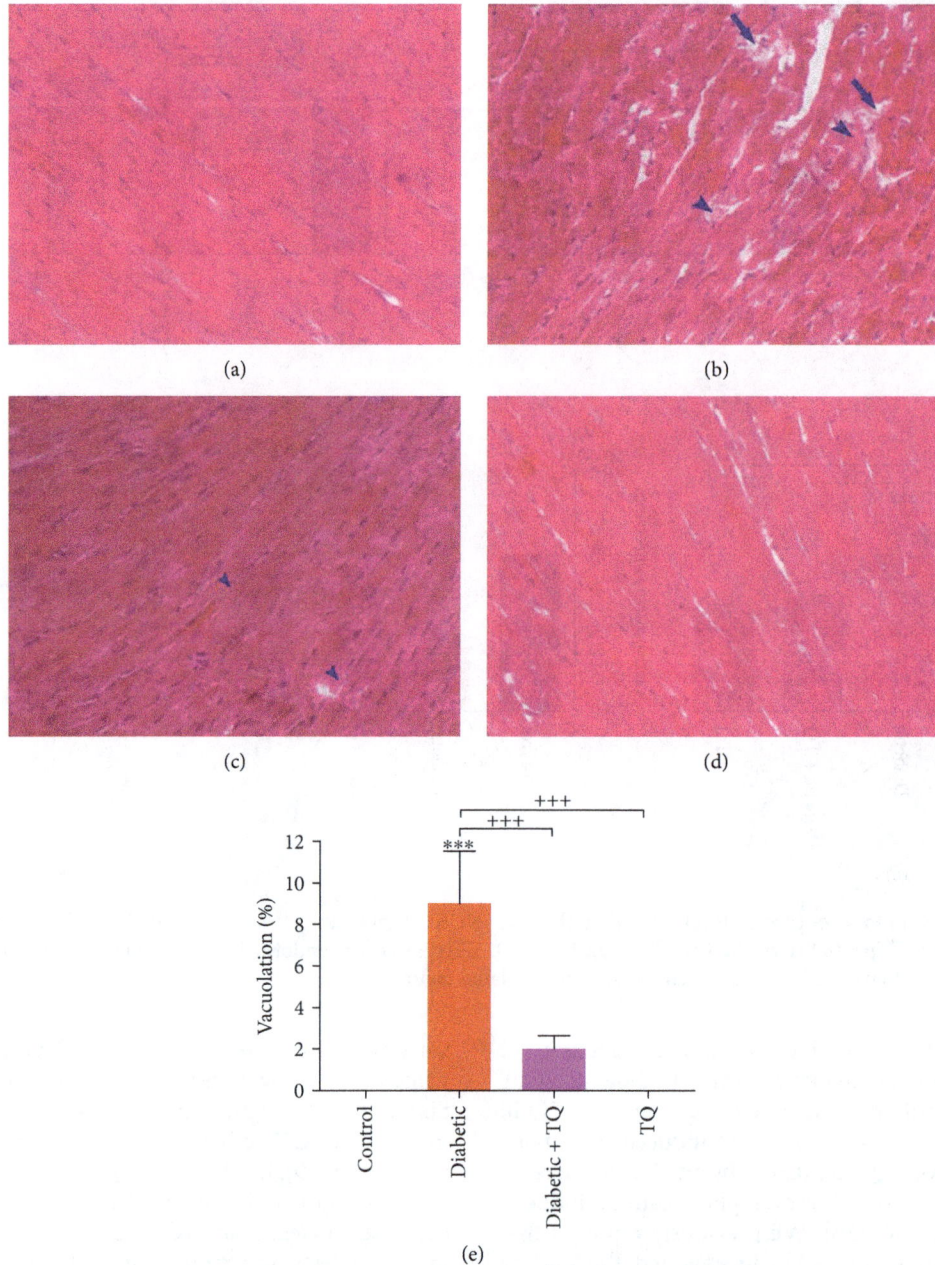

FIGURE 5: Photomicrograph of the rat myocardium showed normal myocardial fiber architecture in the negative control group (a) and TQ group (d). Photomicrograph of diabetic (b) and diabetic + TQ groups (c) showed myocardial degeneration (arrowhead) and vacuolation (arrow). H&E, ×200. (e) Vacuolation percentages. $^{***}p < 0.001$ vs. control. $^{+++}p < 0.001$ vs. diabetic.

Here, the results revealed significant decreases of EPO and VEGF expressions in diabetic rats, while iNOS gene expression fold was significantly increased due to oxidative injuries of cardiac muscles. In the same context, diabetic rats had decreased renal mRNA expression of EPO as a result of oxidative stress due to diabetes [35]. Also, the VEGF gene was downregulated in cardiac tissue of diabetic rats, leading to impairment of angiogenesis [36]. Furthermore, iNOS expression was increased in STZ-diabetic group as shown by Nagareddy et al. [37]. Diabetic rats orally given TQ showed significant improvement of EPO and VEGF and

reduction in iNOS genes that led to enhancement of heart angiogenesis and antioxidant status [13, 38].

A major function of Nrf2 is defeating the oxidant stress that enhances the expression of cellular antioxidant molecules that guard against oxidative injury [39]. Nrf2 defeats ROS through induction of SOD and glutathione peroxidase (GPx) along with regeneration of oxidized glutathione (GSSG) [40]. Also, Nrf2 direct substrate and effector of protein kinase R- (PKR-) like endoplasmic reticulum kinase (PERK) mediated cell survival through amelioration of the endoplasmic reticulum and unfolded protein response

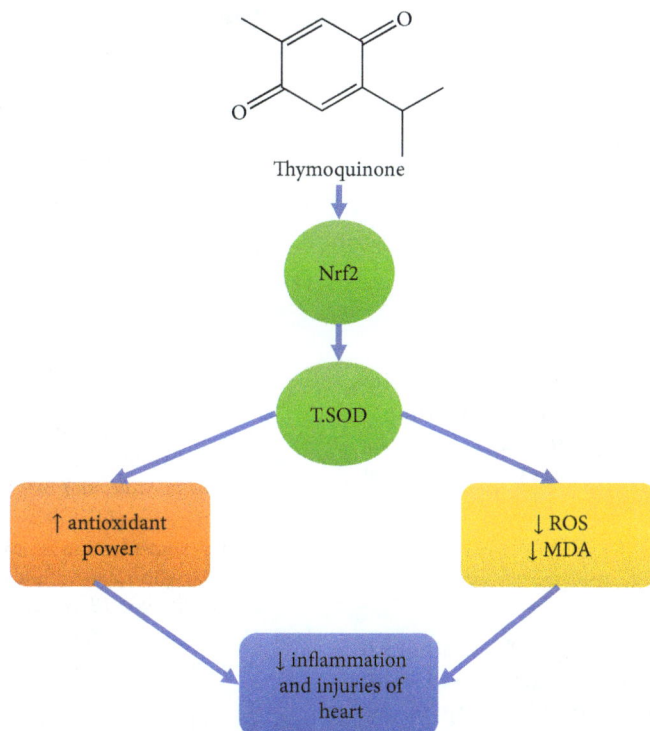

FIGURE 6: Scheme summarizing pathways involved in TQ attenuation of cardiomyopathy.

(UPR) oxidative stresses [41]. Therefore, Nrf2 counteracts the cellular damages due to numerous injuries. The current study showed a considerable decrease in the Nrf2 protein level in diabetic rats relative to normal, control rats. High glucose-induced apoptosis in cardiomyocytes leads to depletion of Nrf2 and antioxidant status of STZ-diabetic rats [42]. Liu et al. [43] found that mulberry granules, a traditional Chinese medicine prescription, protect against STZ-induced cardiomyopathy by suppressing the oxidative stress through Nrf2. The current study displayed the defensive role of TQ counter to the oxidative stress caused by STZ through induction of Nrf2 and antioxidant enzymes (Figure 6). In a like manner, it was shown that the antioxidant potential of TQ through upregulation of Nrf2 consequently augmented the cellular antioxidant status and defeated the cellular oxidative injury [44]. Also, TQ has a crucial shielding role against DNA oxidative damage [45]. The upregulation of Nrf2 due to TQ is considered as a core of the TQ protective effect against cardiomyopathy in diabetic rats. Additionally, Liu et al. [46] suggested that the protective effect of the TQ on cardiovascular function might be due to downregulation of cyclooxygenase-2 levels and the increased phosphorylated-protein kinase B (p-Akt) expression levels in diabetic rats. These findings are mutually supportive to the cardioprotective effect of TQ against diabetic cardiomyopathy demonstrated in our study.

STZ induces oxidative injuries in cardiac muscles through increased production of ROS that leads to myolysis and degeneration in cardiac muscles and finally to failure. Wu et al. [47] reported a significant lessening in antioxidant enzymes with an increased concentration of MDA, leading to heart disease. On the contrary, TQ ameliorates the

histopathological changes induced in rat cardiac muscles due to diabetes oxidative injuries and inflammation. Similarly, TQ protects the cardiac cells against injurious effect induced by different toxicants [48].

5. Conclusions

Diabetes exerts oxidative stress on the cardiac tissues by increasing the oxidative damage, mostly through elevated plasma NO and upregulation of cardiac tissue iNOS mRNA expression. Diabetes decreases the antioxidant ability of heart tissue by decreasing plasma and cardiac tissue T.SOD levels and downregulating cardiac tissue EPO and VEGF mRNA expressions, thereby increasing the major cardiac markers plasma troponin I and CK-MB. Oral administration of TQ protects the cardiac tissue from these oxidative stresses as manifested by normalization of the cardiac markers troponin I and CK-MB. This was achieved via improving the antioxidant status of cardiac muscle and upregulating VEGF and EPO expression, in addition to normalizing the protein expression of Nrf2. Briefly, TQ ameliorates the cardiac injuries in diabetic rats through upregulation of Nrf2 that alleviates oxidative stress and induces cell survival.

Abbreviations

ACP: Acid phosphatase
ALP: Alkaline phosphatase
EPO: Erythropoietin
HDL-C: High-density lipoprotein cholesterol
iNOS: Inducible nitric oxide synthase
LDL-C: Low-density lipoprotein cholesterol

MDA: Malondialdehyde
NO: Nitric oxide
ROS: Reactive oxygen species
STZ: Streptozotocin
T.SOD: Total superoxide dismutase
TAG: Triacylglycerol
TQ: Thymoquinone
VEGF: Vascular endothelial growth factor.

Authors' Contributions

M. S. Atta, A. H. El-Far, F. A. Farrag, and M. M. Abdel-Daim contributed equally to the experimental scheme, experimental work, result analysis, and manuscript writing. S. A. Mousa and S. K. Al Jaouni contributed to the design, manuscript writing, and manuscript modifications.

Acknowledgments

We express thanks to Kelly A. Keating (Pharmaceutical Research Institute, Albany College of Pharmacy and Health Sciences) for the brilliant editing and formatting of the manuscript.

References

[1] L. Yin, W. J. Cai, X. Y. Chang et al., "Association between fetuin-a levels with insulin resistance and carotid intima-media thickness in patients with new-onset type 2 diabetes mellitus," *Biomedical Reports*, vol. 2, no. 6, pp. 839–842, 2014.

[2] D. N. Tziakas, G. K. Chalikias, and J. C. Kaski, "Epidemiology of the diabetic heart," *Coronary Artery Disease*, vol. 16, Supplement 1, pp. S3–S10, 2005.

[3] J. W. Baynes, "Role of oxidative stress in development of complications in diabetes," *Diabetes*, vol. 40, no. 4, pp. 405–412, 1991.

[4] P. S. Tappia, T. Hata, L. Hozaima, M. S. Sandhu, V. Panagia, and N. S. Dhalla, "Role of oxidative stress in catecholamine-induced changes in cardiac sarcolemmal Ca2+ transport," *Archives of Biochemistry and Biophysics*, vol. 387, no. 1, pp. 85–92, 2001.

[5] W. Li, W. Zhao, Q. Wu, Y. Lu, J. Shi, and X. Chen, "Puerarin improves diabetic aorta injury by inhibiting NADPH oxidase-derived oxidative stress in STZ-induced diabetic rats," *Journal of Diabetes Research*, vol. 2016, 9 pages, 2016.

[6] W. Cui, X. Min, X. Xu, B. Du, and P. Luo, "Role of nuclear factor erythroid 2-related factor 2 in diabetic nephropathy," *Journal of Diabetes Research*, vol. 2017, 14 pages, 2017.

[7] M. E. Cooper, D. Vranes, S. Youssef et al., "Increased renal expression of vascular endothelial growth factor (VEGF) and its receptor VEGFR-2 in experimental diabetes," *Diabetes*, vol. 48, no. 11, pp. 2229–2239, 1999.

[8] O. Asghar, A. Al-Sunni, K. Khavandi et al., "Diabetic cardiomyopathy," *Clinical Science*, vol. 116, no. 10, pp. 741–760, 2009.

[9] E. Lipšic, R. G. Schoemaker, P. van der Meer, A. A. Voors, D. J. van Veldhuisen, and W. H. van Gilst, "Protective effects of erythropoietin in cardiac ischemia," *Journal of the American College of Cardiology*, vol. 48, no. 11, pp. 2161–2167, 2006.

[10] B. D. Westenbrink, H. Oeseburg, L. Kleijn et al., "Erythropoietin stimulates normal endothelial progenitor cell-mediated endothelial turnover, but attributes to neovascularization only in the presence of local ischemia," *Cardiovascular Drugs and Therapy*, vol. 22, no. 4, pp. 265–274, 2008.

[11] A. El-Far, "Thymoquinone anticancer discovery: possible mechanisms," *Current Drug Discovery Technologies*, vol. 12, no. 2, pp. 80–89, 2015.

[12] R. B. Kassab and R. E. El-Hennamy, "The role of thymoquinone as a potent antioxidant in ameliorating the neurotoxic effect of sodium arsenate in female rat," *Egyptian Journal of Basic and Applied Sciences*, vol. 4, no. 3, pp. 160–167, 2017.

[13] M. Atta, E. Almadaly, A. El-Far et al., "Thymoquinone defeats diabetes-induced testicular damage in rats targeting antioxidant, inflammatory and aromatase expression," *International Journal of Molecular Sciences*, vol. 18, no. 5, p. 919, 2017.

[14] W. T. Friedewald, R. I. Levy, and D. S. Fredrickson, "Estimation of the concentration of low-density lipoprotein cholesterol in plasma, without use of the preparative ultracentrifuge," *Clinical Chemistry*, vol. 18, no. 6, pp. 499–502, 1972.

[15] H. Ohkawa, N. Ohishi, and K. Yagi, "Assay for lipid peroxides in animal tissues by thiobarbituric acid reaction," *Analytical Biochemistry*, vol. 95, no. 2, pp. 351–358, 1979.

[16] M. Nishikimi, N. Appaji Rao, and K. Yagi, "The occurrence of superoxide anion in the reaction of reduced phenazine methosulfate and molecular oxygen," *Biochemical and Biophysical Research Communications*, vol. 46, no. 2, pp. 849–854, 1972.

[17] K. M. Miranda, M. G. Espey, and D. A. Wink, "A rapid, simple spectrophotometric method for simultaneous detection of nitrate and nitrite," *Nitric Oxide*, vol. 5, no. 1, pp. 62–71, 2001.

[18] M. M. Bradford, "A rapid and sensitive method for the quantitation of microgram quantities of protein utilizing the principle of protein-dye binding," *Analytical Biochemistry*, vol. 72, no. 1–2, pp. 248–254, 1976.

[19] J. Lu, Y.-y. Yao, Q.-m. Dai et al., "Erythropoietin attenuates cardiac dysfunction by increasing myocardial angiogenesis and inhibiting interstitial fibrosis in diabetic rats," *Cardiovascular Diabetology*, vol. 11, no. 1, p. 105, 2012.

[20] A. Grilli, M. A. de Lutiis, A. Patruno et al., "Inducible nitric oxide synthase and heme oxygenase-1 in rat heart: direct effect of chronic exposure to hypoxia," *Annals of Clinical & Laboratory Science*, vol. 33, no. 2, pp. 208–215, 2003.

[21] J. D. Bancroft and C. Layton, "The hematoxylin and eosin," in *Bancroft's Theory and Practice of Histological Techniques*, S. K. Suvarna, C. Layton, and J. D. Bancroft, Eds., pp. 173–186, Churchill Livingstone of Elsevier, Philadelphia, USA, 7th edition, 2013.

[22] I. Hameed, S. R. Masoodi, S. A. Mir, M. Nabi, K. Ghazanfar, and B. A. Ganai, "Type 2 diabetes mellitus: from a metabolic disorder to an inflammatory condition," *World Journal of Diabetes*, vol. 6, no. 4, pp. 598–612, 2015.

[23] O. M. Ighodaro, O. A. Akinloye, R. N. Ugbaja, and S. O. Omotainse, "*Sapium ellipticum* (hochst.) pax ethanol leaf extract maintains lipid homeostasis in streptozotocin-induced diabetic rats," *International Scholarly Research Notices*, vol. 2017, 5 pages, 2017.

[24] S. Zhang, H. Xu, X. Yu, Y. Wu, and D. Sui, "Metformin ameliorates diabetic nephropathy in a rat model of low-dose streptozotocin-induced diabetes," *Experimental and Therapeutic Medicine*, vol. 14, no. 1, pp. 383–390, 2017.

[25] P. Prabhakar, K. H. Reeta, S. K. Maulik, A. K. Dinda, and Y. K. Gupta, "Protective effect of thymoquinone against high-fructose diet-induced metabolic syndrome in rats," *European Journal of Nutrition*, vol. 54, no. 7, pp. 1117–1127, 2015.

[26] M. N. Nagi, O. A. Al-Shabanah, M. M. Hafez, and M. M. Sayed-Ahmed, "Thymoquinone supplementation attenuates cyclophosphamide-induced cardiotoxicity in rats," *Journal of Biochemical and Molecular Toxicology*, vol. 25, no. 3, pp. 135–142, 2011.

[27] N. Giribabu, J. Roslan, S. S. Rekha, and N. Salleh, "Methanolic seed extract of *Vitis vinifera* ameliorates oxidative stress, inflammation and atpase dysfunction in infarcted and non-infarcted heart of streptozotocin–nicotinamide induced male diabetic rats," *International Journal of Cardiology*, vol. 222, pp. 850–865, 2016.

[28] R. B. Nawale, G. S. Mate, and B. S. Wakure, "Ethanolic extract of *Amaranthus paniculatus* Linn. Ameliorates diabetes-associated complications in alloxan-induced diabetic rats," *Integrative Medicine Research*, vol. 6, no. 1, pp. 41–46, 2017.

[29] N. E. Abdelmeguid, R. Fakhoury, S. M. Kamal, and R. J. Al Wafai, "Effects of *Nigella sativa* and thymoquinone on biochemical and subcellular changes in pancreatic β-cells of streptozotocin-induced diabetic rats," *Journal of Diabetes*, vol. 2, no. 4, pp. 256–266, 2010.

[30] A. Festa and S. M. Haffner, "Inflammation and cardiovascular disease in patients with diabetes: lessons from the diabetes control and complications trial," *Circulation*, vol. 111, no. 19, pp. 2414-2415, 2005.

[31] R. Saklani, S. K. Gupta, I. R. Mohanty, B. Kumar, S. Srivastava, and R. Mathur, "Cardioprotective effects of rutin via alteration in TNF-α, CRP, and BNP levels coupled with antioxidant effect in STZ-induced diabetic rats," *Molecular and Cellular Biochemistry*, vol. 420, no. 1-2, pp. 65–72, 2016.

[32] C. G. Liu, Y. P. Ma, and X. J. Zhang, "Effects of mulberry leaf polysaccharide on oxidative stress in pancreatic β-cells of type 2 diabetic rats," *European Review for Medical and Pharmacological Sciences*, vol. 21, no. 10, pp. 2482–2488, 2017.

[33] G. Karaca, O. Aydin, F. Pehlivanli, C. Altunkaya, H. Uzun, and O. Guler, "Effectiveness of thymoquinone, zeolite, and platelet-rich plasma in model of corrosive oesophagitis induced in rats," *Annals of Surgical Treatment and Research*, vol. 92, no. 6, pp. 396–401, 2017.

[34] R. Bargi, F. Asgharzadeh, F. Beheshti, M. Hosseini, H. R. Sadeghnia, and M. Khazaei, "The effects of thymoquinone on hippocampal cytokine level, brain oxidative stress status and memory deficits induced by lipopolysaccharide in rats," *Cytokine*, vol. 96, pp. 173–184, 2017.

[35] Z. S. Ibrahim, M. E. Alkafafy, M. M. Ahmed, and M. M. Soliman, "Renoprotective effect of curcumin against the combined oxidative stress of diabetes and nicotine in rats," *Molecular Medicine Reports*, vol. 13, no. 4, pp. 3017–3026, 2016.

[36] L. Chodari, M. Mohammadi, V. Ghorbanzadeh, H. Dariushnejad, and G. Mohaddes, "Testosterone and voluntary exercise promote angiogenesis in hearts of rats with diabetes by enhancing expression of VEGF-A and SDF-1a," *Canadian Journal of Diabetes*, vol. 40, no. 5, pp. 436–441, 2016.

[37] P. R. Nagareddy, J. H. McNeill, and K. M. MacLeod, "Chronic inhibition of inducible nitric oxide synthase ameliorates cardiovascular abnormalities in streptozotocin diabetic rats," *European Journal of Pharmacology*, vol. 611, no. 1-3, pp. 53–59, 2009.

[38] M. Abd-Elbaset, E. S. A. Arafa, G. A. el Sherbiny, M. S. Abdel-Bakky, and A. N. A. M. Elgendy, "Thymoquinone mitigate ischemia-reperfusion-induced liver injury in rats: a pivotal role of nitric oxide signaling pathway," *Naunyn-Schmiedeberg's Archives of Pharmacology*, vol. 390, no. 1, pp. 69–76, 2017.

[39] R. Gold, L. Kappos, D. L. Arnold et al., "Placebo-controlled phase 3 study of oral BG-12 for relapsing multiple sclerosis," *New England Journal of Medicine*, vol. 367, no. 12, pp. 1098–1107, 2012.

[40] Q. Ma, "Role of Nrf2 in oxidative stress and toxicity," *Annual Review of Pharmacology and Toxicology*, vol. 53, no. 1, pp. 401–426, 2013.

[41] T. Ma, M. A. Trinh, A. J. Wexler et al., "Suppression of eif2α kinases alleviates Alzheimer's disease–related plasticity and memory deficits," *Nature Neuroscience*, vol. 16, no. 9, pp. 1299–1305, 2013.

[42] H. Yang, Y. Mao, B. Tan, S. Luo, and Y. Zhu, "The protective effects of endogenous hydrogen sulfide modulator, s-propargyl-cysteine, on high glucose-induced apoptosis in cardiomyocytes: a novel mechanism mediated by the activation of Nrf2," *European Journal of Pharmacology*, vol. 761, pp. 135–143, 2015.

[43] Y. Liu, Y.-B. Zhao, S.-W. Wang, Y. Zhou, Z.-S. Tang, and F. Li, "Mulberry granules protect against diabetic cardiomyopathy through the AMPK/Nrf2 pathway," *International Journal of Molecular Medicine*, vol. 40, no. 3, pp. 913–921, 2017.

[44] Y. Y. Shao, B. Li, Y. M. Huang, Q. Luo, Y. M. Xie, and Y. H. Chen, "Thymoquinone attenuates brain injury via an antioxidative pathway in a status epilepticus rat model," *Translational Neuroscience*, vol. 8, pp. 9–14, 2017.

[45] B. Babazadeh, H. R. Sadeghnia, E. Safarpour Kapurchal, H. Parsaee, S. Nasri, and Z. Tayarani-Najaran, "Protective effect of *Nigella sativa* and thymoquinone on serum/glucose deprivation-induced DNA damage in pc12 cells," *Avicenna Journal of Phytomedicine*, vol. 2, no. 3, pp. 125–132, 2012.

[46] H. Liu, H. Y. Liu, Y. N. Jiang, and N. Li, "Protective effect of thymoquinone improves cardiovascular function, and attenuates oxidative stress, inflammation and apoptosis by mediating the PI3k/Akt pathway in diabetic rats," *Molecular Medicine Reports*, vol. 13, no. 3, pp. 2836–2842, 2016.

[47] B. Wu, J. Lin, J. Luo et al., "Dihydromyricetin protects against diabetic cardiomyopathy in streptozotocin-induced diabetic mice," *BioMed Research International*, vol. 2017, Article ID 3764370, 13 pages, 2017.

[48] K. M. A. Hassanein and Y. O. El-Amir, "Protective effects of thymoquinone and avenanthramides on titanium dioxide nanoparticles induced toxicity in Sprague-Dawley rats," *Pathology-Research and Practice*, vol. 213, no. 1, pp. 13–22, 2017.

9

Formulated Chinese Medicine Shaoyao Gancao Tang Reduces Tau Aggregation and Exerts Neuroprotection through Anti-Oxidation and Anti-Inflammation

I-Cheng Chen ⓘ,[1] Te-Hsien Lin ⓘ,[2] Yu-Hsuan Hsieh,[2] Chih-Ying Chao,[1] Yih-Ru Wu ⓘ,[1] Kuo-Hsuan Chang ⓘ,[1] Ming-Chung Lee,[3] Guey-Jen Lee-Chen ⓘ,[2] and Chiung-Mei Chen ⓘ[1]

[1]Department of Neurology, Chang Gung Memorial Hospital, Chang Gung University College of Medicine, Taipei 10507, Taiwan
[2]Department of Life Science, National Taiwan Normal University, Taipei 11677, Taiwan
[3]Sun Ten Pharmaceutical Co. Ltd., New Taipei City 23143, Taiwan

Correspondence should be addressed to Guey-Jen Lee-Chen; t43019@ntnu.edu.tw
and Chiung-Mei Chen; cmchen@adm.cgmh.org.tw

Academic Editor: Francisco Jaime Bezerra Mendonça Júnior

Misfolded tau proteins induce accumulation of free radicals and promote neuroinflammation by activating microglia-releasing proinflammatory cytokines, leading to neuronal cell death. Traditional Chinese herbal medicines (CHMs) have been widely used in clinical practice to treat neurodegenerative diseases associated with oxidative stress and neuroinflammation. This study examined the neuroprotection effects of formulated CHMs Bai-Shao (made of *Paeonia lactiflora*), Gan-Cao (made of *Glycyrrhiza uralensis*), and Shaoyao Gancao Tang (SG-Tang, made of *P. lactiflora* and *G. uralensis* at 1 : 1 ratio) in cell model of tauopathy. Our results showed that SG-Tang displayed a greater antioxidative and antiaggregation effect than Bai-Shao and Gan-Cao and a stronger anti-inflammatory activity than Bai-Shao but similar to Gan-Cao. In inducible 293/SH-SY5Y cells expressing proaggregant human tau repeat domain (ΔK280 tau$_{RD}$), SG-Tang reduced tau misfolding and reactive oxygen species (ROS) level in ΔK280 tau$_{RD}$ 293 cells and promoted neurite outgrowth in ΔK280 tau$_{RD}$ SH-SY5Y cells. Furthermore, SG-Tang displayed anti-inflammatory effects by reducing nitric oxide (NO) production in mouse BV-2 microglia and increased cell viability of ΔK280 tau$_{RD}$-expressing SH-SY5Y cells inflamed by BV-2 conditioned medium. To uncover the neuroprotective mechanisms of SG-Tang, apoptosis protein array analysis of inflamed tau expressing SH-SY5Y cells was conducted and the suppression of proapoptotic proteins was confirmed. In conclusion, SG-Tang displays neuroprotection by exerting antioxidative and anti-inflammatory activities to suppress neuronal apoptosis in human tau cell models. The study results lay the base for future applications of SG-Tang on tau animal models to validate its effect of reducing tau misfolding and potential disease modification.

1. Introduction

Neurodegenerative diseases including Alzheimer's disease (AD) and tauopathy are characterized by the presence of hyperphosphorylated, insoluble, and filamentous tau protein, which leads to neuronal dysfunction and loss [1]. Tau is an ubiquitously distributed microtubule-associated protein that promotes and stabilizes microtubule assembly. Aside from helping microtubule assembly, tau also interacts with other cytoskeleton components to play a role in axonal transport

[2]. Tau is encoded by *MAPT* (microtubule-associated protein tau) gene located on chromosome 17q21, containing 16 exons [3]. By alternative splicing, tau proteins exist as six different isoforms in human central nervous system (CNS). Exons 9–12 encode four C-terminal microtubule binding motifs which are imperfect copies of an 18-amino-acid tau repeat domain (tau$_{RD}$). Different point mutations found in tau$_{RD}$ reduced the ability of tau to promote microtubule assembly [4] and accelerated aggregation of tau into filaments [5]. In addition, a single amino acid deletion

(ΔK280) was found in patients with frontotemporal dementia and AD [6–8]. ΔK280 is extremely fibrillogenic and frequently used to model tau aggregation [9–11].

Emerging evidence has shown protein aggregation as a trigger for inflammation and neurodegeneration [12]. Activated microglia are found in the postmortem brain tissues of human tauopathy, and microglial burden correlated with tau burden in most of the pathologically afflicted areas [13, 14]. Chronic activation of microglia may enhance the hyperphosphorylation of tau and the subsequent development of neurofibrillary tangles [15]. Activated microglia contribute to neurofibrillary pathology in AD through production of interleukin (IL)-1 and activation of neuronal p38-MAPK (mitogen-activated protein kinase 1) *in vitro* [16] and *in vivo* [17]. In transgenic mice that develop both tau and amyloid pathologies ($3 \times$Tg-AD line), lipopolysaccharide- (LPS-) induced activation of glia exacerbates tau pathology [18]. Tau oligomers colocalize with astrocytes and microglia to induce inflammation, leading to neuronal damage and eventual cell death [19]. Being a critical component in pathogenesis, neuroinflammation provides an attractive therapeutic target in the treatment and prevention of AD and other tauopathy [20, 21].

Traditional Chinese herbal medicines (CHMs) have accumulated several lines of beneficial evidence in the treatment of AD [22–24]. However, treatment approaches addressing inflammatory processes in tauopathy have not been well investigated. Bai-Shao and Gan-Cao are formulated CHMs prepared from herbs *Paeonia lactiflora* (*P. lactiflora*) and *Glycyrrhiza uralensis* (*G. uralensis*), respectively. Total glucosides of paeony extracted from *P. lactiflora* may exert anti-inflammatory activities that contribute to its analgesic effect through modulating production of proinflammatory cytokines from macrophage-like synoviocytes [25]. In addition, ethanol extracts of *G. uralensis* possess inhibitory effects against NF-κB-mediated inflammatory response and strong activation of the Nrf2-ARE-antioxidative stress signaling pathways [26]. In this study, Bai-Shao, Gan-Cao, and Shaoyao Gancao Tang (SG-Tang), a formulated CHM made of *P. lactiflora* and *G. uralensis* at 1 : 1 ratio, were tested in a tau aggregation model [27] to reveal underlying pathogenesis and develop therapeutic strategy targeting neuroinflammation in tauopathy.

2. Materials and Methods

2.1. Preparation of Formulated CHMs. Bai-Shao (Code: 5722), Gan-Cao (Code: 5536), and SG-Tang (Code: 0703H) were provided by Sun Ten Pharmaceutical Co. Ltd. (New Taipei City, Taiwan). To prepare the CHM stock solution, 5 g powder was dissolved in 10 ml ddH$_2$O, vortexed to mix well, and then centrifuged at 4000 rpm for 10 min at room temperature. The supernatant was collected and used for further experiments.

2.2. HPLC Analysis. High-performance liquid chromatography (HPLC) was performed using a LaChrom Elite HPLC system (Hitachi, Tokyo, Japan) equipped with photodiode array detector. The chromatographic separation of Bai-Shao, Gan-Cao, and SG-Tang (500 mg/ml) was achieved using a Hypersil ODS (C18) column (250×4.6 mm, 5μm). The mobile phase consisted of 0.1% phosphoric acid in water (A) and acetonitrile (B). The linear gradient elution was used as follows: 10~50% B (0~40 min), 50~90% B (40~45 min), 90% B (45~55 min), 90~10% B (55~60 min), and 10% B (60~70 min). The flow rate was 0.8 ml/min. The column and autosampler were maintained at 30°C and 20°C, respectively. Reference compounds were paeoniflorin and ammonium glycyrrhizinate (Sigma-Aldrich, St. Louis, MO, USA) and absorbance was monitored at 230 nm and 250 nm, respectively. The scan range for photo diode array was 190~600 nm. 3-(4,5-Dimethylthiazol-2-yl)-2,5-diphenyltetrazolium bromide (MTT), 1,1-diphenyl-2-picrylhydrazyl (DPPH), LPS, and Congo red were purchased from Sigma-Aldrich. Interferon- (IFN-) γ was obtained from Santa Cruz.

2.3. Cell Culture. Two mouse cell lines, RAW 264.7 macrophage (BCRC 60001, Food Industry Research and Development Institute, Taiwan) and BV-2 microglia (kind gift from Dr. Han-Min Chen, Catholic Fu-Jen University, New Taipei City, Taiwan), were used in this study. The murine RAW 264.7 and microglial BV-2 cells were routinely maintained in DMEM supplemented with 10% FBS (Invitrogen, Waltham, MA, USA) at 37°C under 5% CO$_2$ and 95% relative humidity.

Four human cell lines, HEK-293 cells (ATCC no. CRL-1573), SH-SY5Y neuronal cells (ATCC no. CRL-2266) and Tet-on ΔK280 tau$_{RD}$-DsRed 293/SH-SY5Y cells [27] were used. HEK-293 cells were grown in DMEM with 10% FBS, and SH-SY5Y cells were maintained in DMEM-F12 with 10% FBS. In addition to the basal media for HEK-293 and SH-SY5Y, 5 μg/ml blasticidin and 100 μg/ml hygromycin (InvivoGen, San Diego, CA, USA) were applied for Tet-On ΔK280 tau$_{RD}$-DsRed cells.

2.4. MTT Assay. To evaluate cell viability, 5×10^4 HEK-293/SH-SY5Y cells were plated into 48-well dishes, grown for 20 h, and treated with tested Chinese medicine formulas (0.1~1000 μg/ml Bai-Shao, Gan-Cao, or SG-Tang). After 1 day, 20 μl of 5 mg/ml MTT was added onto each 48-well containing cells with 200 μl of cultured medium at 37°C for 3 h. 200 μl of lysis buffer (10% Triton X-100, 0.1 N HCl, 18% isopropanol) was then added onto 48-well and the absorbance at OD 570 nm was read by a microplate reader (FLx800 fluorescence microplate reader, Bio-Tek, Winooski, VT, USA). The half maximal inhibitory concentration (IC$_{50}$) were calculated using the interpolation method.

2.5. DPPH Assay. The DPPH radical-scavenging activity was measured in a reaction mixture containing 0.1 ml of 0.2 mM DPPH radical solution and 0.1 ml of each tested formulas (100~1000 μg/ml). The solution was rapidly mixed and incubated for 30 min at 25°C. The scavenging capacity was measured by monitoring the absorbance at 517 nm with a microplate reader (Multiskan GO, Thermo Scientific, Waltham, MA, USA). The half maximal effective concentrations (EC$_{50}$) were calculated using the interpolation method.

2.6. Detection of Inflammatory Mediators. Murine RAW 264.7 macrophage cells were seeded in DMEM containing 1% FBS and pretreated with tested formulas (0.5~2 mg/ml) or celecoxib (50 μM) for 8 h followed by LPS (1 μg/ml) stimulation. The release of NO was evaluated by Griess assay according to the manufacturer's protocol (Sigma-Aldrich). The levels of tumor necrosis factor- (TNF-) α, IL-1β, and IL-6 were determined using a mouse enzyme-linked immunosorbent assay (ELISA) system (R&D Systems, Minneapolis, MN, USA) following the manufacturer's protocol. The optical density at 450 nm was detected using a microplate reader (ELISA Reader: SpectraMAX340PC; Molecular Devices, Sunnyvale, CA, USA). In addition, the immortalized murine microglial BV-2 cells, an alternative model system for primary microglia, were used. BV-2 cells were seeded in DMEM containing 1% FBS. Next day, cells were pretreated with SG-Tang for 8~24 h, stimulated with LPS (1 μg/ml) for 20 h, and released of NO in the media determined.

2.7. ΔK280 tau$_{RD}$-DsRed Fluorescence Assay. DsRed fluorescence was evaluated to reflect tau aggregation. On the first day, ΔK280 tau$_{RD}$-DsRed 293 cells were seeded into the 96-well dish in a density of 0.8×10^4 cells/well and one day after seeding, 5~20 μM Congo red or 50~200 μg/ml Bai-Shao, Gan-Cao, and SG-Tang were added. After 8 h of culture, doxycycline (1 μg/ml; Sigma-Aldrich) was added to induce misfolded tau expression. On the fifth day, cells were stained with Hoechst 33342 (0.1 μg/ml) for 30 min, and fluorescence intensities (543 nm excitation and 593 nm emission for DsRed; 377 nm excitation and 447 nm emission for Hoechst 33342) were measured using a high content analysis (HCA) system (ImageXpressMICRO, Molecular Devices). All images were analyzed by MetaXpress Image Acquisition and Analysis Software (Molecular Devices).

2.8. ROS Assay. Cellular ROS of the above Tet-On ΔK280 tau$_{RD}$-DsRed 293 cells was measured by fluorogenic reagent (CellROX™ Deep Red, Molecular Probes, Eugene, OR, USA) with final concentration of 5 μM and incubated at 37°C for 30 min. Then, cells were washed with PBS and analyzed by flow cytometer (Becton-Dickinson, Franklin Lakes, NJ, USA) with excitation/emission wavelengths at 640/665 nm. For each sample, 5×10^4 cells are analyzed.

2.9. Neurite Outgrowth Analysis. 3×10^4 of ΔK280 tau$_{RD}$-DsRed SH-SY5Y cells/well were seeded in a 24-well plate, and 10 μM retinoic acid (Sigma-Aldrich) was added to initiate neuronal differentiation. On the second day, cells were treated with SG-Tang (200 μg/ml) or Congo red (20 μM) for 8 h before tau expression induction by adding doxycycline (1 μg/ml). On day 9, cells were fixed in 4% paraformaldehyde in PBS for 15 min, permeabilized in 0.1% Triton X-100 in PBS for 10 min, and blocked in 3% bovine serum albumin (BSA) in PBS for 20 min. Primary TUBB3 antibody (1 : 1000 dilution in PBS with 1% BSA, 0.05% Tween 20, and 0.02% NaN$_3$; Covance, Princeton, NJ, USA) was used to stain neuronal cells, followed by secondary goat anti-rabbit Alexa Fluor ®555 antibody (1 : 1000 dilution; Molecular probes)

at room temperature. After nuclei staining by 4′-6-diami-dino-2-phenylindole (DAPI), images of cells were taken via the HCA system and analyzed as described.

2.10. Cell Viability/Cytotoxicity Assays of Inflamed SH-SY5Y Cells. Previously, cell-free media obtained from LPS/IFN-γ-exposed microglia-like cells resulted in the highest toxicity on cell viability of SH-SY5Y cells [28]. To prepare conditioned medium (CM) with inflammatory factors, BV-2 cells were stimulated with a combination of LPS (1 μg/ml) and IFN-γ (100 ng/ml) for 24 h. After morphology examination, the BV-2 CM were collected, pooled, and centrifuged to remove cell debris. The induced inflammation was confirmed by release of NO, TNF-α, IL-1β, and IL-6 in the media and increased Iba1 expression in the cell lysate.

For SH-SY5Y cell viability assay, DMEM-F12 was then mixed with two times volume of BV-2 CM (a final FBS concentration at 10%) and added to undifferentiated ΔK280 tau$_{RD}$-DsRed SH-SY5Y cells for 2 days to induce inflammation. Cell viability was determined by MTT assay as described. For SH-SY5Y cytotoxicity assay, neuronal-differentiated ΔK280 tau$_{RD}$-DsRed SH-SY5Y cells were treated with BV-2 CM for 5 days as described and media were collected. 100 μl of supernatant from each sample was transferred to 96-well plate to examine the release of lactate dehydrogenase (LDH) by using LDH cytotoxicity assay kit (Cayman, Ann Arbor, MI, USA). The absorbance was read at 490 nm with a microplate reader (Multiskan GO, Thermo Scientific).

2.11. Human Apoptosis Antibody Array. Protein samples from ΔK280 tau$_{RD}$-DsRed SH-SY5Y cells with different treatments (Dox uninduced/induced, CM unstimulated/ stimulated, and SG-Tang unpretreated/pretreated) were prepared and incubated with apoptosis antibody array membranes (RayBiotech, Norcross, GA, USA). The relative levels of 43 apoptosis-related proteins in human cell lysates were measured with the array. The detected changes in protein levels were confirmed by Western blot or caspase 3 activity assay.

2.12. Western Blot Analysis. Cells were lysed in hypotonic buffer (20 mM HEPES pH 7.4, 1 mM MgCl$_2$, 10 mM KCl, 1 mM DTT, 1 mM EDTA pH 8.0) containing the protease inhibitor mixture (Sigma-Aldrich). After sonication and sitting on ice for 20 min, the lysates were centrifuged at $14000 \times g$ for 30 min at 4°C. Protein concentrations were determined using the Bio-Rad protein assay kit (Bio-Rad, Hercules, CA, USA), with albumin as standards. Total proteins (25 μg) were electrophoresed on 10% or 12% SDS-polyacrylamide gel and transferred onto nitrocellulose membrane (Bio-Rad) by reverse electrophoresis. After being blocked, the membrane is stained with Iba1 (1 : 500; Wako, Osaka, Japan), Tau (1 : 200; Dako, Santa Clara, CA, USA), p-Tau Ser202 (1 : 200; Fremont, CA, USA), p-Tau Thr231 (1 : 500, Invitrogen), p-Tau Ser396 (1 : 500; Invitrogen), BID (1 : 1000; Cell Signaling, Danvers, MA, USA), BAD (1 : 500; Santa Cruz, Dallas, TX, USA), CYCS (1 : 500; Biovision, Milpitas, CA, USA), CASP8 (1 : 1000; Cell Signaling), DsRed

(1:500; Santa Cruz), tubulin (1:1000; Sigma-Aldrich), or GAPDH (1:1000, MDBio) primary antibodies. The immune complexes are detected using horseradish peroxidase-conjugated goat anti-mouse (Jackson ImmunoResearch, West Grove, PA, USA) or goat anti-rabbit (Rockland, Pottstown, PA, USA) IgG antibody (1:10000 dilution) and ImmobilonTM Western Chemiluminescent HRP substrate (Millipore, Billerica, MA, USA).

2.13. Caspase 3 Activity Measurement. Cells were lysed in $1 \times$ lysis buffer by repeated cycles of freezing and thawing. Caspase 3 activity was measured with the caspase 3 assay kit according to the manufacturer's instructions (Sigma-Aldrich).

2.14. Statistical Analysis. For each set of values, data are represented as mean ± SD of three independent experiments. Differences between groups were evaluated by two-tailed Student's *t*-test or ANOVA (one-way and two-way) with post hoc LSD test where appropriate. *p* values < 0.05 were considered significant.

3. Results

3.1. Formulated CHMs and Cytotoxicity. Three formulated CHMs, Bai-Shao, Gan-Cao, and SG-Tang were studied. To examine the cytotoxicity of these CHM formulas, MTT assay was performed on HEK-293 or SH-SY5Y cells after treatment with the tested formulas for 24 h. As shown in Figure 1(a), Bai-Shao, Gan-Cao, and SG-Tang exhibited very low cytotoxicity in HEK-293 and SH-SY5Y cells.

Next, the amounts of active constituents, paeoniflorin and ammonium glycyrrhizinate, in these CHM formulas were analyzed by full-spectrum analytic HPLC. As shown in Figure 1(b), chromatographic patterns showed peaks at 230 and 250 nm corresponding to the retention time compatible with paeoniflorin and ammonium glycyrrhizinate, respectively. The amounts of active constituents in these CHM formulas (0.5 g/ml) were 4.06% (42.25 mM) for paeoniflorin in Bai-Shao, 5.78% (34.41 mM) for ammonium glycyrrhizinate in Gan-Cao, and 2.81% (29.33 mM) for paeoniflorin and 2.43% (14.52 mM) for ammonium glycyrrhizinate in SG-Tang.

3.2. Radical-Scavenging Activity and Anti-Inflammatory Activity of the Tested Formulas. To evaluate the radical-scavenging activity of these CHM formulas, DPPH scavenging assay was conducted. As shown in Figure 2(a), Bai-Shao, Gan-Cao, and SG-Tang displayed free radical-scavenging activities with EC_{50} at 305 μg/ml, 794 μg/ml, and 292 μg/ml, respectively, indicating SG-Tang has a greater radical-scavenging activity than Bai-Shao or Gan-Cao. The anti-inflammatory responses of formulated CHMs were examined using RAW 264.7 cells, as LPS induced NO, TNF-α, and IL-6 production in murine macrophages [29, 30]. As shown in Figure 2(b), the exposure of RAW 264.7 cells to LPS resulted in a significant increase of NO, TNF-α, IL-1β, and IL-6 after 24 h of incubation (100% vs. 1~12%, *p* < 0.001). The elevations in NO, TNF-α, IL-1β, and IL-6 were reduced significantly in the presence of the nonsteroidal anti-inflammatory

drug (NSAID) celecoxib (a selective cyclooxygenase (COX) inhibitor as a positive control) (NO: 39%, *p* < 0.001; TNF-α: 23%, *p* = 0.003; IL-1β: 20%, *p* = 0.001; IL-6: 29%, *p* = 0.002). Similar inhibitory phenomena were observed in the cells treated with Gan-Cao and SG-Tang (NO: 72~16%, *p* = 0.023~<0.001; TNF-α: 66~42%, *p* = 0.044~0.001; IL-1β: 44~26%, *p* = 0.004~<0.001; IL-6: 51~20%, *p* = 0.003 ~<0.001). Our results demonstrated that formulated CHMs Gan-Cao and SG-Tang possess anti-inflammatory effects by reducing production of inflammatory mediators.

3.3. Reduction of Tau Misfolding and Promotion of Neurite Outgrowth of the Tested Formulas. Previously, we generated a proaggregant (ΔK280) tau_{RD} cell model targeting tau misfolding [27]. Inhibition of tau aggregation may improve DsRed misfolding, leading to increased fluorescence in tau_{RD}-DsRed expressing cells. Utilizing the established Tet-on ΔK280 tau_{RD}-DsRed 293 cells, Bai-Shao, Gan-Cao, and SG-Tang were tested for effects of reducing tau misfolding and antioxidation (Figure 3(a)). Fluorescent images of the cells were automatically recorded by a HCA system. As a positive control, Congo red (5~20 μM) significantly increased the ΔK280 tau_{RD}-DsRed fluorescence compared to no treatment (113~127% vs. 100%, *p* = 0.023~0.004). Significantly increased DsRed fluorescence was observed with Bai-Shao (109~117% for 100~200 μg/ml treatment, *p* = 0.028~0.023), Gan-Cao (109~123% for 50~200 μg/ml treatment, *p* = 0.017 ~0.003), and SG-Tang (108~130% for 50~200 μg/ml treatment, *p* = 0.003~ < 0.001) compared to no treatment (Figure 3(b)). Representative fluorescent images of ΔK280 tau_{RD}-DsRed cells untreated or treated with Congo red (20 μM) or SG-Tang (200 μg/ml) are shown in Figure 3(c). The results indicated that Bai-Shao, Gan-Cao, and SG-Tang reduced tau misfolding in our tauopathy 293 cell model and SG-Tang demonstrated a better antiaggregation function than Bai-Shao or Gan-Cao.

Misfolded tau may increase the production of reactive oxygen species (ROS) [31]. To examine whether these CHM formulas display antioxidative effects, ROS level was evaluated in Tet-On ΔK280 tau_{RD}-DsRed 293 cells. As Figure 3(d) shows, pretreatment with Congo red (10 μM, a positive control) or formulas (100 μg/ml) significantly reversed the ROS level elevated by misfolded tau production compared to no treatment (88~95% vs. 100%, *p* = 0.045 ~<0.001). These data showed the anti-oxidative effects of Bai-Shao, Gan-Cao, and SG-Tang, and SG-Tang possesses a greater anti-oxidative effect than Bai-Shao or Gan-Cao.

Since our study showed that SG-Tang has greater effects in free radical scavenging, antioxidation, and antiaggregation than Bai-Shao or Gan-Cao, we focused on SG-Tang treatment in subsequent experiments. The neuroprotective potential of SG-Tang was examined (Figure 4(a)). As Figure 4(b) shows, misfolded tau induction significantly reduced the length of neurites as compared to the absence of induction (93% vs. 100%, *p* = 0.030) and 20 μM Congo red (positive control) or 200 μg/ml SG-Tang pretreatment ameliorated this negative effect (103% vs. 93%, *p* = 0.041 for Congo red; 101% vs. 93%, *p* = 0.039 for SG-Tang). Representative neurite outgrowth images uninduced (− Dox), untreated

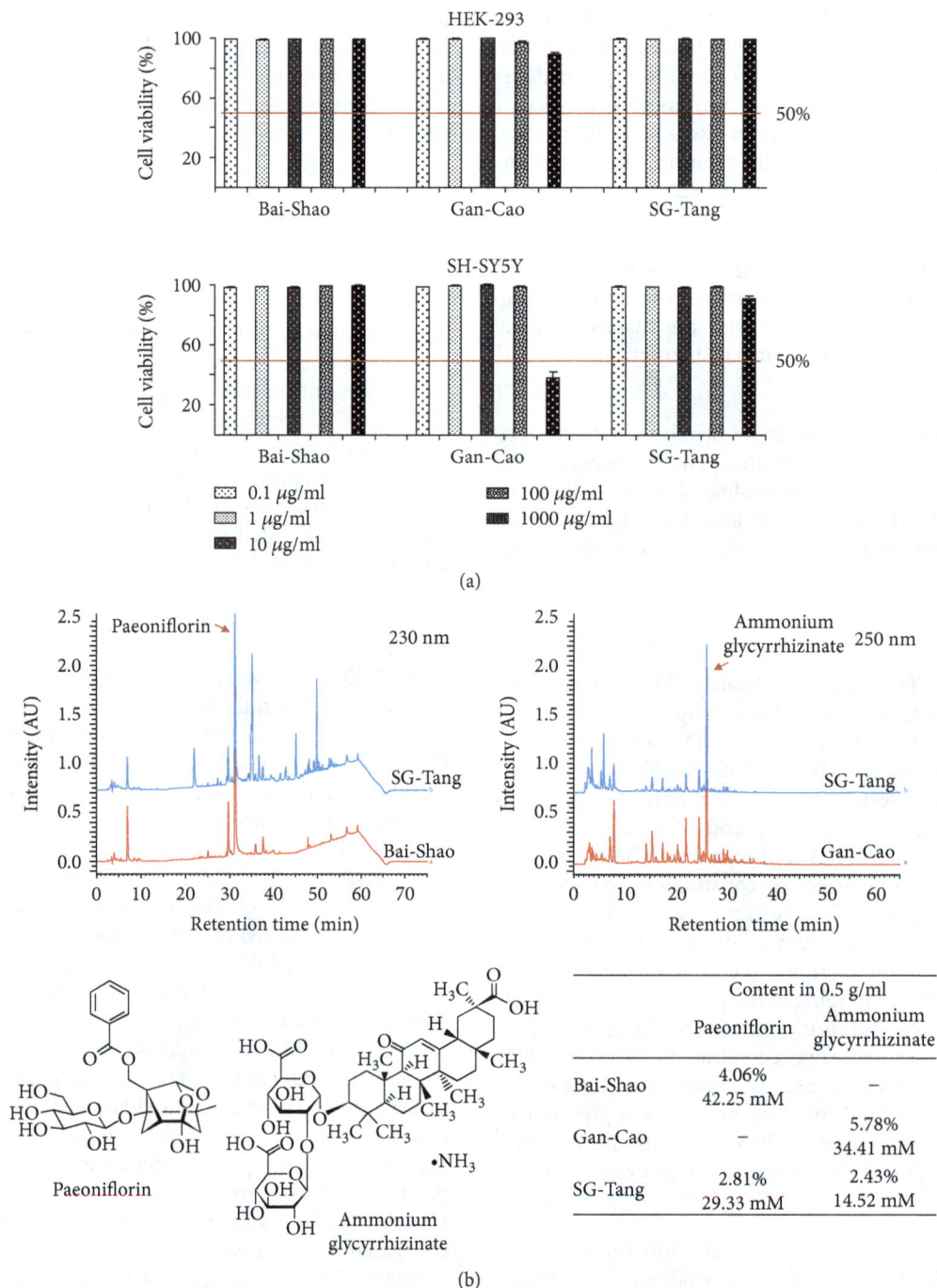

FIGURE 1: Cytotoxicity and chemical profiles of Bai-Shao, Gan-Cao, and SG-Tang. (a) MTT cell viability assay of HEK-293 and SH-SY5Y cells after treatment with Bai-Shao, Gan-Cao, and SG-Tang (0.1~1000 μg/ml) for 24 h. To normalize, the relative viability of untreated cells was set as 100%. The red line represents 50% viability. (b) HPLC analysis of Bai-Shao, Gan-Cao, and SG-Tang. Chromatographic patterns (230 and 250 nm) show peaks compatible with paeoniflorin and ammonium glycyrrhizinate. Also shown below are chemical structures of paeoniflorin and ammonium glycyrrhizinate and the relative amounts (in % and mM) of these molecules in Bai-Shao, Gan-Cao, and SG-Tang (0.5 g/ml).

(+ Dox), and after treatment with Congo red and SG-Tang are shown in Figure 4(c). Thus, SG-Tang exerts neuroprotective effect by rescuing the reduction of neurite outgrowth induced by tau misfolding.

3.4. Anti-Inflammatory Effects of SG-Tang in LPS-Stimulated BV-2 Microglia. In the brain, activated microglia release proinflammatory mediators such as NO and cytokines as a response to inflammation [32]. Thus, the anti-inflammatory effects of SG-Tang were determined using LPS-stimulated BV-2 microglia (Figure 5(a)). Figure 5(b) demonstrates that NO production of BV-2 cells significantly increased by LPS stimulation (33.9 μM vs. 4.8 μM, $p < 0.001$) and pretreatment of 100~500 μg/ml SG-Tang for 8~24 h significantly reduced

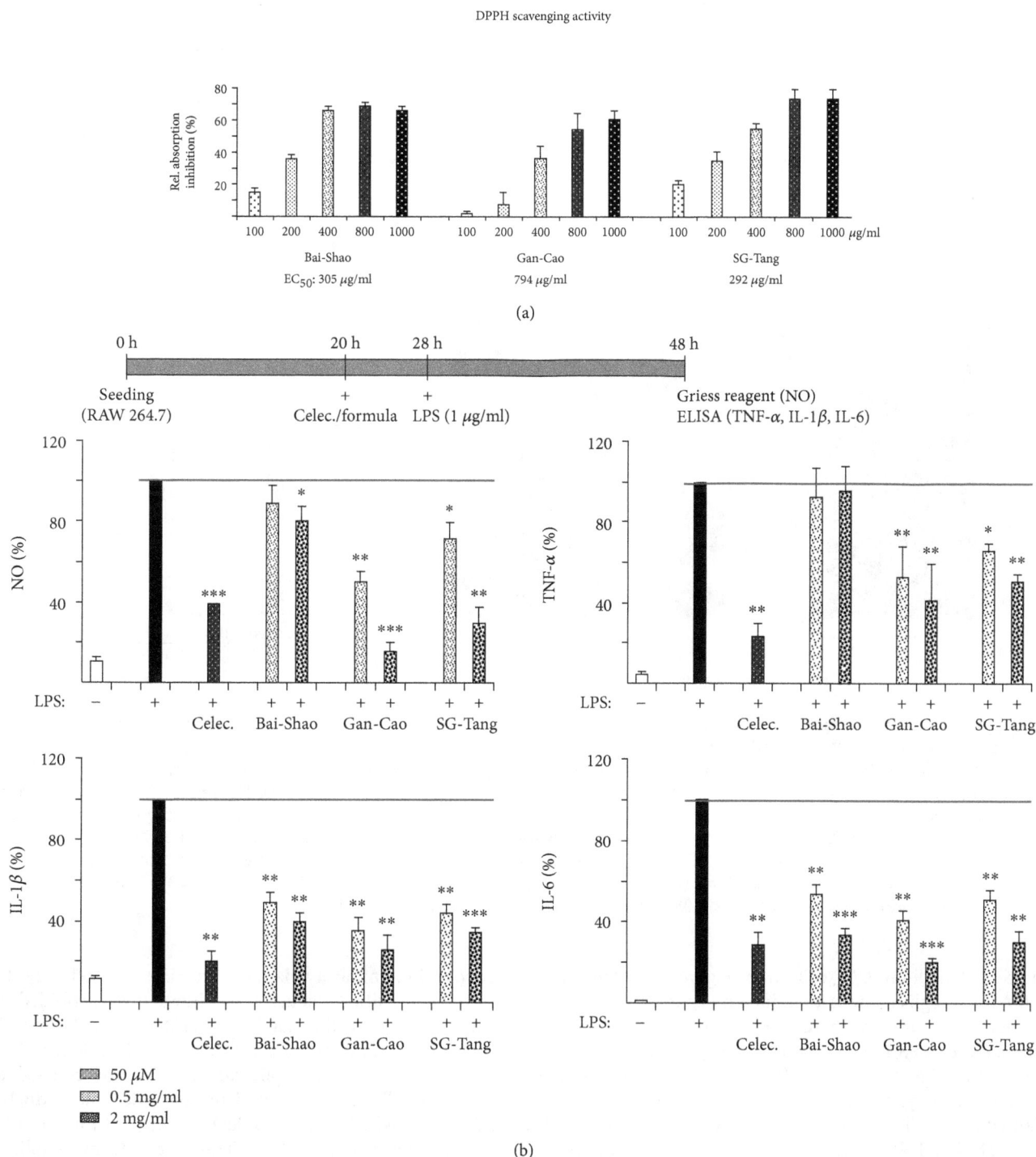

FIGURE 2: Antioxidative and anti-inflammatory activities of Bai-Shao, Gan-Cao, and SG-Tang. (a) DPPH radical-scavenging activities of the tested CHM formulas (100~1000 μg/ml). The EC_{50} of each formula is shown under the columns. (b) Anti-inflammatory activities of the tested formulas on RAW 264.7 macrophages. Cells (10^6) were pretreated with formulas (0.5~2 mg/ml) or compound celecoxib (Celec., 50 μM) as a positive control for 8 h, and LPS (1 μg/ml) was applied to induce inflammation. After 20 h, the levels of NO (assessed by Griess reagent), TNF-α, IL-1β, and IL-6 (assessed by ELISA) released into cultured media were determined ($n = 3$). For normalization, the relative NO, TNF-α, IL-1β, and IL-6 levels of LPS-treated cells were set as 100%. $^* p < 0.05$, $^{**} p < 0.01$, and $^{***} p < 0.001$, celecoxib/formulas treated vs. untreated cells.

NO production (100 μg/ml for 8 h: 23.7 μM, $p = 0.008$; 500 μg/ml for 8 h: 19.4 μM, $p = 0.002$; 100 μg/ml for 24 h: 17.5 μM, $p = 0.001$; 500 μg/ml for 24 h: 12.2 μM, $p = 0.002$).

The results indicate that SG-Tang displayed anti-inflammatory effects by reducing NO production in microglia. We then applied LPS and IFN-γ to BV-2 cells for 24 h for

(a)

(b)

(c)

(d)

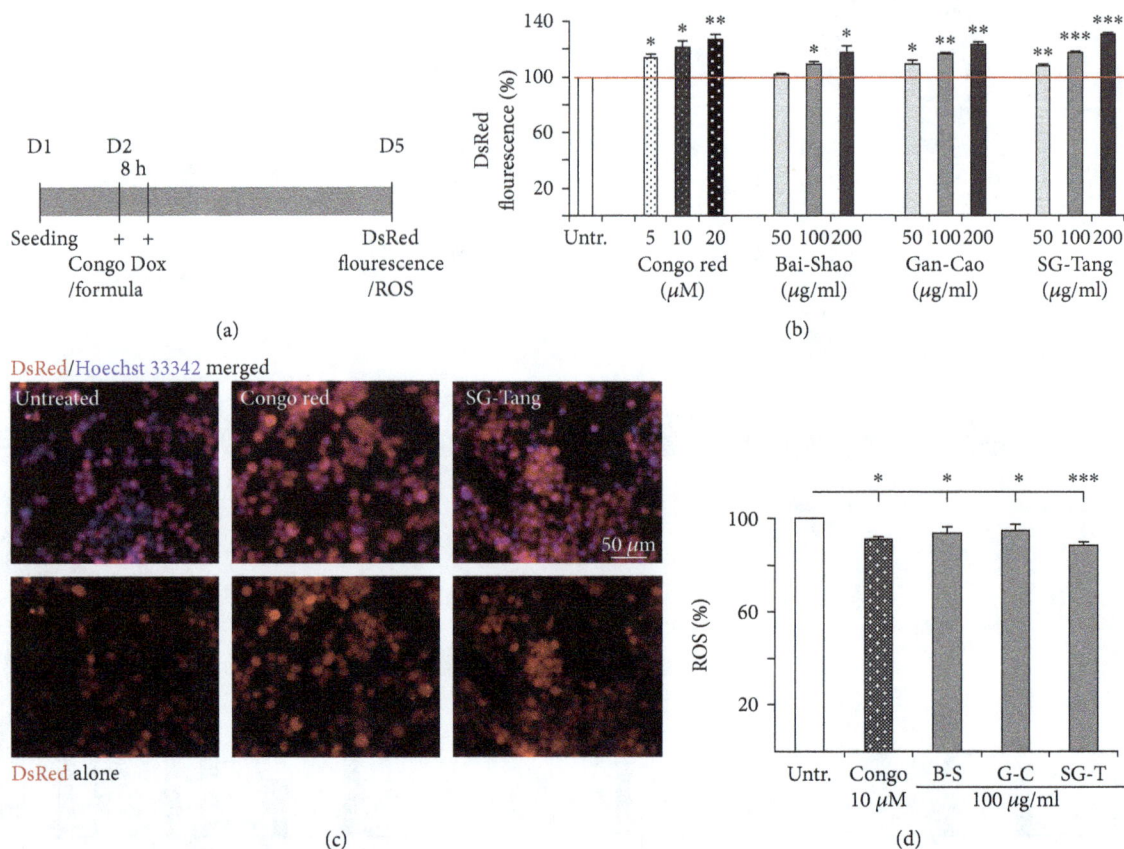

FIGURE 3: The effects of Bai-Shao, Gan-Cao, and SG-Tang on tau misfolding and ROS production in Tet-on ΔK280 tau_{RD}-DsRed 293 cells. (a) Experiment flow chart. ΔK280 tau_{RD}-DsRed 293 cells were pretreated with the tested formulas or Congo red (Congo, as a positive control) for 8 h before misfolded tau induction by doxycycline (Dox, 1 μg/ml) for three days. (b) DsRed fluorescence analysis with Congo red (5~20 μM) or the Chinese medicine formulas Bai-Shao, Gan-Cao, and SG-Tang (50~200 μg/ml) treatment ($n = 3$). The relative DsRed fluorescence of untreated cells is normalized (100%). * $p < 0.05$, ** $p < 0.01$, and *** $p < 0.001$, treated vs. untreated cells. (c) Representative microscopy images (upper row: merged DsRed and Hoechst 33342 signals; low row: DsRed signal alone) of ΔK280 tau_{RD}-DsRed 293 cells untreated or treated with Congo red (20 μM) or SG-Tang (200 μg/ml). (d) ROS assay of ΔK280 tau_{RD}-DsRed 293 cells untreated or treated with Congo red (10 μM) or the tested formulas Bai-Shao (B-S), Gan-Cao (G-C), and SG-Tang (SG-T) (100 μg/ml) ($n = 3$). The relative ROS of untreated cells was normalized as 100%. * $p < 0.05$ and *** $p < 0.001$, treated vs. untreated cells.

conditioned medium (CM) collection (Figure 5(b)). The resting BV-2 microglia showed a ramified morphology but more extended processes with elongated morphology were observed after LPS/IFN-γ treatment for 24 h (Figure 5(d)). As shown in Figures 5(e) and 5(f), elevated Iba1 (induction of brown adipocytes 1, a microglial marker) expression in inflamed BV-2 cells (100% vs. 240%, $p = 0.042$) and increased release of NO, TNF-α, IL-1β, and IL-6 in BV-2 CM (NO: 0.5 μM vs. 49.6 μM, $p = 0.001$; TNF-α: 0.9 ng/ml vs. 28.1 ng/ml, $p = 0.002$; IL-1β: 2.9 pg/ml vs. 8.9 pg/ml, $p < 0.001$; IL-6: 0 ng/ml vs. 33.6 ng/ml, $p = 0.021$) were confirmed. The collected CM was then used to provide inflammatory mediators to ΔK280 tau_{RD}-DsRed SH-SY5Y cells.

3.5. Effects of SG-Tang on BV-2 Conditioned Medium-Inflamed ΔK280 tau_{RD}-DsRed SH-SY5Y Cells. Undifferentiated (without retinoic acid, − RA) or differentiated (with retinoic acid, + RA) ΔK280 tau_{RD}-DsRed SH-SY5Y cells were pretreated with SG-Tang (200 μg/ml) for 8 h before misfolded tau induction and then BV-2 CM was added to

provoke inflammatory damage on SH-SY5Y cells for two days (Figure 6(a)). Figure 6(b) shows that misfolded tau induction reduced the viability of ΔK280 tau_{RD}-DsRed SH-SY5Y cells (− RA: 91% vs. 100%, $p = 0.012$; + RA: 90% vs. 100%, $p = 0.035$) and application of SG-Tang rescued the decreased cell viability caused by misfolded tau induction and BV-2 CM addition (− RA: 122% vs. 88%, $p = 0.015$; + RA: 122% vs. 91%, $p = 0.014$). Thus, the reduced viability of inflamed ΔK280 tau_{RD}-DsRed SH-SY5Y cells was not influenced by retinoic acid.

Differentiated SH-SY5Y cells expressing ΔK280 tau_{RD}-DsRed were further evaluated on day 8 for LDH release, neurite outgrowth, and tau phosphorylation (Figure 6(c)). Both addition of Dox (118% vs. 100%, $p = 0.019$) and BV-2 CM (184% vs. 118%, $p < 0.001$) increased the LDH release of ΔK280 tau_{RD}-DsRed SH-SY5Y cells and application of SG-Tang attenuated the LDH release (156% vs. 184%, $p = 0.010$) (Figure 6(d)). Misfolded tau induction significantly reduced the length of neurites compared to the uninduced cells (94% vs. 100%, $p = 0.005$), and addition of BV-2 CM

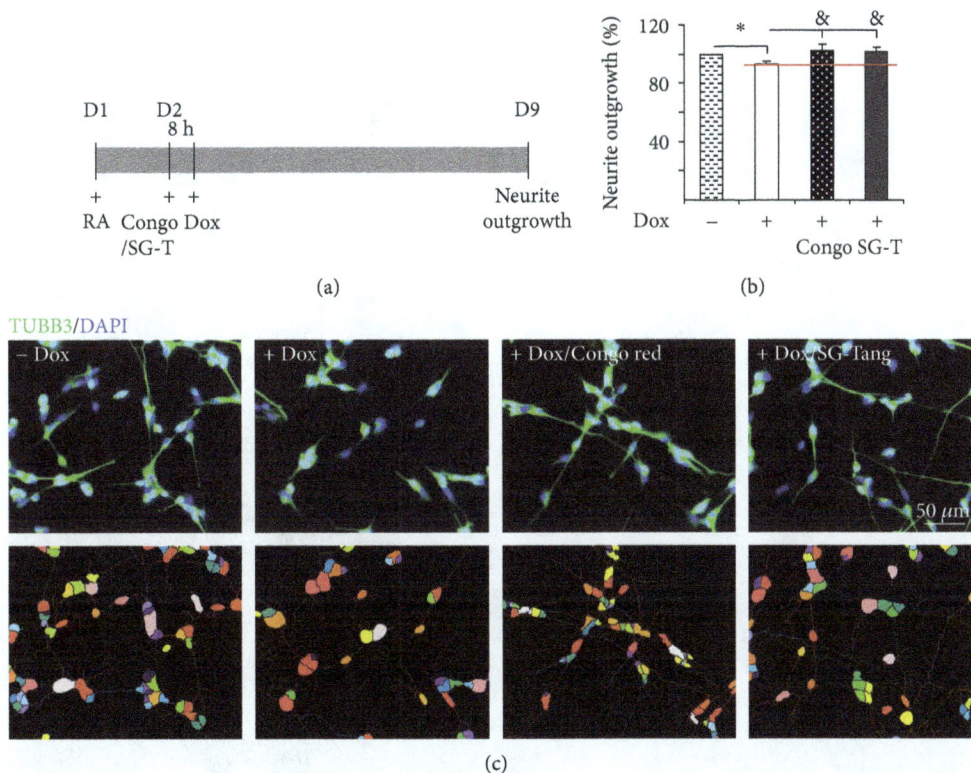

FIGURE 4: The effects of Bai-Shao, Gan-Cao and SG-Tang on neurite outgrowth in Tet-on ΔK280 tau$_{RD}$-DsRed SH-SY5Y cells. (a) Experiment flow chart. ΔK280 tau$_{RD}$-DsRed SH-SY5Y cells were seeded in 24-well (3×10^4/well) plate with all *trans* retinoic acid (RA, $10\,\mu M$). On day 2, cells were treated with Congo red ($20\,\mu M$) or SG-Tang ($200\,\mu g/ml$) for 8 h, induced tau$_{RD}$-DsRed expression with doxycycline (Dox, $1\,\mu g/ml$), and neurite outgrowth assayed on day 9. (b) Neurite outgrowth assay ($n = 3$) with Congo red or SG-Tang (SG-T) treatment. To normalize, the relative neurite outgrowth of untreated cells is set as 100%. $^*p < 0.05$, induced vs. un-induced cells; $^\&p < 0.05$, treated vs. untreated cells. (c) Representative microscopy images of neuronally differentiated ΔK280 tau$_{RD}$-DsRed SH-SY5Y cells uninduced (− Dox), untreated (+ Dox), and after treatment with Congo red (+ Dox/Congo red) or SG-Tang (+ Dox/SG-Tang). Neurites were stained with TUBB3 (neuronal class III β-tubulin, green) antibody. Nuclei were detected using (DAPI, blue). Upper row, merged TUBB3 and DAPI signals; lower row, images of the neurites and the body of individual cells being outlined by the same color for outgrowth quantification.

aggravated this condition (88% vs. 94%, $p < 0.001$). Pretreatment of SG-Tang resulted in significant increase of neurite outgrowth (98% vs. 88%, $p = 0.004$) (Figure 6(e)). Representative images of neurite outgrowth of the above cells are shown in Figure 6(f).

The abnormal hyperphosphorylation of tau plays a role in the molecular pathogenesis of AD and other tauopathies. Therefore, the amount of phosphorylated tau was examined and Western blot showed that misfolded tau induction increased tau phosphorylation at residue Ser202, Thr231, and Ser396 compared to uninduced cells (Ser202: 130% vs. 100%, $p = 0.020$; Thr231: 119% vs. 100%, $p = 0.016$; Ser396: 127% vs. 100%, $p = 0.012$). Although addition of BV-2 CM in misfolded tau-expressing cells did not cause further increase of tau phosphorylation at Ser202, Thr231, and Ser396, pretreatment of SG-Tang could reverse abnormal tau hyperphosphorylation at Ser202 (76% vs. 107%, $p = 0.022$) and Thr231 (79% vs. 122%, $p = 0.021$) (Figure 6(g)). Our results demonstrate that SG-Tang could protect cells from cell death, increase neurite outgrowth, and reduce hyperphosphorylation of tau in inflamed misfolded tau-expressing ΔK280 tau$_{RD}$-DsRed cells.

3.6. Identification of SG-Tang Targets by Human Apoptosis Antibody Array.

TNF-α has been long considered as an effecter of inflammation-induced cell death. It has been shown that TNF-α binds to receptor TNFR1 to permit the release of silencer of death domain (SODD) and the recruitment of intracellular death signaling inducing signaling complex (DISC) proteins, including TNFR-associated death domain protein (TRADD) and Fas-associated protein with death domain (FADD), which then activates caspase 8 leading to apoptosis [33]. Caspase 8 is also a key mediator of inflammation and processing of pro-IL-1β to IL-1β [34]. Since we have found SG-Tang decreased TNF-α and IL-1β in CM of BV-2, we proposed that SG-Tang may also act on the inflammation-induced cell death. To elucidate the molecular mechanisms underlying the rescue from inflammation-induced cell death by SG-Tang, proteins from uninduced (− Dox), induced (+ Dox), inflamed (+ Dox/CM), and SG-Tang-pretreated inflamed (+ Dox/CM/SG-Tang) ΔK280 tau$_{RD}$-DsRed SH-SY5Y cells were examined by using human apoptosis array to evaluate expression levels of 43 apoptosis-related proteins (Figure 7(a)). Among these targets, expression of proapoptotic Bcl2-associated agonist of cell death

(a)

(b)

(c)

(d)

(e)

(f)

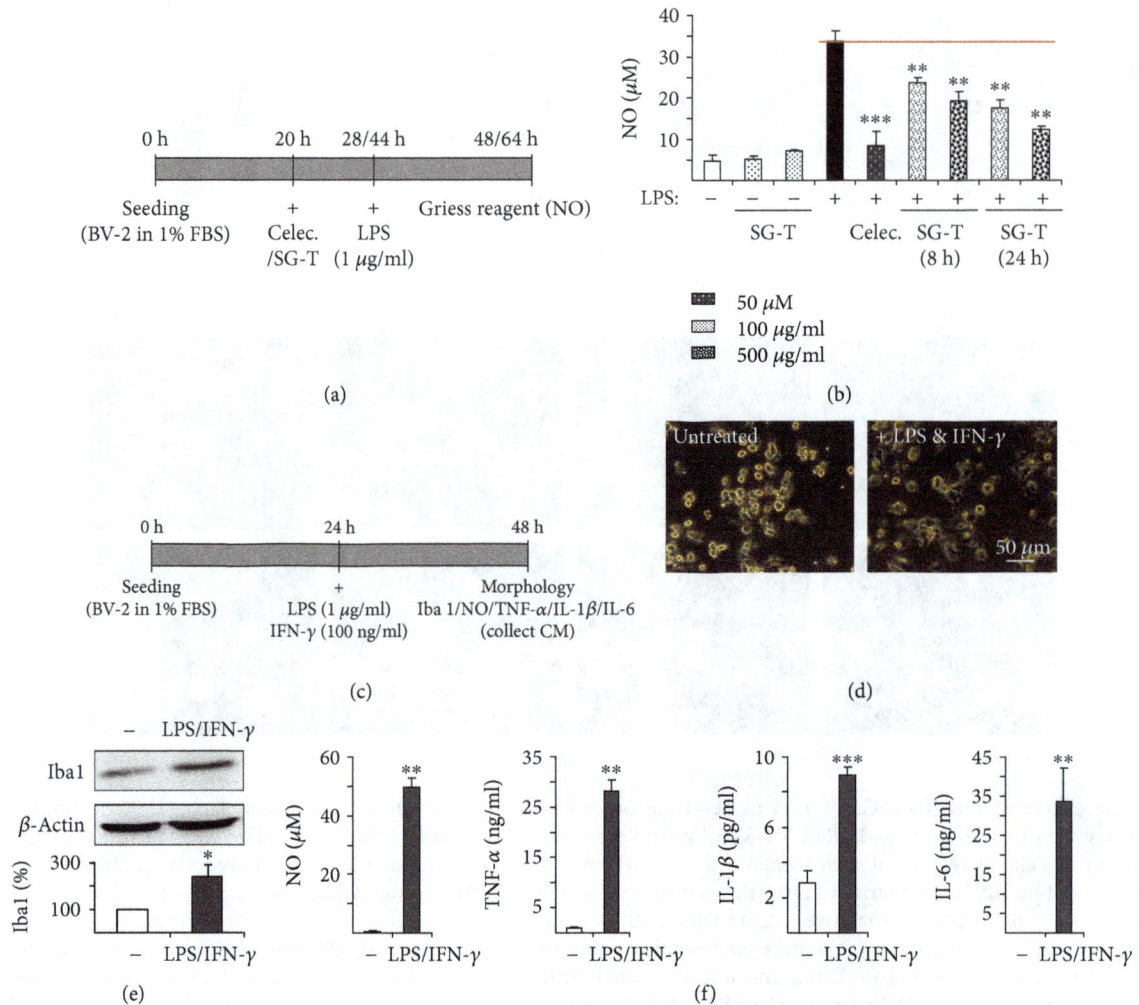

FIGURE 5: Anti-inflammatory effects of SG-Tang and BV-2 conditioned medium preparation. (a) Experiment flow chart for LPS stimulation. BV-2 cells were seeded in 1% fetal bovine serum (FBS) and pretreated with $50 \mu M$ celecoxib (Celec.) for 8 h or $100 \sim 500 \mu g/ml$ SG-Tang (SG-T) $8 \sim 24$ h followed by $1 \mu g/ml$ LPS stimulation 20 h. NO level was evaluated with Griess reagent. (b) Anti-inflammatory effect of celecoxib (Celec.) and SG-Tang (SG-T) on BV-2 cells ($n = 3$). $^{**} p < 0.01$ and $^{***} p < 0.001$, treated vs. untreated cells. (c) Experiment flow chart for LPS/IFN-γ stimulation. For preparation of BV-2 conditioned medium (CM), BV-2 cells were seeded in Dulbecco's modified Eagle's medium (DMEM) with 1% FBS medium. Next day, cells were stimulated with a combination of LPS ($1 \mu g/ml$) and IFN-γ (100 ng/ml). After 24 h stimulation, the BV-2 CM was collected and examined for inflammation by morphology, Iba1 Western blotting and NO/TNF-α/IL-1β/IL-6 determination. (d) Morphology of BV-2 cells. (e) Western blot analysis of Iba1 expression in inflamed BV-2 cells ($n = 3$). To normalize, Iba1 expression level in uninflamed cells was set as 100%. $^{*} p < 0.05$, stimulated vs. unstimulated cells. (f) Secretion of NO, TNF-α, IL-1β, and IL-6 in BV-2 CM. $^{**} p < 0.01$ and $^{***} p < 0.001$, stimulated vs. unstimulated cells.

(BAD), BH3-interacting domain death agonist (BID), caspase 3 (CASP3), caspase 8 (CASP8) and cytochrome c, and somatic (CYCS) were apparently reduced by SG-Tang treatment (Table 1). Western blot analysis of BAD, BID, CASP8, and CYCS expression changes and caspase 3 activity assay further confirmed that pretreatment of SG-Tang could significantly decrease these identified targets (BAD: from 228% to 157%, $p = 0.023$; BID: from 139% to 110%, $p = 0.038$; CASP8: from 118% to 104%, $p = 0.024$; CYCS: from 163% to 96%, $p = 0.040$; caspase 3 activity: from 165% to 103%, $p = 0.005$). Moreover, addition of SG-Tang improved ΔK280 tau$_{RD}$-DsRed misfolding and enhanced soluble tau$_{RD}$-DsRed protein level in inflamed ΔK280 tau$_{RD}$-DsRed SH-SY5Y cells (from 90% to 115%, $p = 0.004$) (Figure 7(b)). Our results indicated that SG-Tang may protect inflamed

ΔK280 tau$_{RD}$-DsRed SH-SY5Y cells by inhibiting production of proapoptotic proteins.

4. Discussion

In this study, we demonstrated neuroprotection, antioxidative and anti-inflammatory effects of formulated CHM SG-Tang. Our results showed that SG-Tang displayed a greater antioxidative and antiaggregation effect than Bai-Shao and Gan-Cao and a stronger anti-inflammatory activity than Bai-Shao but similar to Gan-Cao (Figures 2 and 3). Moreover, SG-Tang showed neuroprotective effect of promoting neurite outgrowth probably by ameliorating tau misfolding and oxidative stress in our tauopathy model (Figures 3 and 4). The anti-inflammatory effects of SG-Tang were further

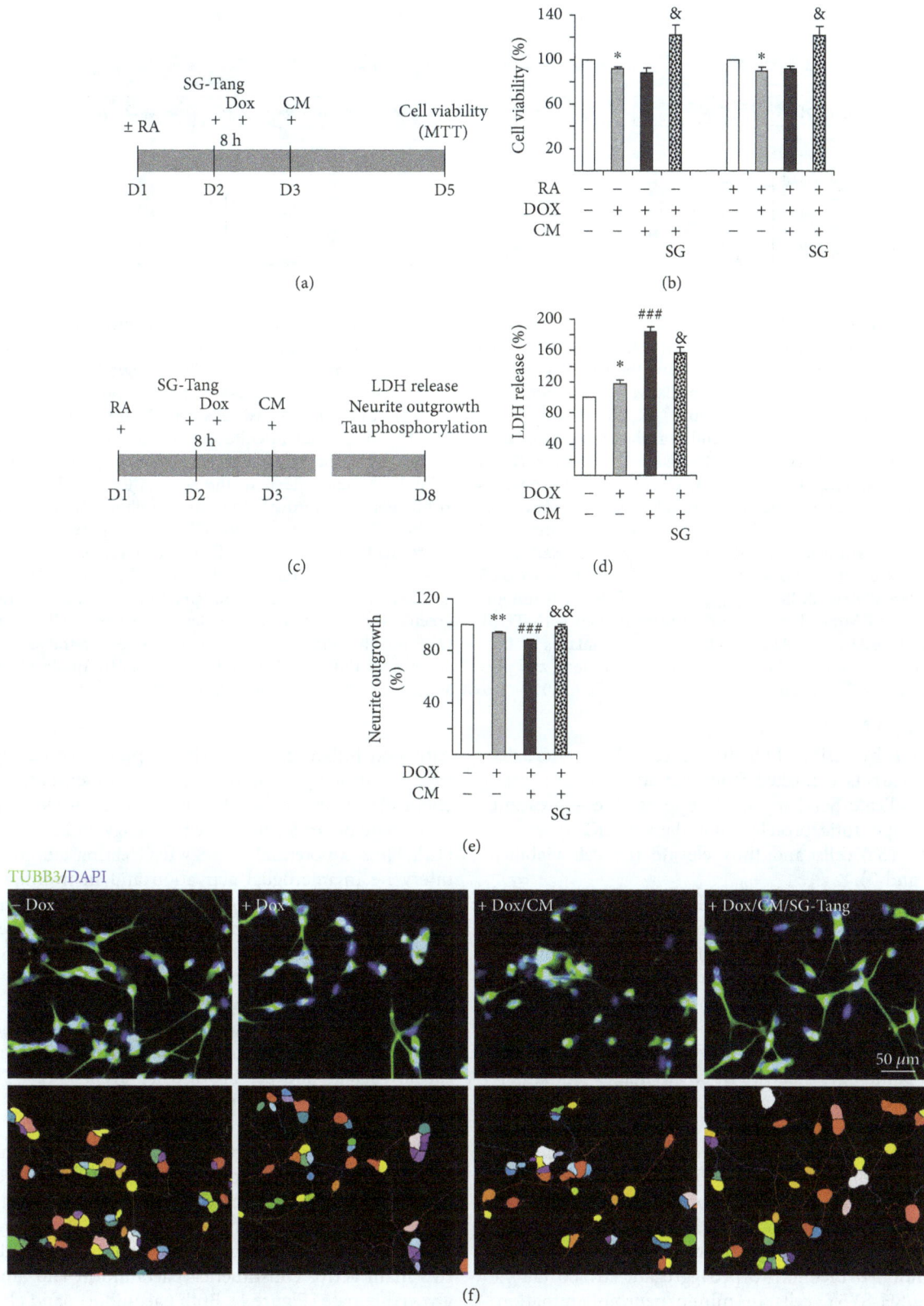

(a)

(b)

(c)

(d)

(e)

TUBB3/DAPI

(f)

FIGURE 6: Continued.

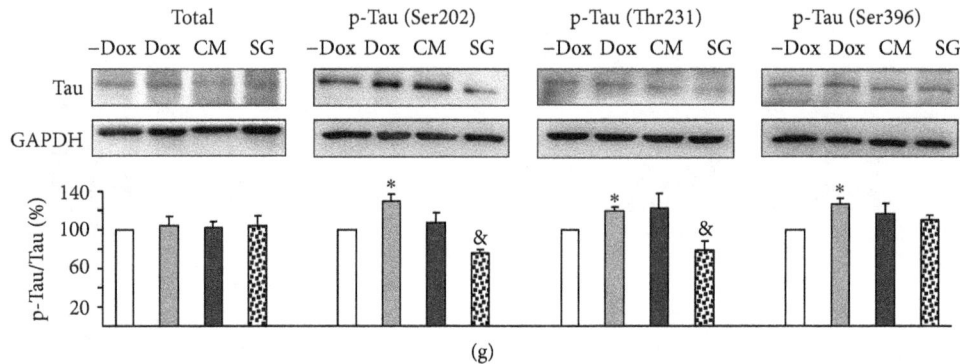

FIGURE 6: Neuroprotection of SG-Tang on ΔK280 tau$_{RD}$-DsRed SH-SY5Y cells from BV-2 conditioned medium-induced cell death. (a) Experiment flow chart for cell viability assay. ΔK280 tau$_{RD}$-DsRed SH-SY5Y cells were plated in media with/without retinoic acid ($\pm$ RA, 10 μM) on day 1 and pretreated with SG-Tang the next day for 8 h, followed by doxycycline addition (Dox, 1 μg/ml) to induce misfolded tau expression. On day 3, DMEM-F12 media was mixed with BV-2 CM and cell viability was assessed by MTT assay on day 5. (b) Cell viability assay (* $p < 0.05$, $-$ Dox vs. $+$ Dox; $^{\&}p < 0.05$, $+$ Dox/CM vs. $+$ Dox/CM/SG-Tang-treated cells) ($n = 3$). (c) Experiment flow chart for LDH release, neurite outgrowth, and tau phosphorylation assays. RA (10 μM, present in cultures throughout) differentiated ΔK280 tau$_{RD}$-DsRed SH-SY5Y cells were pretreated with SG-Tang (200 μg/ml) on day 2 for 8 h, followed by inducing ΔK280 tau$_{RD}$-DsRed expression ($+$ Dox, 1 μg/ml). On day 3, DMEM-F12 was mixed with BV-2 CM and added to the cells. After five days, media were collected for LDH release examination. In addition, cells were examined for neurite outgrowth and tau phosphorylation. (d) LDH assay (*$p < 0.05$, $-$ Dox vs. $+$ Dox; $^{\#\#\#}p < 0.001$, $+$ Dox vs. $+$Dox/CM; $^{\&}p < 0.05$, $+$ Dox/CM vs. $+$ Dox/CM/SG-Tang treated cells) ($n = 3$). (e) Neurite outgrowth assay ($n = 3$). To normalize, the relative neurite outgrowth of uninduced cells is set as 100%. ** $p < 0.01$, $-$ Dox vs. $+$ Dox; $^{\#\#\#}p < 0.001$, $+$ Dox vs. $+$ Dox/CM; $^{\&\&}p < 0.01$, $+$ Dox/CM vs. $+$ Dox/CM/SG-Tang-treated cells. (f) Representative microscopy images of differentiated ΔK280 tau$_{RD}$-DsRed SH-SY5Y cells uninduced ($-$ Dox), induced ($+$ Dox), inflamed ($+$ Dox/CM), or treated with SG-Tang ($+$ Dox/CM/SG-Tang). Neurites were stained with TUBB3 (green) antibody. Nuclei were detected using DAPI (blue). Upper row, merged TUBB3 and DAPI signals; lower row, images of the neurites and the body of a cell being outlined by the same color for outgrowth quantification. (g) Western blot analysis of total and phosphorylated (Ser202, Thr231, and Ser396) tau (normalized to GAPDH internal control, $n = 3$). * $p < 0.05$, $-$ Dox vs. $+$ Dox; $^{\&}p < 0.05$, $+$ Dox/CM vs. $+$ Dox/CM/SG-Tang-treated cells.

demonstrated by using LPS-stimulated BV-2 microglia (Figure 5). Targets identified from human apoptosis protein array indicate SG-Tang may suppress the expression levels of proapoptotic proteins in inflamed ΔK280 tau$_{RD}$-DsRed SH-SY5Y cells and thus elevate the cell viability (Figures 6 and 7).

In human tauopathy, substantial activated microglia are found in regions of phosphorylated tau accumulation [35]. In tau P301S transgenic mice, prominent glial activation precedes tangle formation and the pattern of activated glia correlates closely with the distribution and density of NFTs [36]. As neuroinflammation is linked to the progression of tauopathy, anti-inflammatory strategy may be effective at reducing tau-related pathology. Indeed, FK506 attenuates tau pathology and increased lifespan in tau P301S mouse model [36]. Treatment of 3xTg-AD mice with anti-inflammatory drug ibuprofen reduces tau phosphorylation and memory impairment [37]. Administration of potent anti-inflammatory minocycline reduces the development of disease-associated tau species in the htau mouse model [38] by reducing several inflammatory factors [39]. In the present study, we applied BV-2 conditioned medium to proaggregant ΔK280 tau$_{RD}$-DsRed 293/SH-SY5Y cells to mimic neuroinflammation. The study results reveal that CHM formula SG-Tang displays neuroprotection by exerting anti-inflammatory and antiapoptotic activities.

Inflammation is a double-edged sword. Inflammatory response could lead to activation of immune system and elimination of pathogens thereby reducing further cell loss.

Although inflammation might be protective and beneficial to cells, prolonged or dysregulated inflammatory process could also result in production of neurotoxic factors that exacerbate neurodegenerative pathology and cause cell death [12]. Thus, a potential strategy for treating tauopathies is to intervene in microglial activation and neuroinflammation. NSAID has been commonly used as treatment of inflammation and known to be neuroprotective [40]. The mechanism of NSAID has been shown to inhibit the synthesis or activity of inflammatory mediators such as prostaglandin and COX isoforms 1 and 2. Although NSAID could effectively suppress the inflammatory symptoms, these agents may also induce significant side effects such as increased risk of thrombotic cardiovascular and cerebrovascular events [41]. Therefore, more safely, anti-inflammatory drugs need to be explored and developed.

There is a growing interest in natural compounds/products with anti-inflammatory activities which have long been used for treating inflammation-related diseases. In this study, SG-Tang used was formulated with Bai-Shao (*P. lactiflora*) and Gan-Cao (*G. uralensis*) and analyzed by HPLC using two main active constituents, paeoniflorin and ammonium glycyrrhizinate (Figure 1). Both paeoniflorin and glycyrrhizinic acid were demonstrated to be able to cross the blood-brain barrier (BBB) in middle cerebral artery occlusion rats [42]. However, multiplicity of the components *in P. lactiflora and G. uralensis* contributes to the effects *of* antioxidation and anti-inflammation. In the root of *P. lactiflora*, a total of 40 components including 29 monoterpene glycosides,

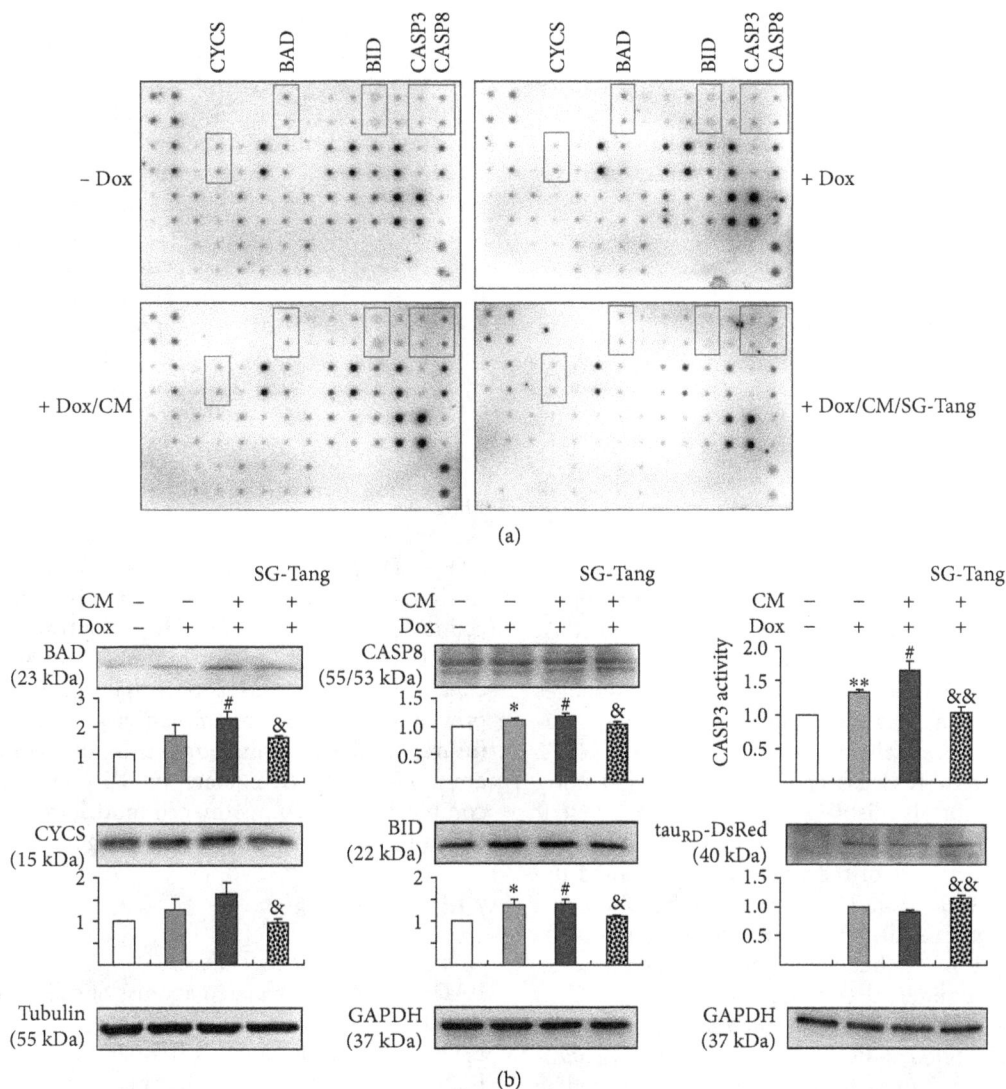

FIGURE 7: Apoptosis-related protein targets of SG-Tang in BV-2 conditioned medium-stimulated ΔK280 tau$_{RD}$-DsRed SH-SY5Y cells. (a) Representative images of apoptosis antibody array of proteins collected from Figure 6(c). (b) Western blot analysis of BAD, CYCS, CASP8, BID, and tau$_{RD}$-DsRed protein levels (normalized to tubulin or GAPDH internal control, $n = 3$) and caspase 3 activity assay from each sample. $^*p < 0.05$ and $^{**}p < 0.01$, − Dox vs. + Dox; $^{\#}p < 0.05$, + Dox vs. + Dox/CM; $^{\&}p < 0.05$ and $^{\&\&}p < 0.01$, + Dox/CM vs. + Dox/CM/SG-Tang-treated cells.

TABLE 1: Proteins identified by human apoptosis antibody array.

Gene symbol	UniProt accession number	Protein	Fold change (+ Dox/CM vs. − Dox)	Fold change (+ Dox/CM/SG-T vs. + Dox/CM)
BAD	Q92934	Bcl2-associated agonist of cell death	1.16	0.63
BID	P55957	BH3-interacting domain death agonist	1.33	0.41
CASP3	P42574	Caspase 3	1.49	0.71
CASP8	Q14790	Caspase 8	1.34	0.62
CYCS	P99999	Cytochrome c, somatic	0.92	0.62

8 galloyl glucoses, and 3 phenolic compounds were identified [43]. Among them, paeoniflorin, a monoterpene glycoside, is known to possess anti-inflammatory effect and has been applied to cerebral ischemic injury [44]. Paeoniflorin also exhibits neuroprotective effects via inhibiting

neuroinflammation in APP/PS1 and in PS2 mutant mice [45, 46]. Paeoniflorin and the isomer albiflorin attenuated neuropathic pain by inhibiting the activation of p38 MAPK pathway in spinal microglia and subsequent upregulated IL-1β and TNF-α [47]. Benzoylpaeoniflorin, another paeoniflorin-related glycoside in *P. lactiflora* root, protected primary rat cortical cells against H$_2$O$_2$-induced oxidative stress [48]. In addition to monoterpene glycosides, gallic acid, a phenolic compound in *P. lactiflora* root, displayed antioxidative effect by scavenging free radicals, inhibiting lipid peroxidation, and protecting against oxidative DNA damage [49]. Paeonol, another phenolic compound in *P. lactiflora* root, exerted neuroprotective effect in the model of ischemia through reducing proinflammatory receptors/mediators [50].

The main bioactive components of *G. uralensis* are triterpene saponins and various types of flavonoids, including glycyrrhetinic acid, glycyrrhizic acid, liquiritigenin, isoliquiritigenin, liquiritin, and licochalcone A [51]. Glycyrrhizin and related compounds were found to show anti-inflammatory activity *in vitro* [52] and *in vivo* [53]. Although diammonium glycyrrhizinate rescues neurotoxicity in Aβ$_{1-42}$-induced mice [54], its effect in tauopathy models is not known. Isoliquiritigenin, isoliquiritin, and liquiritigenin significantly suppressed iNOS, TNF-α, and IL-6 expression in IL-1β-treated rat hepatocytes [55]. Interestingly, the purified glycyrrhiza polysaccharides increased the pinocytic activity, the production of NO, IL-1, IL-6, and IL-12 in macrophages of mice [56]. Glycyrrhetinic acid, liquiritigenin, isoliquiritigenin, and liquiritin were also found to be all potent NRF2 inducers [57]. Moreover, Calzia et al. has shown that polyphenolic phytochemicals displayed a potent antioxidant action by modulating the ectopic F$_0$F$_1$-ATP synthase activity of the rod outer segments of the retina and prevented the induction of apoptosis [58]. Therefore, polyphenolic compounds from Bai-Shao and Gan-Cao may also exert antioxidative activities not only in but also outside of mitochondria. Given that multiple different compounds in both Bai-Shao and Gan-Cao are exerting effects on different pathways, the combination of Bai-Shao and Gan-Cao may thus have additive protection effects than each alone, which is supported by our study results.

The anti-inflammatory effect of Jakyakgamcho-tang, a formulated *P. lactiflora* and *G. uralensis* in Korea, has been shown by inhibiting the NF-κB signaling pathway in keratinocytes [59]. Aberrant activation of NF-κB signaling may lead to apoptosis and cell death [60]. We found that several proapoptotic proteins including BAD, BID, CASP3, CASP8, and CYCS were induced by misfolded tau expression and/or caused by LPS/IFN-γ-stimulated BV2 microglia. BAD protein is a proapoptotic member of the Bcl-2 gene family involved in initiating apoptosis [61]. BID is also a proapoptotic protein which plays a role as a sentinel for protease-mediated death signals [62]. Caspases are well-studied important mediators of apoptosis. CYCS is known to be released from mitochondria into cytosol to stimulate cell apoptosis [63]. Administration of SG-Tang decreased the production of these proapoptotic proteins, indicating that SG-Tang may target on inhibiting proapoptotic proteins to protect neuron cells from inflammatory damage.

Finally, pretreatment of SG-Tang reversed abnormal hyperphosphorylation at tau Ser202 and Thr231 in inflamed misfolded tau-expressing SH-SY5Y cells (Figure 6). Tau function is regulated by phosphorylation at specific sites,

and tau phosphorylation plays both physiological and pathological roles in the cells. Tau Ser199/202 and Thr205 were found to be locally phosphorylated along the nascent axon during axonogenesis [64]. Phosphorylation of tau Thr231 inhibited tau to bind and stabilize microtubules [65]. Both Ser202 and Thr231 are hyperphosphorylated in degenerating AD brain [66]. Among kinases that regulate tau Ser202 and Thr231 phosphorylation, cyclic AMP-dependent protein kinase (PKA) and cyclin-dependent kinase 2 (CDC2) might be the potential targets of SG-Tang, and SG-Tang treatment may result in activity suppression of these two kinases [66, 67]. The exact mechanism for PKA or CDC2 regulation by SG-Tang remains to be determined in our future work.

5. Conclusions

Plant-derived natural medications have been used for centuries and becoming more popular because of their low side effects. Despite the fact that natural compounds are relatively safe, the complexity of natural products makes nutraceutical preparations difficult to be appropriately designed. In this study, we showed antioxidative and anti-inflammatory effects of SG-Tang as a potential agent for treatment or prevention of neuroinflammation-associated tauopathy. In future, studies of main active compounds paeoniflorin and ammonium glycyrrhizinate in SG-Tang, separately or in combination, in tauopathy cell model are warranted to provide a novel avenue for protection against tauopathy.

Abbreviations

AD:	Alzheimer's disease
BAD:	Bcl2-associated agonist of cell death
BBB:	Blood-brain barrier
BID:	BH3-interacting domain death agonist
BSA:	Bovine serum albumin
CASP3:	Caspase 3
CASP8:	Caspase 8
CDC2:	Cyclin-dependent kinase 2
CHM:	Chinese herbal medicine
CM:	Conditioned medium
CNS:	Central nervous system
COX:	Cyclooxygenase
CYCS:	Cytochrome c, somatic
DAPI:	4'-6-Diamidino-2-phenylindole
Dox:	Doxycycline
DMEM:	Dulbecco's modified Eagle's medium
DPPH:	1,1-Diphenyl-2-picrylhydrazyl
EC$_{50}$:	Half maximal effective concentration
ELISA:	Enzyme-linked immunosorbent assay
FBS:	Fetal bovine serum
HCA:	High-content analysis
HPLC:	High-performance liquid chromatography
Iba1:	Induction of brown adipocytes 1
IC$_{50}$:	Half maximal inhibitory concentration
IFN:	Interferon
IL:	Interleukin
LDH:	Lactate dehydrogenase
LPS:	Lipopolysaccharide

MTT: 3-(4,5-Dimethylthiazol-2-yl)-2,5-diphenyltetrazolium bromide
NO: Nitric oxide
NSAID: Nonsteroidal anti-inflammatory drug
PKA: Cyclic AMP-dependent protein kinase
ROS: Reactive oxygen species
SG-Tang: Shaoyao Gancao Tang
tau_{RD}: Tau repeat domain
TNF: Tumor necrosis factor.

Authors' Contributions

Guey-Jen Lee-Chen and Chiung-Mei Chen designed the research and revised the paper. I-Cheng Chen performed the experiments, analyzed the data, and wrote the manuscript. Te-Hsien Lin conducted experiments and analyzed the data. Yu-Hsuan Hsieh and Chih-Ying Chao performed experiments and assisted in the technical work. Yih-Ru Wu and Kuo-Hsuan Chang commented on the experiment design. Ming-Chung Lee provided CHM materials for this study. All authors approved the final version of the manuscript. I-Cheng Chen and Te-Hsien Lin contributed equally to this work.

Acknowledgments

This work was supported by the grants from the Ministry of Science and Technology (105-2325-B-003-001) and Chang Gung Memorial Hospital (CMRPG3F136, CMRPG3F1611-2, and CMRPG3G052). We thank the Molecular Imaging Core Facility of National Taiwan Normal University for the technical assistance.

References

[1] D. R. Williams, "Tauopathies: classification and clinical update on neurodegenerative diseases associated with microtubule-associated protein tau," *Internal Medicine Journal*, vol. 36, no. 10, pp. 652–660, 2006.

[2] G. Lee and C. J. Leugers, "Tau and tauopathies," *Progress in Molecular Biology and Translational Science*, vol. 107, pp. 263–293, 2012.

[3] R. L. Neve, P. Harris, K. S. Kosik, D. M. Kurnit, and T. A. Donlon, "Identification of cDNA clones for the human microtubule-associated protein tau and chromosomal localization of the genes for tau and microtubule-associated protein 2," *Brain Research*, vol. 387, no. 3, pp. 271–280, 1986.

[4] M. Hasegawa, M. J. Smith, and M. Goedert, "Tau proteins with FTDP-17 mutations have a reduced ability to promote microtubule assembly," *FEBS Letters*, vol. 437, no. 3, pp. 207–210, 1998.

[5] P. Nacharaju, J. Lewis, C. Easson et al., "Accelerated filament formation from tau protein with specific FTDP-17 missense mutations," *FEBS Letters*, vol. 447, no. 2-3, pp. 195–199, 1999.

[6] I. D'Souza, P. Poorkaj, M. Hong et al., "Missense and silent tau gene mutations cause frontotemporal dementia with parkinsonism-chromosome 17 type, by affecting multiple alternative RNA splicing regulatory elements," *Proceedings of the National Academy of Sciences of the United States of America*, vol. 96, no. 10, pp. 5598–5603, 1999.

[7] P. Rizzu, J. C. van Swieten, M. Joosse et al., "High prevalence of mutations in the microtubule-associated protein tau in a population study of frontotemporal dementia in the Netherlands," *The American Journal of Human Genetics*, vol. 64, no. 2, pp. 414–421, 1999.

[8] P. Momeni, A. Pittman, T. Lashley et al., "Clinical and pathological features of an Alzheimer's disease patient with the MAPT ΔK280 mutation," *Neurobiology of Aging*, vol. 30, no. 3, pp. 388–393, 2009.

[9] S. Barghorn, Q. Zheng-Fischhöfer, M. Ackmann et al., "Structure, microtubule interactions, and paired helical filament aggregation by tau mutants of frontotemporal dementias," *Biochemistry*, vol. 39, no. 38, pp. 11714–11721, 2000.

[10] V. Vogelsberg-Ragaglia, J. Bruce, C. Richter-Landsberg et al., "Distinct FTDP-17 missense mutations in tau produce tau aggregates and other pathological phenotypes in transfected CHO cells," *Molecular Biology of the Cell*, vol. 11, no. 12, pp. 4093–4104, 2000.

[11] M. von Bergen, S. Barghorn, L. Li et al., "Mutations of tau protein in frontotemporal dementia promote aggregation of paired helical filaments by enhancing local β-structure," *The Journal of Biological Chemistry*, vol. 276, no. 51, pp. 48165–48174, 2001.

[12] P. J. Khandelwal, A. M. Herman, and C. E. H. Moussa, "Inflammation in the early stages of neurodegenerative pathology," *Journal of Neuroimmunology*, vol. 238, no. 1-2, pp. 1–11, 2011.

[13] P. L. DiPatre and B. B. Gelman, "Microglial cell activation in aging and Alzheimer disease: partial linkage with neurofibrillary tangle burden in the hippocampus," *Journal of Neuropathology and Experimental Neurology*, vol. 56, no. 2, pp. 143–149, 1997.

[14] K. Ishizawa and D. W. Dickson, "Microglial activation parallels system degeneration in progressive supranuclear palsy and corticobasal degeneration," *Journal of Neuropathology and Experimental Neurology*, vol. 60, no. 6, pp. 647–657, 2001.

[15] M. Kitazawa, T. R. Yamasaki, and F. M. Laferla, "Microglia as a potential bridge between the amyloid β-peptide and tau," *Annals of the New York Academy of Sciences*, vol. 1035, no. 1, pp. 85–103, 2004.

[16] Y. Li, L. Liu, S. W. Barger, and W. S. T. Griffin, "Interleukin-1 mediates pathological effects of microglia on tau phosphorylation and on synaptophysin synthesis in cortical neurons through a p38-MAPK pathway," *The Journal of Neuroscience*, vol. 23, no. 5, pp. 1605–1611, 2003.

[17] K. Bhaskar, M. Konerth, O. N. Kokiko-Cochran, A. Cardona, R. M. Ransohoff, and B. T. Lamb, "Regulation of tau pathology by the microglial fractalkine receptor," *Neuron*, vol. 68, no. 1, pp. 19–31, 2010.

[18] M. Kitazawa, S. Oddo, T. R. Yamasaki, K. N. Green, and F. LaFerla, "Lipopolysaccharide-induced inflammation exacerbates tau pathology by a cyclin-dependent kinase 5-mediated pathway in a transgenic model of Alzheimer's disease," *Journal of Neuroscience*, vol. 25, no. 39, pp. 8843–8853, 2005.

[19] A. N. Nilson, K. C. English, J. E. Gerson et al., "Tau oligomers associate with inflammation in the brain and retina of tauopathy mice and in neurodegenerative diseases," *Jour-

nal of Alzheimer's Disease, vol. 55, no. 3, pp. 1083–1099, 2017.

[20] P. D. Wes, F. A. Sayed, F. Bard, and L. Gan, "Targeting microglia for the treatment of Alzheimer's disease," Glia, vol. 64, no. 10, pp. 1710–1732, 2016.

[21] A. Ardura-Fabregat, E. W. G. M. Boddeke, A. Boza-Serrano et al., "Targeting neuroinflammation to treat Alzheimer's disease," CNS Drugs, vol. 31, no. 12, pp. 1057–1082, 2017.

[22] J. Gao, Y. Inagaki, X. Li, N. Kokudo, and W. Tang, "Research progress on natural products from traditional Chinese medicine in treatment of Alzheimer's disease," Drug Discoveries & Therapeutics, vol. 7, no. 2, pp. 46–57, 2013.

[23] Z. Y. Wang, J. G. Liu, H. Li, and H. M. Yang, "Pharmacological effects of active components of Chinese herbal medicine in the treatment of Alzheimer's disease: a review," The American Journal of Chinese Medicine, vol. 44, no. 08, pp. 1525–1541, 2016.

[24] T. Y. Wu, C. P. Chen, and T. R. Jinn, "Traditional Chinese medicines and Alzheimer's disease," Taiwanese Journal of Obstetrics & Gynecology, vol. 50, no. 2, pp. 131–135, 2011.

[25] Y. Q. Zheng and W. Wei, "Total glucosides of paeony suppresses adjuvant arthritis in rats and intervenes cytokine-signaling between different types of synoviocytes," International Immunopharmacology, vol. 5, no. 10, pp. 1560–1573, 2005.

[26] T.-Y. Wu, T. O. Khor, C. L. L. Saw et al., "Anti-inflammatory/anti-oxidative stress activities and differential regulation of Nrf2-mediated genes by non-polar fractions of tea Chrysanthemum zawadskii and licorice Glycyrrhiza uralensis," The AAPS Journal, vol. 13, no. 1, pp. 1–13, 2011.

[27] K.-H. Chang, I.-C. Chen, H.-Y. Lin et al., "The aqueous extract of Glycyrrhiza inflata can upregulate unfolded protein response-mediated chaperones to reduce tau misfolding in cell models of Alzheimer's disease," Drug Design, Development and Therapy, vol. 10, pp. 885–896, 2016.

[28] D. Brown, A. Tamas, D. Reglodi, and Y. Tizabi, "PACAP protects against inflammatory-mediated toxicity in dopaminergic SH-SY5Y cells: implication for Parkinson's disease," Neurotoxicity Research, vol. 26, no. 3, pp. 230–239, 2014.

[29] Y. C. Park, C. H. Lee, H. S. Kang, H. T. Chung, and H. D. Kim, "Wortmannin, a specific inhibitor of phosphatidylinositol-3-kinase, enhances LPS-induced NO production from murine peritoneal macrophages," Biochemical and Biophysical Research Communications, vol. 240, no. 3, pp. 692–696, 1997.

[30] H. Fang, R. A. Pengal, X. Cao et al., "Lipopolysaccharide-induced macrophage inflammatory response is regulated by SHIP," Journal of Immunology, vol. 173, no. 1, pp. 360–366, 2004.

[31] M. Cente, P. Filipcik, M. Pevalova, and M. Novak, "Expression of a truncated tau protein induces oxidative stress in a rodent model of tauopathy," The European Journal of Neuroscience, vol. 24, no. 4, pp. 1085–1090, 2006.

[32] P. L. McGeer, T. Kawamata, D. G. Walker, H. Akiyama, I. Tooyama, and E. G. McGeer, "Microglia in degenerative neurological disease," Glia, vol. 7, no. 1, pp. 84–92, 1993.

[33] L. M. Sedger and M. F. McDermott, "TNF and TNF-receptors: from mediators of cell death and inflammation to therapeutic giants - past, present and future," Cytokine & Growth Factor Reviews, vol. 25, no. 4, pp. 453–472, 2014.

[34] T. P. Monie and C. E. Bryant, "Caspase-8 functions as a key mediator of inflammation and pro-IL-1β processing via both

canonical and non-canonical pathways," Immunological Reviews, vol. 265, no. 1, pp. 181–193, 2015.

[35] A. Sasaki, T. Kawarabayashi, T. Murakami et al., "Microglial activation in brain lesions with tau deposits: comparison of human tauopathies and tau transgenic mice TgTauP301L," Brain Research, vol. 1214, pp. 159–168, 2008.

[36] Y. Yoshiyama, M. Higuchi, B. Zhang et al., "Synapse loss and microglial activation precede tangles in a P301S tauopathy mouse model," Neuron, vol. 53, no. 3, pp. 337–351, 2007.

[37] A. C. McKee, I. Carreras, L. Hossain et al., "Ibuprofen reduces Aβ, hyperphosphorylated tau and memory deficits in Alzheimer mice," Brain Research, vol. 1207, pp. 225–236, 2008.

[38] W. Noble, C. Garwood, J. Stephenson, A. M. Kinsey, D. P. Hanger, and B. H. Anderton, "Minocycline reduces the development of abnormal tau species in models of Alzheimer's disease," The FASEB Journal, vol. 23, no. 3, pp. 739–750, 2009.

[39] C. J. Garwood, J. D. Cooper, D. P. Hanger, and W. Noble, "Anti-inflammatory impact of minocycline in a mouse model of tauopathy," Frontiers in Psychiatry, vol. 1, p. 136, 2010.

[40] M. A. Ajmone-Cat, A. Bernardo, A. Greco, and L. Minghetti, "Non-steroidal anti-inflammatory drugs and brain inflammation: effects on microglial functions," Pharmaceuticals (Basel), vol. 3, no. 6, pp. 1949–1965, 2010.

[41] J. C. Maroon, J. W. Bost, and A. Maroon, "Natural anti-inflammatory agents for pain relief," Surgical Neurology International, vol. 1, no. 1, p. 80, 2010.

[42] H. Li, M. Ye, Y. Zhang et al., "Blood-brain barrier permeability of Gualou Guizhi granules and neuroprotective effects in ischemia/reperfusion injury," Molecular Medicine Reports, vol. 12, no. 1, pp. 1272–1278, 2015.

[43] S. L. Li, J. Z. Song, F. F. K. Choi et al., "Chemical profiling of Radix Paeoniae evaluated by ultra-performance liquid chromatography/photo-diode-array/quadrupole time-of-flight mass spectrometry," Journal of Pharmaceutical and Biomedical Analysis, vol. 49, no. 2, pp. 253–266, 2009.

[44] Y. Zhang, H. Li, M. Huang et al., "Paeoniflorin, a monoterpene glycoside, protects the brain from cerebral ischemic injury via inhibition of apoptosis," The American Journal of Chinese Medicine, vol. 43, no. 03, pp. 543–557, 2015.

[45] H. R. Zhang, J. H. Peng, X. B. Cheng, B. Z. Shi, M. Y. Zhang, and R. X. Xu, "Paeoniflorin atttenuates amyloidogenesis and the inflammatory responses in a transgenic mouse model of Alzheimer's disease," Neurochemical Research, vol. 40, no. 8, pp. 1583–1592, 2015.

[46] X. Gu, Z. Cai, M. Cai et al., "Protective effect of paeoniflorin on inflammation and apoptosis in the cerebral cortex of a transgenic mouse model of Alzheimer's disease," Molecular Medicine Reports, vol. 13, no. 3, pp. 2247–2252, 2016.

[47] J. Zhou, L. Wang, J. Wang et al., "Paeoniflorin and albiflorin attenuate neuropathic pain via MAPK pathway in chronic constriction injury rats," Evidence-Based Complementary and Alternative Medicine, vol. 2016, Article ID 8082753, 11 pages, 2016.

[48] S. H. Kim, M. K. Lee, K. Y. Lee, S. H. Sung, J. Kim, and Y. C. Kim, "Chemical constituents isolated from Paeonia lactiflora roots and their neuroprotective activity against oxidative stress in vitro," Journal of Enzyme Inhibition and Medicinal Chemistry, vol. 24, no. 5, pp. 1138–1140, 2009.

[49] S. C. Lee, Y. S. Kwon, K. H. Son, H. P. Kim, and M. Y. Heo,

"Antioxidative constituents from *Paeonia lactiflora*," *Archives of Pharmacal Research*, vol. 28, no. 7, pp. 775–783, 2005.

[50] W. Y. Liao, T. H. Tsai, T. Y. Ho, Y. W. Lin, C. Y. Cheng, and C. L. Hsieh, "Neuroprotective effect of paeonol mediates anti-inflammation via suppressing toll-like receptor 2 and toll-like receptor 4 signaling pathways in cerebral ischemia-reperfusion injured rats," *Evidence-Based Complementary and Alternative Medicine*, vol. 2016, Article ID 3704647, 12 pages, 2016.

[51] Q. Zhang and M. Ye, "Chemical analysis of the Chinese herbal medicine Gan-Cao (licorice)," *Journal of Chromatography. A*, vol. 1216, no. 11, pp. 1954–1969, 2009.

[52] S. Matsui, H. Matsumoto, Y. Sonoda et al., "Glycyrrhizin and related compounds down-regulate production of inflammatory chemokines IL-8 and eotaxin 1 in a human lung fibroblast cell line," *International Immunopharmacology*, vol. 4, no. 13, pp. 1633–1644, 2004.

[53] T. Genovese, M. Menegazzi, E. Mazzon et al., "Glycyrrhizin reduces secondary inflammatory process after spinal cord compression injury in mice," *Shock*, vol. 31, no. 4, pp. 367–375, 2009.

[54] H. Zhao, S. L. Wang, L. Qian et al., "Diammonium glycyrrhizinate attenuates $A\beta_{1-42}$-induced neuroinflammation and regulates MAPK and NF-κB pathways *in vitro* and *in vivo*," *CNS Neuroscience & Therapeutics*, vol. 19, no. 2, pp. 117–124, 2013.

[55] R. Tanemoto, T. Okuyama, H. Matsuo, T. Okumura, Y. Ikeya, and M. Nishizawa, "The constituents of licorice (*Glycyrrhiza uralensis*) differentially suppress nitric oxide production in interleukin-1β-treated hepatocytes," *Biochemistry and Biophysics Reports*, vol. 2, pp. 153–159, 2015.

[56] A. Cheng, F. Wan, J. Wang, Z. Jin, and X. Xu, "Macrophage immunomodulatory activity of polysaccharides isolated from *Glycyrrhiza uralensis* fish," *International Immunopharmacology*, vol. 8, no. 1, pp. 43–50, 2008.

[57] H. Gong, B. K. Zhang, M. Yan et al., "A protective mechanism of licorice (*Glycyrrhiza uralensis*): isoliquiritigenin stimulates detoxification system via Nrf2 activation," *Journal of Ethnopharmacology*, vol. 162, pp. 134–139, 2015.

[58] D. Calzia, M. Oneto, F. Caicci et al., "Effect of polyphenolic phytochemicals on ectopic oxidative phosphorylation in rod outer segments of bovine retina," *British Journal of Pharmacology*, vol. 172, no. 15, pp. 3890–3903, 2015.

[59] S. J. Jeong, H. S. Lim, C. S. Seo et al., "Traditional herbal formula Jakyakgamcho-tang (*Paeonia lactiflora* and *Glycyrrhiza uralensis*) impairs inflammatory chemokine production by inhibiting activation of STAT1 and NF-κB in HaCaT cells," *Phytomedicine*, vol. 22, no. 2, pp. 326–332, 2015.

[60] B. Kaltschmidt, C. Kaltschmidt, T. G. Hofmann, S. P. Hehner, W. Droge, and M. L. Schmitz, "The pro- or anti-apoptotic function of NF-κB is determined by the nature of the apoptotic stimulus," *European Journal of Biochemistry*, vol. 267, no. 12, pp. 3828–3835, 2000.

[61] E. Yang, J. Zha, J. Jockel, L. H. Boise, C. B. Thompson, and S. J. Korsmeyer, "Bad, a heterodimeric partner for Bcl-XL and Bcl-2, displaces Bax and promotes cell death," *Cell*, vol. 80, no. 2, pp. 285–291, 1995.

[62] K. Wang, X. M. Yin, D. T. Chao, C. L. Milliman, and S. J. Korsmeyer, "BID: a novel BH3 domain-only death agonist," *Genes & Development*, vol. 10, no. 22, pp. 2859–2869, 1996.

[63] X. Liu, C. N. Kim, J. Yang, R. Jemmerson, and X. Wang, "Induction of apoptotic program in cell-free extracts: requirement for dATP and cytochrome c," *Cell*, vol. 86, no. 1, pp. 147–157, 1996.

[64] J. W. Mandell and G. A. Banker, "A spatial gradient of tau protein phosphorylation in nascent axons," *The Journal of Neuroscience*, vol. 16, no. 18, pp. 5727–5740, 1996.

[65] J.-H. Cho and G. V. W. Johnson, "Glycogen synthase kinase 3β phosphorylates tau at both primed and unprimed sites: differential impact on microtubule binding," *Journal of Biological Chemistry*, vol. 278, no. 1, pp. 187–193, 2003.

[66] J. Z. Wang and F. Liu, "Microtubule-associated protein tau in development, degeneration and protection of neurons," *Progress in Neurobiology*, vol. 85, no. 2, pp. 148–175, 2008.

[67] D. P. Hanger, B. H. Anderton, and W. Noble, "Tau phosphorylation: the therapeutic challenge for neurodegenerative disease," *Trends in Molecular Medicine*, vol. 15, no. 3, pp. 112–119, 2009.

10

Effects of Redox Disturbances on Intestinal Contractile Reactivity in Rats Fed with a Hypercaloric Diet

Iara L. L. de Souza,[1,2] Elba dos S. Ferreira,[1] Anderson F. A. Diniz,[1]
Maria Thaynan de L. Carvalho,[3] Fernando R. Queiroga,[1] Lydiane T. Toscano,[4]
Alexandre S. Silva,[4] Patrícia M. da Silva,[5] Fabiana de A. Cavalcante ⓘ,[1,2]
and Bagnólia A. da Silva ⓘ[1,6]

[1]*Programa de Pós-graduação em Produtos Naturais e Sintéticos Bioativos, Centro de Ciências da Saúde, Universidade Federal da Paraíba, João Pessoa, PB, Brazil*
[2]*Departamento de Fisiologia e Patologia, Centro de Ciências da Saúde, Universidade Federal da Paraíba, João Pessoa, PB, Brazil*
[3]*Centro de Ciências da Saúde, Universidade Federal da Paraíba, João Pessoa, PB, Brazil*
[4]*Departamento de Educação Física, Centro de Ciências da Saúde, Universidade Federal da Paraíba, João Pessoa, PB, Brazil*
[5]*Programa de Pós-graduação em Biologia Celular e Molecular, Centro de Ciências Exatas e da Natureza, Universidade Federal da Paraíba, João Pessoa, PB, Brazil*
[6]*Departamento de Ciências Farmacêuticas, Centro de Ciências da Saúde, Universidade Federal da Paraíba, João Pessoa, PB, Brazil*

Correspondence should be addressed to Bagnólia A. da Silva; bagnolia@ltf.ufpb.br

Academic Editor: Jeferson L. Franco

Few studies have associated the effects of changes in caloric intake and redox disturbances in the gastrointestinal tract. Therefore, the present study aimed at evaluating the hypercaloric diet consumption influence on the contractile reactivity of intestinal smooth muscle, morphology, and oxidative stress of rat ileum. Wistar rats were randomly divided into groups that received a standard diet and fed with a hypercaloric diet for 8 weeks. Animals were euthanized, and the ileum was isolated to isotonic contraction monitoring. Morphology was evaluated by histological staining and oxidative stress by quantification of malondialdehyde levels and total antioxidant activity. Cumulative concentration-response curves to KCl and carbachol were attenuated in rats fed with a hypercaloric diet compared to those that received a standard diet. In addition, an increase in caloric intake promotes a rise in the thickness of the longitudinal smooth muscle layer of rat ileum and tissue malondialdehyde levels, characterizing lipid peroxidation, as well as a decrease in the antioxidant activity. Thus, it was concluded that the consumption of a hypercaloric diet impairs rat intestinal contractility due to mechanisms involving modifications in the intestinal smooth muscle architecture triggered by redox disturbances.

1. Introduction

World Health Organization (WHO) defines obesity as a chronic condition characterized by an excessive accumulation of adipose tissue that causes health risk [1]. Therefore, obesity is categorized in the 10th revision of the International Classification of Diseases (ICD-10) at endocrine, nutritional, and metabolic diseases section [2].

Currently, several models develop obesity in animals through genetic mutations. However, most cases of human obesity are considered polygenic because of several gene integration. Thus, when analyzing the genesis of obesity in humans, the induction of this disease in animals through the consumption of highly palatable and hypercaloric diets is indicated as the most appropriate [3].

Recently, our research group established a model of erectile dysfunction in Wistar rat associated to a hypercaloric diet consumption and characterized by an increase in body adiposity, endothelial dysfunction, and systemic oxidative stress [4]. The integral role of oxidative stress in the genesis of diseases affecting smooth muscle cells has been highlighted, mainly due to evidence of free radicals influence on contractility and/or relaxation of smooth muscle cells [5, 6].

The reactive oxygen species (ROS) are signaling agents under physiological conditions and control healing processes, apoptosis, and maintenance of smooth muscle tone and proliferation of this tissue, among others [7, 8]. ROS include a variety of free radicals, such as superoxide anion (O^{2-}) and hydroxyl radicals (OH^-), as well as nonradical oxygen derivatives such as hydrogen peroxide (H_2O_2), hypochlorous acid ($HClO$), peroxynitrite ($ONOO^-$), and ozone (O_3) [9].

An imbalance resulting from overproduction of ROS can damage proteins, lipids, DNA, and other cellular components [10, 11]. In order to contain the formation of these ROS, the organism presents enzymatic and nonenzymatic antioxidant systems, and both play a fundamental role in the prevention of oxidation resulting from ROS [12]. The enzymatic antioxidant system comprises superoxide dismutase (SOD), glutathione peroxidase (GSH-PX) and reductase (GSH-Rd), and catalase, which are the enzymes responsible for removing O^{2-}, organic hydroperoxides, and H_2O_2, respectively [13, 14]. The nonenzymatic system involves a group of antioxidants that can be complexed in compounds produced *in vivo*, such as glutathione, ubiquinone, and uric acid, and in compounds obtained directly from the diet such as α-tocopherol (vitamin E), β-carotene, ascorbic acid (vitamin C), and phenolic compounds such as flavonoids [11, 15].

In view of this information, changes in the balance between oxidative stress and body antioxidant defenses, with a predominance of ROS, observed when there is an increase in caloric intake, raise the probability of the development of organic dysfunctions. However, few studies have reported the effect of a change in dietary pattern on intestinal disorders; despite the abnormalities on intestinal contraction are related to pathophysiological processes, such as constipation, diarrhea, and intestinal colic [16]. Therefore, the aim of this study was to investigate the influence of hypercaloric diet consumption on the contractile reactivity of intestinal smooth muscle, morphology, and oxidative stress on rat ileum.

2. Materials and Methods

2.1. Animals. Wistar rats (*Rattus norvegicus*), 2 months old (approximately 150 g), were obtained from the Bioterium Professor Thomas George from Universidade Federal da Paraíba (UFPB). The animals were maintained under controlled ventilation and temperature ($21 \pm 1°C$) with water *ad libitum* in a 12 h light-dark cycle (light on from 6 to 18 h).

The experimental procedures were performed following the principles of guidelines for the ethical use of animals in applied etiology studies [17] and from the Conselho Nacional de Controle de Experimentação Animal of Brazil [18] and were previously approved by the Ethics Committee on Animal Use of UFPB (protocol no. 0201/14).

2.2. Groups and Diets. Animals were randomly divided into two groups (10 rats/group): rats that received a standard diet (Presence®) containing by weight 23% protein, 63% carbohydrate, and 4% lipids with energy density 3.8 kcal/g (SD) and rats fed with a hypercaloric diet composed by a standard diet (Presence®), milk chocolate, peanuts, and sweet biscuit in the proportion of $3:2:2:1$ (HD) [19]. The hypercaloric diet containing by weight 23% protein, 45% carbohydrate, and 16% lipids with the energy density of 4.2 kcal/g was prepared weekly and supplied to animals as pellets [4]. The experimental groups were fed for 8 weeks.

2.3. Drugs. Potassium chloride (KCl), calcium chloride ($CaCl_2$), magnesium chloride ($MgCl_2$), sodium chloride (NaCl), and formaldehyde were purchased from Vetec Química Fina Ltda. (Brazil). Sodium bicarbonate ($NaHCO_3$) and glucose ($C_6H_{12}O_6$) were purchased from Dinâmica (Brazil). Sodium monobasic phosphate (NaH_2PO_4), sodium hydroxide (NaOH), and hydrochloric acid (HCl) were purchased from Nuclear (Brazil). These substances, except glucose, NaCl, and $NaHCO_3$, were diluted in distilled water to obtain each solution, which was maintained under refrigeration.

Carbamylcholine hydrochloride (CCh) was purchased from Merck (USA). Cremophor®, thiobarbituric acid, tetramethoxypropane, perchloric acid, Mayer's hematoxylin, and eosin were acquired from Sigma-Aldrich (Brazil). All substances were diluted in distilled water as needed for each experimental protocol. The carbogen mixture (95% O_2 and 5% CO_2) was obtained from White Martins (Brazil).

2.4. Ileum Isolation. Animals were euthanized by guillotine and the ileum was removed, cleaned of connective tissue and fat, immersed in physiological solution at room temperature, and bubbled with carbogen mixture (95% O_2 and 5% CO_2). In order to record the isotonic contractions, ileum segments (2–3 cm) were individually suspended in organ baths (5 mL) by cotton yarn and registered on the smoked drum through levers coupled to kymographs (DTF) with a thermostatic pump model Polystat 12002 Cole-Parmer (Vernon Hills) that controlled the organ bath temperature.

The physiological solution of Tyrode was used and has the composition (in mM) as follows: NaCl (150.0), KCl (2.7), $CaCl_2$ (1.8), $MgCl_2$ (2.0), $NaHCO_3$ (12.0), NaH_2PO_4 (0.4), and D-glucose (5.5). The pH was adjusted to 7.4, and the ileum was stabilized for 1 h under a resting tension of 1 g at 37°C and bubbled with a carbogen mixture [20].

2.5. Contractile Reactivity Measurement. The ileum was assembled as previously described. After a stabilization period of 30 min to verify the organ functionality, a contraction was induced with 30 mM KCl. Subsequently, cumulative concentration-response curves were obtained to KCl (10^{-3}–3×10^{-1} M) and CCh (10^{-9}–3×10^{-5} M).

The contractile reactivity was evaluated based on the values of the maximum effect (E_{max}) and the negative logarithm of the molar concentration of a substance that produced 50% of its maximal effect (pCE_{50}) of both contractile agents, calculated from the concentration-response curves obtained. The maximum amplitude obtained from the SD group concentration-response curve was elected as 100%, and the HD was assessed referring to it.

2.6. Histological Analysis. Ileum segments were assembled as previously described fixed in 10% formaldehyde solution and subjected to a standard histological procedure. This process was composed of the following steps: (1) tissue dehydration at increasing alcohol series of 70% for 24 h and 80, 96, and 100% (third bath) during 1 h each; (2) tissue diaphanization/bleaching with immersion in 100% xylene alcohol (1 : 1) during 1 h, followed by two baths in pure xylene during 1 h each; (3) tissue embedding in paraffin, wherein the sample was immersed in two baths of liquid paraffin (heated to 50°C) during 1 h each. Then, samples were embedded in new paraffin.

The blocks obtained were cut to 5 μm thick in cross-section of the ileum and stained with Mayer's hematoxylin/eosin [21]. Digital images of histological sections were obtained and analyzed with an optical microscope with an attached camera. In this analysis, two cross-sections per animal were photographed, and the second quadrant of the ileum circumference was used to measure both circular and longitudinal muscle layers using the Leica Qwin 3.1 software [22].

2.7. Assessment of Lipidic Peroxidation Levels. Lipid peroxidation was measured by the chromogenic product of 2-thiobarbituric acid (TBA) reaction with malondialdehyde (MDA) that is a product formed as a result of membrane lipid peroxidation [23]. Therefore, ileum segments were homogenized with KCl (1 : 1), and samples of tissue homogenate (250 μL) were incubated at 37°C for 60 min. After that, the mixture was precipitated with 35% perchloric acid and centrifuged at 1207g for 20 min at 4°C. Then, the supernatant was collected and 400 μL of 0.6% TBA was added and incubated at 95–100°C for 1 h. After cooling, the samples were read in a spectrophotometer at a wavelength of 532 nm (Biospectro, SP-220 model-Brazil). The determination of the MDA concentration was made by substituting the absorbance values in the MDA standard curve obtained on the basis of a standard solution (1 μL of 1,1,3,3- tetramethoxypropane in 70 mL distilled water) diluted in series of 250, 500, 750, 1000, 1250, 1500, 1750, 2000, 2250, 2500, 2750, and 3000 μL of distilled water.

2.8. Antioxidant Activity Assay. The ileum homogenate was assembled as previously described. In addition, an aliquot of 1.25 mg of DPPH was diluted in ethanol (100 mL), kept under refrigeration, and protected from light. Then, 3.9 mL of DPPH solution was added with 100 μL of the supernatant ileum homogenate on appropriate centrifuge tubes. These tubes were vortexed and left to stand for 30 min, centrifuged at 1207g for 15 min at 20°C. Then, the samples were read in a spectrophotometer at a wavelength of 515 nm (Biospectro, SP-220 model-Brazil) [24].

Results were expressed as the percentage of the oxidation inhibition: AOA = 100 − (((DPPH· R) S/(DPPH· R) W) × 100), where (DPPH· R) S and (DPPH· R) W correspond to the concentration of DPPH· remaining after 30 min, measured in the sample (S) and white (W) prepared with distilled water.

2.9. Statistical Analysis. Results were expressed as the mean and standard error of the mean (S.E.M.) and statistically analyzed using Student's *t*-test to the intergroup comparison. Cumulative concentration-response curves were fitted, and pCE_{50} values were obtained by nonlinear regression [25]. Values were significantly different when $p < 0.05$. All data were analyzed by GraphPad Prism® version 5.01 (GraphPad Software Inc., USA), and the visualization of histological sections was performed on Q-Capture® Pro version 7.0 software.

3. Results

3.1. Contractile Reactivity Measurement. In the HD group, cumulative concentration-response curves to KCl (10^{-3}–3×10^{-1} M) were attenuated with the reduction on E_{max} from 100% (SD) to 42.7 ± 3.1%. However, the pCE_{50} value of the HD group ($pCE_{50} = 1.8 \pm 0.8$) showed no statistical difference compared to the SD group ($pCE_{50} = 1.8 \pm 0.2$) (Figure 1(a), Table 1, $n = 5$).

Meanwhile, cumulative concentration-response curves to CCh (10^{-9}–3×10^{-5} M) were shifted to the right in rats fed with a hypercaloric diet ($pCE_{50} = 6.6 \pm 0.1$) compared to the SD group ($pCE_{50} = 6.3 \pm 0.05$). In addition, E_{max} value was decreased on HD related to SD ($E_{max} = 32.7 \pm 7.5$ and 100%, respectively), changing both potency and efficacy of CCh (Figure 1(b), Table 1, $n = 5$).

3.2. Histological Analysis. The circular smooth muscle layer thickness of rat ileum has no significant difference between HD (48.3 ± 4.0 μm) and SD groups (47.0 ± 1.8 μm). However, the longitudinal smooth muscle layer of rat ileum presented an increased thickness on rats fed with a hypercaloric diet compared to that in the SD group (36.53 ± 4.6 and 29.0 ± 1.9 μm, respectively) (Figure 2, $n = 5$).

3.3. Assessment of Lipidic Peroxidation Levels. The MDA levels in rat ileum were increased from 5.4 ± 0.2 μM/L (SD) to 7.0 ± 0.3 μM/L in rats fed with a hypercaloric diet (Figure 3(a), $n = 5$).

3.4. Antioxidant Activity Assay. The antioxidant activity in rat ileum was decreased from 93.0 ± 1.4% (SD) to 77.5 ± 1.5% in rats fed with a hypercaloric diet (Figure 3(b), $n = 5$).

4. Discussion

In this work, the influence of hypercaloric diet consumption on the contractile reactivity, morphology, and oxidative

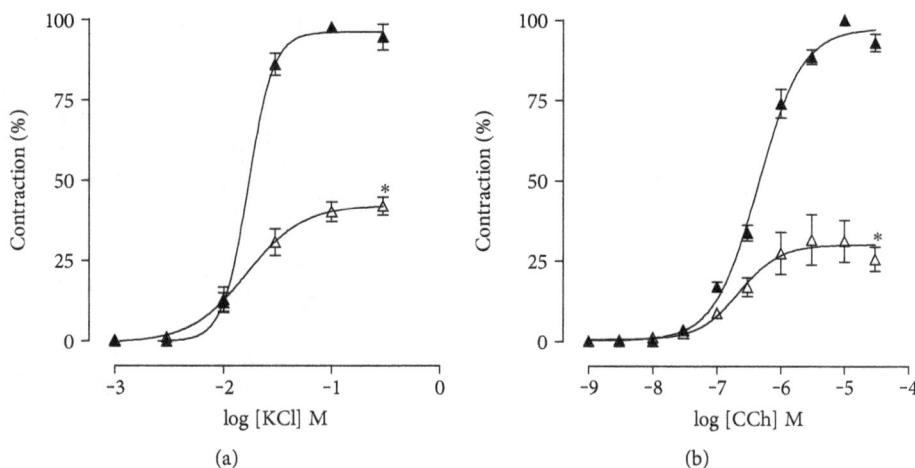

FIGURE 1: Cumulative concentration-response curves to KCl (a) and CCh (b) in rat ileum from both SD (▲) and HD groups (Δ). The symbols and vertical bars represent the mean and S.E.M., respectively ($n = 5$). Student's t-test, $^*p < 0.05$ (SD $vs.$ HD).

TABLE 1: Values of E_{max} (%) and pCE_{50} of KCl and CCh in rat ileum from both SD and HD groups. Student's t-test, $^*p < 0.05$ (SD $vs.$ HD) ($n = 5$).

Groups	KCl		CCh	
	E_{max} (%)	pCE_{50}	E_{max} (%)	pCE_{50}
SD	100	1.8 ± 0.2	100	6.3 ± 0.05
HD	$42.7 \pm 3.1^*$	1.8 ± 0.8	$32.7 \pm 7.5^*$	$6.6 \pm 0.1^*$

stress in rat ileum was investigated, demonstrating that an increase in caloric intake is associated with a decrease in contractile reactivity, an increase in the longitudinal smooth muscle layer thickness, lipid peroxidation, and a decrease in the antioxidant activity of this organ.

Chronic noncommunicable diseases (NCDs), such as type 2 diabetes mellitus, dyslipidemias, hypertension, and obesity, play an important and growing role in global public health due to their disabilities and early mortality. In this view, a central part of the genesis of these diseases is the excessive increase in body adiposity [26].

There are many determinants of obesity, being, therefore, a multifactorial disease characterized by the abnormal or excessive accumulation of adipose tissue [1]. Basically, obesity is caused by genetic and environmental factors, which are associated to an imbalance between energy expenditure and caloric consumption that are often determined by the consumption of diets with high energy density and high levels of fat and sugar [27, 28].

The ethical limitation in studying the mechanisms by which obesity induces physiological disorders in humans has resulted in the creation of experimental models using animals that are induced mainly by dietary and/or endocrine manipulation [29]. In these models, it is known that the consumption of hypercaloric/hyperlipidic diets is directly related to the development of various metabolic and hemodynamic disorders that result in adipose tissue hypertrophy/hyperplasia [30, 31].

Nevertheless, few studies have investigated the association of metabolic dysfunctions arising from the consumption of hypercaloric diets with possible alteration of cavernous smooth muscle reactivity on rats. Newly, Wistar rats fed with a hypercaloric diet, during eight weeks, showed increased systemic oxidative stress as well as impairment of contractile and relaxing reactivity of the corpus cavernosum in both pharmaco- and electromechanical couplings [4]. However, there is a lack of information about possible changes in intestinal contractile reactivity due to hypercaloric diet consumption, regarding the caloric content as well as the diet composition.

In view of these premises, it was decided to investigate whether the consumption of this diet, for eight weeks, would also alter the Wistar rats' intestinal contractile reactivity. Thus, the effect of the consumption of hypercaloric diet on both electro- and pharmacomechanical couplings was tested using KCl and CCh, respectively. The KCl was employed to simulate alterations on the membrane potential, which are physiologically controlled by the pacemaker of interstitial cells of Cajal located at the boundaries and in the substance of the inner circular muscle layer from which they spread to the outer longitudinal muscle layer. The CCh was used to mimic the cholinergic stimulation that happens in the intestinal smooth muscle [32, 33].

In this study, the KCl contractile efficacy was reduced in rats fed with hypercaloric diet in relation to those that received standard diet, with no change in potency (Figure 1(a), Table 1). Rembold [34] that verified an attenuation in cumulative concentration-response curves to KCl in rat ileum, decreasing its efficacy without changing the contractile potency, obtained similar results due to exercise. Thus, it is shown that an increase in caloric intake reduces the contraction elicited by the electromechanical coupling of rat ileum.

In addition, when rats consumed hypercaloric diet, a reduction was observed in both contractile efficacy and potency of CCh (Figure 1(b), Table 1). Data obtained by Araujo et al. [35] have demonstrated a similar decrease in

(a)

(b)

(c)

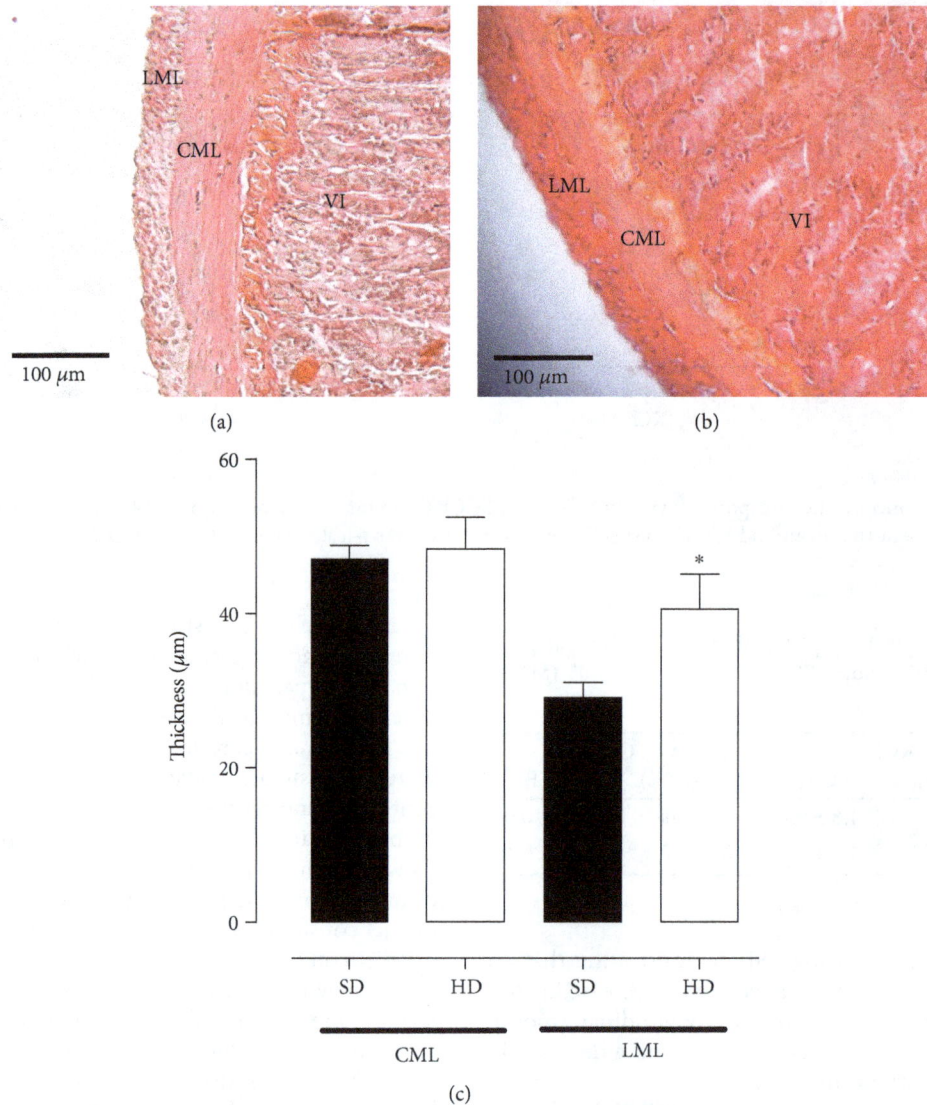

FIGURE 2: Microphotography of rat ileum from both SD (a) and HD groups (b) and thickness of CML and LML (c). Increased lens 20x. The symbols and vertical bars represent the mean and S.E.M., respectively ($n = 5$). Student's t-test, $^*p < 0.05$ (SD $vs.$ HD). CML = circular muscle layer; LML = longitudinal muscle layer; VI = villus.

both efficacy and potency of CCh in the ileum of rats submitted to acute aerobic swimming exercise that were associated to a possible desensitization of intestinal muscarinic receptors. Moreover, the reperfusion process was also correlated to a reduction of ACh-induced contractile response in the ileum of rats submitted to occlusion of superior mesenteric artery plus interruption of collateral blood flow, leading to reperfusion [36]. Therefore, we demonstrate that an increase in caloric intake reduces the contraction elicited by the pharmacomechanical coupling of rat ileum, due to a less response of smooth muscle cell to cholinergic stimulation.

The synchrony between the smooth muscle layers, a circular and a longitudinal layer, modulates the intestinal contractility. In this view, Bertoni et al. [37] showed that hypertrophy of the circular smooth muscle layer is associated to an increase in contractile efficacy, whereas hypertrophy of the longitudinal smooth muscle layer exhibits a greater sensitivity to the relaxing factors, leading to a decrease in

contractile efficacy. Thus, as the present study demonstrated a reduced contractility of rat ileum (Figure 1) due to hypercaloric diet consumption, it was hypothesized that changes in the architecture of the intestinal smooth muscle could be responsible for these results.

Therefore, to verify this hypothesis, histological analyses were performed on rat ileum from both experimental groups. The circular smooth muscle layer thickness was not altered by the consumption of a hypercaloric diet (Figure 2). Interestingly, an increase in the longitudinal smooth muscle layer thickness was observed (Figure 2), characterizing a hypertrophy process. Based on these results, it can be proposed that an increase in caloric intake leads to longitudinal smooth muscle layer hypertrophy and, consequently, reduced the ileum contractility (Figures 1 and 2).

A common problem related to the pathogenesis of intestinal reactivity disorders is the presence of a chronic low-grade inflammation that results in adipose tissue

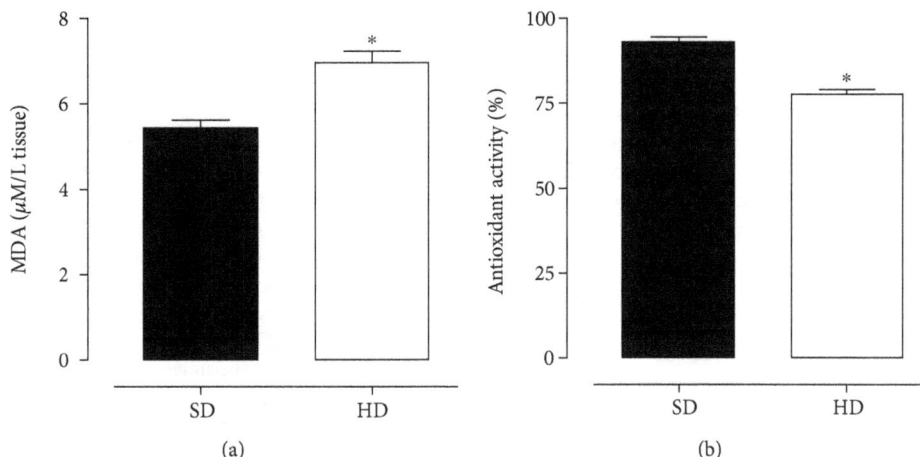

FIGURE 3: Concentration of MDA (a) and antioxidant activity (b) of rat ileum from both SD and HD groups. The symbols and vertical bars represent the mean and S.E.M., respectively ($n = 5$). Student's t-test, $*p < 0.05$ (SD $vs.$ HD). MDA = malondialdehyde.

hypertrophy [38]. Similar to other inflammatory processes, adipose tissue inflammation is a trigger for the oxidative stress and can be started by an increase in caloric intake. Briefly, due to the consumption of hypercaloric/hyperlipidic diets, there is an increase in glucose and circulating lipid levels resulting in the excessive supply of energetic substrates to metabolic routes. In turn, ROS production is raised, especially O^{2-}, H_2O_2, and OH^-, among others [8, 9].

It is consolidated in the literature that an imbalance in tissue peroxidation and antioxidant activity leads to oxidative damage, consequently, modulating both structure and/or function of the tissue [39–41]. Ischemia-reperfusion events in the intestinal musculature are closely related to oxidative stress [42], promoting motor and intestinal mucosa alteration, decrease in nutrient absorption, and gastrointestinal permeability [43, 44]. Other processes that also alter redox homeostasis, such as physical exercise, have already been correlated to increased lipid peroxidation. Specifically, Araujo et al. [45] showed that chronic aerobic swimming exercise increases lipid peroxidation after four weeks of exercise. Based on this information, it was decided to investigate whether the consumption of a hypercaloric diet would also alter lipid peroxidation of rat ileum. For this, the levels of MDA, a lipid peroxidation marker, were evaluated.

In studies involving oxidative stress, MDA represents a compound formed through the oxidative decomposition of polyunsaturated fatty acids from the membrane and is the most frequently quantified systemic and tissue marker [46]. MDA levels are therefore quantified through a calorimetric reaction in which two molecules of thiobarbituric acid are condensed with a molecule of MDA, and the end product is detected by spectrophotometry technique [47].

According to this methodology, it was observed that MDA concentration was increased in rat ileum from the HD group in relation to the SD group (Figure 3(a)). Souza et al. [4], using the same hypercaloric diet, showed that rats had an increase in MDA levels in plasma, characterizing a systemic oxidative stress. The remarkable increase in the level of ileum peroxidation in the HD group (Figure 3(a)) is quite suggestive that hypercaloric diet consumption also promotes

tissue peroxidation. Additionally, it is an important challenge for intestinal redox homeostasis and indicates a possible compromise of the antioxidant defense system of these animals. The peroxidation increase may be a consequence of proinflammatory cytokine production (TNF-α, IL-1, and IL-6), due to excess body adiposity, since these cytokines stimulate ROS production by macrophages [48].

In biological systems, this imbalance in ROS production is counterbalanced by the body's antioxidant capacity, representing the body's ability to sequester free radicals through redox systems [49]. Knowing this, it was investigated whether the consumption of a hypercaloric diet would alter the antioxidant activity of these rats. For this, the DPPH reduction colorimetric method was used, which is based on the sample's ability to reduce the DPPH radical (purple) to 1,1-diphenyl 2-picryl hydrazine (translucent), detected by spectrophotometry technique [50].

In this study, the HD group presented a reduction in tissue antioxidant activity in relation to the SD group (Figure 3(b)). The decrease of systemic antioxidant activity was demonstrated by Souza et al. [4] using the same hypercaloric diet. Therefore, the reduction of the ileum antioxidant capacity observed in the HD group (Figure 3(b)) reinforces the idea of an imbalance between ROS production and antioxidant defense systems, correlated with an increase in MDA levels in these rats (Figure 3(a)). Since free radicals are regulators in several cellular processes, such as transcriptional factor activation, gene expression, and cell proliferation [7], it was proposed that an oxidative stress caused by the consumption of a hypercaloric diet may underlie the hypertrophy process of intestinal smooth muscle cells in rats (Figures 2 and 3).

In conclusion, the current study showed initial evidence that the consumption of a hypercaloric diet impairs rat intestinal contractility due to mechanisms involving modifications in the intestinal smooth muscle architecture triggered by redox disturbances. Thus, we provide a model to understand biochemical and metabolic processes involved in the pathophysiological changes caused by the increase in caloric intake, as well as to help to reduce the impact of the various diseases related to it.

Acknowledgments

The authors thank Coordenação de Aperfeiçoamento de Pessoal de Nível Superior (CAPES) and Conselho Nacional de Desenvolvimento Científico e Tecnológico (CNPq) for financial support. The authors thank José Crispim Duarte and Luís C. Silva for providing technical assistance and Camila Leão Luna de Souza for English review.

References

[1] WHO, *Health Topics – Obesity*, WHO, 2018.

[2] WHO, *Obesity: Preventing and Managing the Global Epidemic*, WHO, 2000.

[3] T. A. LUTZ and S. C. WOODS, "Overview of animal models of obesity," *Current Protocols in Pharmacology*, vol. 58, no. 1, pp. 5.61.1–5.61.18, 2012.

[4] I. L. L. de Souza, B. C. Barros, G. A. de Oliveira et al., "Hypercaloric diet establishes erectile dysfunction in rat: mechanisms underlying the endothelial damage," *Frontiers in Physiology*, vol. 8, 2017.

[5] A. Castela, P. Gomes, V. F. Domingues et al., "Role of oxidative stress-induced systemic and cavernosal molecular alterations in the progression of diabetic erectile dysfunction," *Journal of Diabetes*, vol. 7, no. 3, pp. 393–401, 2015.

[6] F. B. M. Priviero, H. A. F. Toque, K. P. Nunes, D. G. Priolli, C. E. Teixeira, and R. C. Webb, "Impaired corpus cavernosum relaxation is accompanied by increased oxidative stress and up-regulation of the rho-kinase pathway in diabetic (Db/Db) mice," *PLoS One*, vol. 11, no. 5, article e0156030, 2016.

[7] H. Suenaga and K. Kamata, "Lysophosphatidylcholine activates extracellular-signal-regulated protein kinase and potentiates vascular contractile responses in rat aorta," *Journal of Pharmacological Sciences*, vol. 92, no. 4, pp. 348–358, 2003.

[8] F. Mcmurray, D. A. Patten, and M. E. Harper, "Reactive oxygen species and oxidative stress in obesity-recent findings and empirical approaches," *Obesity*, vol. 24, no. 11, pp. 2301–2310, 2016.

[9] B. Halliwell, "Reactive species and antioxidants. Redox biology is a fundamental theme of aerobic life," *Plant Physiology*, vol. 141, no. 2, pp. 312–322, 2006.

[10] T. Finkel and N. J. Holbrook, "Oxidants, oxidative stress and the biology of ageing," *Nature*, vol. 408, no. 6809, pp. 239–247, 2000.

[11] B. Halliwell and J. M. C. Gutteridge, *Free Radicals in Biology and Medicine*, Oxford University Press, USA, 5 edition, 2015.

[12] P. R. B. Broinizi, E. R. S. d. Andrade-Wartha, A. M. d. O. e. Silva et al., "Propriedades antioxidantes em subproduto do pedúnculo de caju (*Anacardium occidentale* L.): efeito sobre a lipoperoxidação e o perfil de ácidos graxos poliinsaturados em ratos," *Revista Brasileira de Ciências Farmacêuticas*, vol. 44, no. 4, pp. 773–781, 2008.

[13] B. P. Yu, "Cellular defenses against damage from reactive oxygen species," *Physiological Reviews*, vol. 74, no. 1, pp. 139–162, 1994.

[14] P. G. Pietta, "Flavonoids as antioxidants," *Journal of Natural Products*, vol. 63, no. 7, pp. 1035–1042, 2000.

[15] C. De Moraes and R. C. Sampaio, "Estresse oxidativo e envelhecimento: papel do exercício físico," *Motriz. Revista de Educação Física. UNESP*, vol. 16, no. 2, pp. 506–515, 2010.

[16] Y. Sato, J. X. He, H. Nagai, T. Tani, and T. Akao, "Isoliquiritigenin, one of the antispasmodic principles of *Glycyrrhiza ularensis* roots, acts in the lower part of intestine," *Biological and Pharmaceutical Bulletin*, vol. 30, no. 1, pp. 145–149, 2007.

[17] C. M. Sherwin, S. B. Christiansen, I. J. Duncan et al., "Guidelines for the ethical use of animals in applied ethology studies," *Applied Animal Behaviour Science*, vol. 81, no. 3, pp. 291–305, 2003.

[18] BRASIL, Ministério da Ciência, Tecnologia e Inovação, and Conselho Nacional de Experimentação Animal, *Guia Brasileiro de Produção, Manutenção ou Utilização de Animais em Atividades de Ensino ou Pesquisa Científica: Fascículo 1: Introdução Geral*, Ministério da Ciência, Tecnologia e Inovação, Brasília–DF, 2016.

[19] D. Estadella, L. M. Oyama, A. R. Dâmaso, E. B. Ribeiro, and C. M. Oller Do Nascimento, "Effect of palatable hyperlipidic diet on lipid metabolism of sedentary and exercised rats," *Nutrition*, vol. 20, no. 2, pp. 218–224, 2004.

[20] M. Radenkovic, V. Ivetic, M. Popovic, N. Mimica-Dukic, and S. Veljkovic, "Neurophysiological effects of mistletoe (*Viscum album* L.) on isolated rat intestines," *Phytotherapy Research*, vol. 20, no. 5, pp. 374–377, 2006.

[21] D. W. Howard, E. J. Lewis, B. J. Keller, and C. Smith, *Histological Techniques for Marine Bivalve Molluscs and Crustaceans*, NOAA/National Centers for Coastal Ocean Science, Oxford, MD, USA, 2nd edition, 2004.

[22] C. A. B. de Lira, R. L. Vancini, S. S. M. Ihara, A. C. da Silva, J. Aboulafia, and V. L. A. Nouailhetas, "Aerobic exercise affects C57BL/6 murine intestinal contractile function," *European Journal of Applied Physiology*, vol. 103, no. 2, pp. 215–223, 2008.

[23] C. C. Winterbourn, J. M. C. Gutteridge, and B. Halliwell, "Doxorubicin-dependent lipid peroxidation at low partial pressures of O_2," *Journal of Free Radicals in Biology & Medicine*, vol. 1, no. 1, pp. 43–49, 1985.

[24] W. Brand-Williams, M. E. Cuvelier, and C. Berset, "Use of a free radical method to evaluate antioxidant activity," *LWT - Food Science and Technology*, vol. 28, no. 1, pp. 25–30, 1995.

[25] R. R. Neubig, M. Spedding, T. Kenakin, A. Christopoulos, and International Union of Pharmacology Committee on Receptor Nomenclature and Drug Classification., "International union of pharmacology committee on receptor nomenclature and drug classification. XXXVIII. Update on terms and symbols in quantitative pharmacology," *Pharmacological Reviews*, vol. 55, no. 4, pp. 597–606, 2003.

[26] F. Bäckhed, H. Ding, T. Wang et al., "The gut microbiota as an environmental factor that regulates fat storage," *Proceedings of the National Academy of Sciences of the United States of America*, vol. 101, no. 44, pp. 15718–15723, 2004.

[27] D. W. Haslam and W. P. T. James, "Obesity," *The Lancet*, vol. 366, no. 9492, pp. 1197–1209, 2005.

[28] J. J. Patel, M. D. Rosenthal, K. R. Miller, P. Codner, L. Kiraly, and R. G. Martindale, "The critical care obesity paradox and implications for nutrition support," *Current Gastroenterology Reports*, vol. 18, no. 9, p. 45, 2016.

[29] L. O. Pereira, R. P. d. Francischi, and A. H. Lancha Jr, "Obesidade: hábitos nutricionais, sedentarismo e resistência à insulina," *Arquivos Brasileiros de Endocrinologia e Metabologia*, vol. 47, no. 2, pp. 111–127, 2003.

[30] L. A. Velloso, "The brain is the conductor: diet-induced inflammation overlapping physiological control of body mass and metabolism," *Arquivos Brasileiros de Endocrinologia & Metabologia*, vol. 53, no. 2, pp. 151–158, 2009.

[31] A. Tchernof and J. P. Després, "Pathophysiology of human visceral obesity: an update," *Physiological Reviews*, vol. 93, no. 1, pp. 359–404, 2013.

[32] J. C. Bornstein, M. Costa, and J. R. Grider, "Enteric motor and interneuronal circuits controlling motility," *Neurogastroenterology & Motility*, vol. 16, no. s1, pp. 34–38, 2004.

[33] K. M. Sanders, S. D. Koh, T. Ordog, and S. M. Ward, "Ionic conductances involved in generation and propagation of electrical slow waves in phasic gastrointestinal muscles," *Neurogastroenterology & Motility*, vol. 16, no. s1, pp. 100–105, 2004.

[34] C. M. Rembold, "Electromechanical and pharmacomechanical coupling," in *Biochemistry of Smooth Muscle Contraction*, M. Bárány, Ed., pp. 227–239, Elsevier, San Diego, CA, USA, 1996.

[35] L. C. da Cunha Araujo, I. L. L. de Souza, L. H. C. Vasconcelos et al., "Acute aerobic swimming exercise induces distinct effects in the contractile reactivity of rat ileum to KCl and carbachol," *Frontiers in Physiology*, vol. 7, 2016.

[36] V. Ballabeni, E. Barocelli, S. Bertoni, and M. Impicciatore, "Alterations of intestinal motor responsiveness in a model of mild mesenteric ischemia/reperfusion in rats," *Life Sciences*, vol. 71, no. 17, pp. 2025–2035, 2002.

[37] S. Bertoni, V. Ballabeni, L. Flammini, T. Gobbetti, M. Impicciatore, and E. Barocelli, "Intestinal chronic obstruction affects motor responsiveness of rat hypertrophic longitudinal and circular muscles," *Neurogastroenterology & Motility*, vol. 20, no. 11, pp. 1234–1242, 2008.

[38] S. P. Weisberg, D. McCann, M. Desai, M. Rosenbaum, R. L. Leibel, and A. W. Ferrante Jr, "Obesity is associated with macrophage accumulation in adipose tissue," *The Journal of Clinical Investigation*, vol. 112, no. 12, pp. 1796–1808, 2003.

[39] K. P. Davies and A. Melman, "Markers of erectile dysfunction," *Indian Journal of Urology*, vol. 24, no. 3, pp. 320–328, 2008.

[40] K. M. Azadzoi, T. Golabek, Z. M. Radisavljevic, S. V. Yalla, and M. B. Siroky, "Oxidative stress and neurodegeneration in penile ischaemia," *BJU International*, vol. 105, no. 3, pp. 404–410, 2010.

[41] C. Vlachopoulos, N. Ioakeimidis, and C. Stefanadis, "Biomarkers, erectile dysfunction, and cardiovascular risk prediction: the latest of an evolving concept," *Asian Journal of Andrology*, vol. 17, no. 1, pp. 17–20, 2015.

[42] V. H. Ozacmak, H. Sayan, S. O. Arslan, S. Altaner, and R. G. Aktas, "Protective effect of melatonin on contractile activity and oxidative injury induced by ischemia and reperfusion of rat ileum," *Life Sciences*, vol. 76, no. 14, pp. 1575–1588, 2005.

[43] J. Liu, H. C. Yeo, E. Overvik-Douki et al., "Chronically and acutely exercised rats: biomarkers of oxidative stress and endogenous antioxidants," *Journal of Applied Physiology*, vol. 89, no. 1, pp. 21–28, 2000.

[44] M. L. Marquezi, H. A. Roschel, A. d. S. Costa, L. A. Sawada, and A. H. Lancha Jr, "Effect of aspartate and asparagine supplementation on fatigue determinants in intense exercise," *International Journal of Sport Nutrition and Exercise Metabolism*, vol. 13, no. 1, pp. 65–75, 2003.

[45] L. C. da Cunha Araujo, I. L. L. de Souza, L. H. C. Vasconcelos et al., "Chronic aerobic swimming exercise promotes functional and morphological changes in rat ileum," *Bioscience Reports*, vol. 35, no. 5, article e00259, 2015.

[46] D. del Rio, A. J. Stewart, and N. Pellegrini, "A review of recent studies on malondialdehyde as toxic molecule and biological marker of oxidative stress," *Nutrition, Metabolism and Cardiovascular Diseases*, vol. 15, no. 4, pp. 316–328, 2005.

[47] M. Giera, H. Lingeman, and W. M. A. Niessen, "Recent advancements in the LC- and GC-based analysis of malondialdehyde (MDA): a brief overview," *Chromatographia*, vol. 75, no. 9-10, pp. 433–440, 2012.

[48] J. D. Morrow, "Is oxidant stress a connection between obesity and atherosclerosis?," *Arteriosclerosis, Thrombosis and Vascular Biology*, vol. 23, no. 3, pp. 368–370, 2003.

[49] F. Brighenti, S. Valtueña, N. Pellegrini et al., "Total antioxidant capacity of the diet is inversely and independently related to plasma concentration of high-sensitivity C-reactive protein in adult Italian subjects," *British Journal of Nutrition*, vol. 93, no. 05, pp. 619–625, 2005.

[50] A. Floegel, D. O. Kim, S. J. Chung, S. I. Koo, and O. K. Chun, "Comparison of ABTS/DPPH assays to measure antioxidant capacity in popular antioxidant-rich US foods," *Journal of Food Composition and Analysis*, vol. 24, no. 7, pp. 1043–1048, 2011.

11

An Overview on the Anti-inflammatory Potential and Antioxidant Profile of Eugenol

Joice Nascimento Barboza,[1] Carlos da Silva Maia Bezerra Filho,[1] Renan Oliveira Silva,[2] Jand Venes R. Medeiros ⓘ,[3] and Damião Pergentino de Sousa ⓘ[1]

[1]*Department of Pharmaceutical Sciences, Universidade Federal da Paraíba, 58051-970 João Pessoa, Paraíba, Brazil*
[2]*Department of Biomedicine, University Center INTA-UNINTA, 62050-130 Sobral, Ceará, Brazil*
[3]*Laboratory of Pharmacology of Inflammation and Gastrointestinal Disorders-LAFIDG, Federal University of Piauí, Parnaíba, Piauí, Brazil*

Correspondence should be addressed to Damião Pergentino de Sousa; damiao_desousa@yahoo.com.br

Guest Editor: Anderson J. Teodoro

The bioactive compounds found in foods and medicinal plants are attractive molecules for the development of new drugs with action against several diseases, such as those associated with inflammatory processes, which are commonly related to oxidative stress. Many of these compounds have an appreciable inhibitory effect on oxidative stress and inflammatory response, and may contribute in a preventive way to improve the quality of life through the use of a diet rich in these compounds. Eugenol is a natural compound that has several pharmacological activities, action on the redox status, and applications in the food and pharmaceutical industry. Considering the importance of this compound, the present review discusses its anti-inflammatory and antioxidant properties, demonstrating its mechanisms of action and therapeutic potential for the treatment of inflammatory diseases.

1. Introduction

Eugenol (4-allyl-2-methoxyphenol) is a phenolic compound from the class of phenylpropanoids and the main component of clove (*Syzygium aromaticum* (L.) Merr. & L. M. Perry.). It consists of 45–90% of its essential oil [1]. It is used in the food industry as a preservative, mainly due to its antioxidant property [2], and as a flavoring agent for foods and cosmetics [3]. It can also be found in soybean (*Glycine max* (L.) Merr.), beans [4], coffee [5], cinnamon (*Cinnamomum verum* J. Presl), basil (*Ocimum basilicum* L.) [6], "canelinha" (*Croton zehntneri* Pax et Hoffm) [7], banana [8, 9], bay laurel (*Laurus nobilis* L.), and other foods [10]. Among the plants that contain eugenol, soybeans, cloves, beans, and cinnamon also present the antioxidant activity, possibly performed by this compound and other constituents [11–14]. In addition, clove is also known by anti-inflammatory activity [15], which may be related to anti-inflammatory action of eugenol (Figure 1).

Inflammation is a complex protective response of the body against harmful agents, such as microorganisms or damaged cells [16, 17], which the biological system objective to remove harmful stimuli from the body and promote healing. However, this response needs to be controlled and last for a short period; otherwise, it may provide the appearance of pathological disorders related to the immune system [18]. Classically, inflammation can be classified in acute and chronic. The acute inflammation is an initial response, which is characterized by resident cell activation, with liberation of proinflammatory cytokines and chemokines, culminating in the recruitment of polymorphonuclear, primarily neutrophils, from the innate immune system to the injury site. This response complex act to promote cardinal signs of inflammation, such as pain, edema, and heat [19]. On the other hand, chronic inflammation is a prolonged response characterized by a gradual change in the cells type found at the inflammatory site, which over time cause both

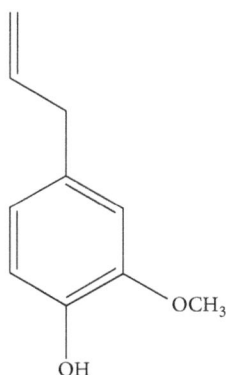

FIGURE 1: Chemical structure of eugenol.

permanent damage and healing of the tissue. In both types of inflammation occur increased local blood flow, vasodilation, fluid extravasation, and liberation of proinflammatory mediators [17, 20].

The nuclear factor-kappa B (NF-κB) signaling pathway is a key part of the immune response. It is essential to inflammatory processes due to its importance in the transcription of cytokines, such as tumor necrosis factor-α (TNF-α), interleukin-1β (IL-1β), interleukin-6 (IL-6), and nitric oxide (NO). Like eugenol, substances that inhibit this pathway are of interest to the pharmaceutical industry [21–23]. In general, patients with inflammatory disorders use clinically glucocorticoids or nonsteroidal anti-inflammatory drugs (NSAIDs). However, these drugs are associated with critical side effects (i.e., gastrointestinal ulcers and bleeding) and limited therapeutic efficacy, which often leads patients to abandon the treatment [24]. In this context, the pharmaceutical industry has directed efforts in the attempt to find new bioactive molecules.

Medicinal plants have been important sources of constituents with pharmacological activities. Phenylpropanoids are considered a group of secondary compounds found in a variety of plants and usually in the oxidized form, presenting a hydroxyl at the aromatic ring [25]. Studies recently demonstrated that phenylpropanoids and their synthetic derivatives have a variety of pharmacologic activities, including anti-inflammatory action [26, 27].

Several pharmacological activities have been reported to eugenol: anti-inflammatory [28], antitumor [29], antibacterial [30], antifungal [31, 32], antipyretic [33], anesthetic [34], and analgesic activities [35]. Considering the importance of eugenol as bioactive molecule and its presence in various foods and medicinal plants, this review discusses its role in the inflammatory response in experimental models, including animals and cell culture tests, demonstrating its antioxidant profile and potential therapeutical application against inflammatory diseases.

2. Methodology

The present review was based on the data search performed in the scientific literature database PubMed, using the publication from January 2008 to January 2018, using the following keywords: eugenol, asthma, antiasthmatic

effect, allergy, antiallergic effect, inflammation, anti-inflammatory, immune response, lymphocytes, cytokines, immunoglobulins, immunoregulatory, and antioxidant. Table 1 shows the studies reported for this review and summarizes the results obtained, indicating the dose/concentration of eugenol administered, experimental model, parameters evaluated, and biological effect.

3. Results and Discussion

3.1. Antioxidant Action of Eugenol. The free radical scavenger effect of diphenyl-1-picrylhydrazyl (DPPH) is due to the ability of certain substances to donate hydrogen, especially those with a phenolic group in their structure. Thus, eugenol's ability to sequester free radicals in the DPPH assay (IC$_{50}$ = 11.7 μg/mL), as well as to inhibit reactive oxygen species (ROS) (IC$_{50}$ = 1.6 μg/mL), H$_2$O$_2$ (IC$_{50}$ = 22.6 μg/mL and 27.1 μg/mL), and NO (IC$_{50}$ < 50.0 μg/mL) [36]. These data corroborate with other studies in which eugenol demonstrated DPPH sequestering activity with EC$_{50}$ of 22.6 μg/mL [37]. In another study, it was able to eliminate about 81% of the DPPH radicals and reduce the potency of the radicals when the concentration decreased from 1.0 μM/mL to 0.1 μM/mL [38]. Similar data were described in the study by Kim et al., in which eugenol performed the elimination of ABTS free radicals (76.9% at a dose of 20 μg/mL) and DPPH (90.8% at a dose of 20 μg/mL) in L-ascorbic acid in 76.9% and 89.9%, respectively [14].

In a comparative study of the antioxidant activity of clove and eugenol, both showed similar activities, with values of sequestering radicals DPPH and ABTS, respectively, IC$_{50}$ = 0.3257 and 0.1595 mg/mL for the clove and of IC$_{50}$ = 0.1967 and 0.1492 mg/mL for eugenol. Therefore, the antioxidant properties of this essential oil are related to the antioxidant action of its chemical constituent, which is eugenol [13]. The biochemical profile of this compound was confirmed in a study in which the antioxidant activity of eugenol was associated with anti-inflammatory activity. In this approach, Yogalakshmi et al. showed that pretreatment with eugenol (10.7 mg/kg.bw/day) in rats for 15 days resulted in a decrease in lipid peroxidation indices, protein oxidation, and inflammatory markers (reduction in the expression of COX-2, TNF-α, and IL-6) and by improving antioxidant status by maintaining antioxidants such as glutathione peroxidase (GPx), superoxide dismutase (SOD), catalase (CAT), and glutathione-S-transferase (GST) [39]. Confirming these findings, a study by Kaur et al. showed that pretreatment with eugenol in male Swiss albino mice inhibited the expression of inflammatory markers such as iNOS and COX-2 and the cytokines IL-6, TNF-α, and PGE2, as well as prevented the depletion of antioxidant enzymes and reduced lipid peroxidation (LPO), acting both as anti-inflammatory and antioxidant agents [40]. In fact, eugenol pretreatment, in addition to reducing inflammation caused by lung exposure to LPS, was also able to significantly improve the levels of SOD1, CAT, Gpx1, and GST. Thus, eugenol can be used as an anti-inflammatory agent, as well as protecting the damage caused by oxidative stress [41].

TABLE 1: Modulation of inflammatory response mediated by eugenol.

Experimental model	Animal and/or cells lines	Dose or concentration of eugenol	Inflammatory parameters evaluated	Biological effect	References
In vitro and *in vivo* leukocyte migration induced by fMLP, LTB4, and carrageenan	BALB/c mice	0.5, 1, 3, 9, or 27 μg/mL 62.5, 125, or 250 mg/kg	Leukocyte migration	Decreased the number of leukocytes that rolled, adhered, and migrated to perivascular tissue	[50]
Model of allergic asthma	BALB/c mice	10 or 20 mg/kg	Cytokines (IL-4 and IL-5) levels, histological assessment, and VDUP1/NF-κB signaling pathways	Inhibited OVA-induced eosinophilia, recovered IL-4 and IL-5 levels, inhibited P-IκBα, NF-κBP65, and p-NF-κBP65 protein levels, and increased VDUP1 and IκBα protein levels.	[51]
LPS-induced inflammatory reaction in acute lung injury	BALB/c mice	5 or 10 mg/kg	Activities of antioxidant enzymes (CAT, SOD, GPx, and GST) and inflammatory markers (MPO, IL-6, and TNF-α) and inflammatory cells recruitment	Reduced the IL-6 and TNF-α expression, suppressed NF-κB signaling, decreased the leukocyte recruitment, and increased the protein levels (SOD, CAT, GPx, and GST)	[41]
LPS-induced lung injury	BALB/c mice	160 mg/kg body	Inflammatory cells, TNF-α, and NF-κB levels	Reduced the neutrophil recruitment, macrophages, TNF-α, and NF-κB expression	[52]
Diesel exhaust particles induced pulmonary damage	BALB/c mice	164 mg/kg	Amounts of polymorpho (PMN) and mononuclear cells, apoptosis, and oxidative stress	Prevented the PMN infiltration, reduced apoptosis through caspase-3 cleavage, but limited the effects on oxidative stress	[53]
Ischemia/reperfusion (I/R) injury	Wistar rats	10 or 100 mg/kg	Inflammatory markers (MPO, TNF-α, and NF-κB p65) and oxidative stress (GSH and MDA)	Reduced MPO, TNF-α, NF-κB, and MDA. Eugenol also increased GSH levels.	[54]
Isoproterenol-induced myocardial infarction	Wistar rats	100 mg/kg	Cells inflammatory infiltration, oxidative stress, and protein biomarker (α1, α2, β1, β2, and γ globulin)	Reduction of inflammatory cells infiltration and mediators proteins, increased SOD, GPx, and GSH, with reduction of TBARS	[55]
LPS-induced inflammatory signalizing	Macrophage RAW 264.7	1, 10, 50, or 100 μM	Inflammatory markers (NO, TNF-α, IL-1β, and NF-κB), regulatory enzymes (iNOS), and signal transduction (Akt, ERK1/2, JNK, and p38 MAPK)	Reduced NO, TNF-α, IL-1β, NF-κB, and iNOS expression. Eugenol also decreased the ERK1/2 and p38 MAPK signaling pathways	[57]
LPS-activated peritoneal macrophages	BALB/c mice	0.31, 0.62, 1.24, or 2.48 μg/mL	COX-2, NF-κB, and TNF-α expression in resting macrophages	Promoted hypoexpression of TNF-α, but not COX-2 or NF-κB	[58]
RANKL-induced osteoclast formation	RAW264.7 murine macrophages	50, 100, or 200 μM	Degradation of IkBα and NF-κB, MAPK activation	Attenuated the degradation of IkBa, activation of NF-κB and MAPK pathways	[5]
Alveolar bone deformities in an ovariectomized (OVX) rodent model	Wistar rats	2.5 or 5 mg/kg	Histopathology and inflammatory mediators (IL-1β, IL-6, and TNF-α)	Reduced the inflammatory cell infiltrate, IL-1β, IL-6, and TNF-α levels	[60]
LPS-induced inflammation	Human dental pulp fibroblasts	13 μM	Genes expression (NF-κB, IL-1β, and TNF-α)	Inhibition of TNF-α expression and NF-κB signaling pathway, but not IL-1β levels	[62]
Cutaneous chemical carcinogenesis	Swiss mice	15% (v/v)	Inflammatory markers (IL-6, TNF-α, PGE$_2$, COX-2, and iNOS) and oxidative stress (MDA, GSH, GPx, GR, CAT, and GST)	Reduced the IL-6, TNF-α, PGE$_2$, COX, and iNOS levels. Eugenol also decreased the MDA levels and increased the GSH content and activities of GR, CAT, GPx, and GST	[40]

TABLE 1: Continued.

Experimental model	Animal and/ or cells lines	Dose or concentration of eugenol	Inflammatory parameters evaluated	Biological effect	References
Ability to interfere with cell growth	HeLa cells	300 μM	Genes expression (COX-2 and IL-1β)	Reduced the COX-2 and IL-1β expression	[63]
Cisplatin-mediated toxicity	MDA-MB-231, MDA-MB-468, and BT-20 cells	0.25, 0.50, 0.75, 1.0, or 1.5 μM	Gene expression (NF-κB, IL-1β, and TNF-α)	Reduced NF-κB, IL-1β, and TNF-α expression	[23]
Postoperative alveolar osteitis in patients having third molars extracted	Human	0.2% chlorhexidine gel, a eugenol-based paste	Postoperative pain, inflammation, infection, and wound healing	Reduced the incidence of alveolar osteitis, pain, inflammation, infection, and better wound healing compared to control group	[65]
Carrageenan-induced paw edema	Rats	1, 2, or 4%	Paw edema	Inhibited the inflammation, reducing the edema	[64]

3.2. Can Eugenol Reduce the Inflammatory Response via Its Antioxidant Action? Oxidative stress is a condition that reflect an imbalance between biological defensive and aggressive system, mediated by excessive production of reactive oxygen species (ROS), e.g., O^{2-} (superoxide radical), $\cdot$OH (hydroxyl radical), and H_2O_2 (hydrogen peroxide), in which there is an inability of the antioxidant mechanisms to neutralize them [42]. This process results in toxic effects and alterations of the normal redox state, which is associated with cellular damage and lipid peroxidation [43].

Studies have shown that inflammation and oxidative stress are interconnected phenomena, which are involved in pathological conditions as cardiovascular [44], kidney [45], liver disease [46], and cancer [47]. In this way, during inflammatory events occur exacerbated production of ROS in the damaged inflammatory tissue, which can stimulate and had a critical role in the signaling pathway for inflammatory mediators production, such as proinflammatory cytokines and chemokines, resulting in inflammatory cell migration [48].

Thus, compounds capable of modulating oxidative stress may contribute to reduce critical mediators in inflammatory events act as anti-inflammatory agents, even by indirect way. So, several research groups have demonstrated that eugenol has anti-inflammatory and antioxidant capacity, and therefore, be more effective in reducing inflammation.

3.3. Eugenol Reduces the Inflammatory Response and Ameliorate the Function of Specific Organ. The anti-inflammatory effect of eugenol has been investigated in the leukocytes migration using different stimuli, such as N-formyl-methionyl-leucyl-phenylalanine (fMLP), leukotriene B4 (LTB4), and carrageenan. Polymorphonuclear (PMN) recruitment to the inflammatory site occurs dependent on a complex response involving the endothelium-leukocyte interactions and subsequent extravasation to the inflamed site [49]. In this background, Estevão-Silva and colleagues [50] demonstrated that eugenol significantly decreased the *in vitro* and *in vivo* leukocytes migration in response to chemotactic factors by the modulation of rolling and adherence to perivascular tissue. In addition, the authors showed that

eugenol did not induce changes in cell viability, which suggest absence of toxic effect [50].

Additionally, Pan and Dong [51], using an experimental model of allergic asthma induced by ovalbumin (OVA), demonstrated that eugenol administration inhibited the OVA-induced eosinophilia in the lung tissue, prevented the increased of IL-4 and IL-5 levels, and reduced the NF-κB signalizing pathways. According to the authors, the inflammatory response reduction had a pivot role in the antiasthmatic effect of eugenol, resulting in the decrease of airway resistance (AWR) [51]. This data suggests that eugenol can be a therapeutic and strategic agent in patients with asthma.

Eugenol also has anti-inflammatory activity on lipopolysaccharide- (LPS-) induced acute lung injury. Pretreatment with eugenol inhibited the inflammatory response and leukocyte recruitment into the lung tissue by the downregulation of proinflammatory cytokines (IL-6 and TNF-α) expression and NF-κB signaling. In addition, eugenol also increased the superoxide dismutase (SOD), catalase (CAT), glutathione peroxidase (GPx), and glutathione-S-transferase (GST), which are important antioxidative enzymes [41]. Similarly, Magalhães and colleagues [52], using an animal model of LPS-induced lung injury for 6 hours, demonstrated that eugenol significantly reduced neutrophil infiltration, TNF-α, and the NF-κB-mediated signalizing pathway, decreasing the lung inflammation, resulting in an improved lung structure and function, which suggest an important drug to treat disorders of lung inflammatory diseases [52].

So, eugenol reduces the inflammatory response in animal model pulmonary damage caused by diesel exhaust particles. Eugenol administration reduced the pulmonary inflammation by inhibiting the PMN infiltration and apoptosis through caspase-3 cleavage but limited the effects against oxidative stress. This resulted in the improvement of airspace collapse and pulmonary mechanics, which are evaluated by pneumotachography and altered by diesel particles [53]. These data demonstrated the potential of eugenol as an agent to treat the damage effects of air pollutant exposure, by mechanisms mediated, at the last in part, of its anti-inflammatory effects.

Motteleb and colleagues (2014) conducted a study using eugenol to assess its efficacy in the prevention of liver damage in a model of ischemia and reperfusion (I/R). In this work, eugenol abolished the inflammation, reduced myeloperoxidase (MPO) activity, TNF-α levels, and NF-κB expression, and altered oxidative marker. It also reduced malondialdehyde (MDA) and increased GSH levels. This potent effect of eugenol resulted in the amelioration of hepatic structural and functional damage [54]. Thus, eugenol reduced the liver damage by the reduction of inflammatory mediators and modulation of redox status, suggesting a possible application against hepatic I/R injury.

Eugenol also was evaluated as preventive agent against cardiac remodeling following myocardial infarction. This pathology was induced using isoproterenol, which eugenol reduced inflammatory mediator's proteins and lipid peroxidation as well as increased antioxidative enzymes markers (i.e., SOD, GPx, and GSH). In this study, eugenol reduced cardiac injury biomarkers, such as troponin-T, creatine kinase-muscle/brain (CK-MB), and LDH, resulting in the improvement of electrocardiographic and hemodynamic parameters, and great potential antithrombotic, anti-inflammatory, and anti-ischemic activities [55].

3.4. Eugenol Inhibits the Liberation of Inflammatory Mediators from Macrophages.

Macrophage is one of the immune system cells that contribute to the production of mediators (i.e., proinflammatory cytokines and nitric oxide), which are important to cellular and vascular events during the installation and progression of inflammatory process [56]. Thus, studies have demonstrated that eugenol can modulate the macrophage functions and regulates negatively the inflammation.

Yeh and colleagues demonstrated that eugenol inhibits the inducible nitric oxide synthase (iNOS) expression from macrophages in response to LPS, culminating in the reduction of NO levels. Additionally, eugenol also reduced the TNF-α and IL-1β as well as the NF-κB, ERK1/2, and p38 MAPK signaling pathways [57]. In other study, de Paula Porto and colleagues [58] also reported that eugenol promotes the downregulation of TNF-α in LPS-activated macrophages, which are associated with antigenotoxic activity when DNA damage was induced with doxorubicin (DXR) [58]. Thus, this data suggests that the molecular mechanisms to anti-inflammatory effects of eugenol are mediated by the regulation of inflammatory mediators production from macrophages.

3.5. Anti-inflammatory Effect of Eugenol Modulates the Bone Remodeling.

Several research groups have described the effect of eugenol as anti-inflammatory agent and its role modulator on bone remodeling. Deepak and colleagues [59], using cell culture preexposed to RANKL (a receptor activator of NF-κB ligand), demonstrated that eugenol prevented the osteoclast differentiation in a dose-dependent manner. Among the molecular mechanisms involved, the authors emphasized the downregulation of NF-κB and MAPKs signaling pathways, which suggest its use in bone remodeling disorders, such as osteoporosis [59]. A recent study demonstrated that eugenol administration for twelve weeks attenuated the alveolar bone loss and remodeling associated with estrogen insufficiency using an ovariectomized (OVX) rat model, which is similar to what occurs after menopause in humans. The authors suggested that anti-inflammatory effect of eugenol had primary importance, since it was accompanied by the reduction of IL-1β, IL-6, and TNF-α levels resulting in the reduction of inflammatory cell [60].

Additionally, the effects of eugenol against inflammatory response also have been investigated in dental pulp fibroblasts from extracted third molars. During permanent teeth extractions arise postoperative complications, such as alveolar osteitis, an inflammatory condition with delayed healing and persistent pain [61]. In this context, Martínez-Herrera and colleagues [62] reported that eugenol inhibited TNF-α expression and NF-κB signaling pathway, but not IL-1β, when fibroblasts was exposed to LPS, confirming its anti-inflammatory property in bone disorders. Curiously, eugenol also induced inflammatory gene mild expression in fibroblasts absence of previous inflammation [62].

3.6. The Antitumor Effect of Eugenol Appears to Be Mediated, in Part, by Its Anti-inflammatory Activity.

Kaur and colleagues [40] demonstrated that eugenol prevents the 7,12-dimethylbenz[a]anthracene- (DMBA-) and 12-O-tetradecanoylphorbol-13-acetate- (TPA-) promoted skin carcinogenesis. According to the authors, the molecular mechanism of eugenol is related to its anti-inflammatory properties, since reduced proinflammatory cytokine levels (i.e., IL-6 and TNF-α) and inflammation enzymes marker (COX and iNOS) are associated with the modulation of redox status (Figure 2) with reduced MDA and increased antioxidative enzymes [40]. Thus, these data strongly suggest the chemotherapeutic potential of eugenol against carcinogenesis. In accordance with these data, studies have evaluated the efficacy of eugenol alone or combined with other agents. Using HeLa cells, a human cervical cancer line, Hussain and colleagues [63] demonstrated that eugenol alone promoted cell growth inhibition and increase the therapeutic efficacy when combined with gemcitabine (a standard drug). In the clinical use, it can decrease the side effects promoted by gemcitabine administration. These beneficial effects appear to be mediated by its antiapoptotic and anti-inflammatory effects, since it were associated with increased caspase-3 activity and reduction of COX-2 and IL-1β expression, respectively [63]. Additionally, a recent study reported that eugenol promotes cytotoxicity against breast cancer cells (TNBC) and animal model and synergistic chemotherapeutic effects with cisplatin. A key point in this effect was the inhibition of the NF-κB signaling pathway, which resulted in the inhibition of the p50 and p65 subunits phosphorylation, and its consequence migration to the cellular nucleus, reducing IL-6 and IL-8 levels [23].

3.7. Eugenol-Based Pharmaceutical Formulation and Its Anti-inflammatory Effects.

From the pharmacological potential of eugenol in the modulation of inflammation, its use has also been tested in pharmaceutical formulations. Experimentally, Esmaeili and colleagues [64], using an animal model of

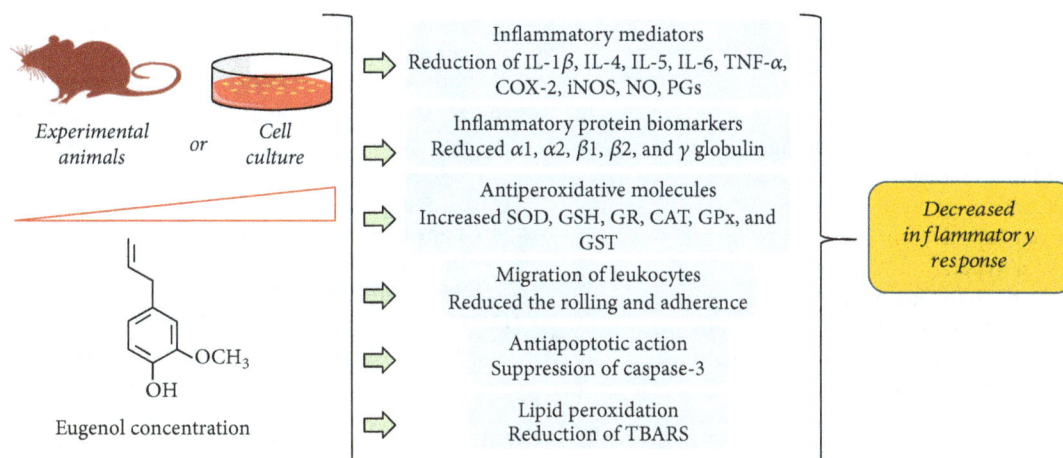

FIGURE 2: The effect of eugenol in the inflammation control.

carrageenan-induced edema, reported that a nano-emulsion containing 1%, 2%, and 4% of eugenol reduced the edema formation and has increased efficacy when combinated with piroxicam, revealing a synergistic anti-inflammatory effect.

Additionally, a clinical dental study involving 270 patients having third molars extracted demonstrated that 0.2% chlorhexidine gel, a eugenol-based paste, reduced postoperative alveolar osteitis, pain, and time of wound healing compared to control group, but with better results when applied in two interventions [65].

3.8. Toxicity of Eugenol. Eugenol is known for its antioxidant, anti-inflammatory, antimicrobial, and antitumor activities; however, it may present some toxicity depending on the type of histological structure exposed to this compound and the concentration used [66]. Thus, eugenol toxicity was observed in human dental pulp fibroblasts from deciduous teeth, with DNA damage at concentrations ranging from $0.06–5.1\,\mu M$, which was not observed at higher interval concentrations of 320 to $818\,\mu M$ [67]. Eugenol was also able to induce genotoxicity by inducing DNA damage of mouse peritoneal macrophages at all concentrations tested (0.62, 1.24, and 2.48 mg/mL). However, it has demonstrated antigenotoxic potential depending on the treatment protocol, which may be interlinked with its effect on drug metabolism [58]. Therefore, eugenol can modulate inflammatory and oxidizing processes. However, its use must be made according to the therapeutic safety evidenced in toxicity.

4. Conclusions

This review demonstrates that eugenol exerts a beneficial action on oxidative stress through the inhibition of enzymes and oxidative processes, which is related to the anti-inflammatory drug profile of this compound. The set of pharmacological studies reported evidences of the clinical potential of eugenol for the treatment of diseases associated with oxidative stress and inflammatory response. Considering the presence of this compound in foods and medicinal plants, the use of these vegetables can result in health benefits and consequently improvement in the quality of life.

However, advanced investigations are needed to understand its metabolism in the body and the contribution of metabolites in antioxidant action and possible interactions in receptors related to inflammation.

Abbreviations

ALDH: Aldehyde dehydrogenase
AP-I: Activating protein 1
AWR: Airway resistance
Bcl-2: B-cell lymphoma 2, apoptosis regulator
CAT: Catalase
CK-MB: Creatine kinase-muscle/brain
COX-2: Cyclooxygenase-2
DNA: Deoxyribonucleic acid
DMBA: 7,12-dimethylbenz[a]anthracene
DXR: Doxorubicin
EC_3: Estimated concentration
fMLP: Formyl-methionyl-leucyl-phenylalanine
GPx: Glutathione peroxidase
GSH: Reduced glutathione
GST: Glutathione-S-transferase
IFN-γ: Interferon gamma
IL-1: Interleukin-1
IL-2: Interleukin-2
IL-4: Interleukin-4
IL-5: Interleukin-5
IL-6: Interleukin-6
IL-8: Interleukin-8
IL-18: Interleukin-18
IL-1β: Interleukin 1 beta
iNOS: Inducible nitric oxide synthase
LPS: Lipopolysaccharide
LTB_4: Leukotriene B_4
MAPK: Mitogen-activated protein kinase pathways
MDA: Malondialdehyde
MPO: Myeloperoxidase
NSAIDs: Nonsteroidal anti-inflammatory drugs
NF-κB: Nuclear factor kappa B
NO: Nitric oxide
OVA: Ovalbumin

OVX: Ovariectomized
PGE: Prostaglandins
PGE2:   Prostaglandins-2
PMN: Polymorphonuclear
RANKL: Receptor activator of NF-κB ligand
SI: Stimulation indices
SOD: Dismutase
TH1:   T helper type 1
TH2:   T helper type 2
TNF-α: Tumor necrosis factor α
TNBC: Cytotoxicity against breast cancer cells
TPA: 12-O-tetradecanoylphorbol-13-acetate
TRAP: Acid phosphatase assay.

Acknowledgments

This work was supported by the Brazilian agencies: Conselho Nacional de Desenvolvimento Científico e Tecnológico (CNPq) and Coordenação de Aperfeiçoamento de Pessoal de Nível Superior (CAPES).

References

[1] P. Zhang, E. Zhang, M. Xiao, C. Chen, and W. Xu, "Study of anti-inflammatory activities of α-d-glucosylated eugenol," *Archives of Pharmacal Research*, vol. 36, no. 1, pp. 109–115, 2013.

[2] H. Zhang, X. Chen, and J. J. He, "Pharmacological action of clove oil and its application in oral care products," *Oral Care Industry*, vol. 19, pp. 23-24, 2009.

[3] D. Chatterjee and P. Bhattacharjee, "Use of eugenol-lean clove extract as a flavoring agent and natural antioxidant in mayonnaise: product characterization and storage study," *Journal of Food Science and Technology*, vol. 52, no. 8, pp. 4945–4954, 2015.

[4] K. G. Lee and T. Shibamoto, "Antioxidant properties of aroma compounds isolated from soybeans and mung beans," *Journal of Agricultural and Food Chemistry*, vol. 48, no. 9, pp. 4290–4293, 2000.

[5] G. Charalambous, Ed., *The Quality of Foods and Beverages V1: Chemistry and Technology*, Elsevier, 2012.

[6] M. Marotti, R. Piccaglia, and E. Giovanelli, "Differences in essential oil composition of basil (*Ocimum basilicum* L.) Italian cultivars related to morphological characteristics," *Journal of Agricultural and Food Chemistry*, vol. 44, no. 12, pp. 3926–3929, 2005.

[7] W. Bin-Nan, H. Tsong-Long, L. Ching-Fong, and C. Ing-Jun, "Vaninolol: a new selective β1-adrenoceptor antagonist derived from vanillin," *Biochemical Pharmacology*, vol. 48, no. 1, pp. 101_109, 1994.

[8] D. P. Bezerra, G. C. G. Militão, M. C. de Morais, and D. P. de Sousa, "The dual antioxidant/prooxidant effect of eugenol and its action in cancer development and treatment," *Nutrients*, vol. 9, no. 12, p. 1367, 2017.

[9] M. J. Jordán, K. Tandon, P. E. Shaw, and K. L. Goodner, "Aromatic profile of aqueous banana essence and banana fruit by gas chromatography-mass spectrometry (GC-MS) and gas chromatography-olfactometry (GC-O)," *Journal of Agricultural and Food Chemistry*, vol. 49, no. 10, pp. 4813–4817, 2001.

[10] M. J. N. Diógenes and F. J. A. Matos, "Dermatite de contato por plantas (DCP)," *Anais Brasileiros De Dermatologia*, vol. 74, no. 6, pp. 629–634, 1999.

[11] M. Sedighi, A. Nazari, M. Faghihi et al., "Protective effects of cinnamon bark extract against ischemia–reperfusion injury and arrhythmias in rat," *Phytotherapy Research*, vol. 32, no. 10, pp. 1983–1991, 2018.

[12] S. J. Lee and K. G. Lee, "Inhibitory effects of volatile antioxidants found in various beans on malonaldehyde formation in horse blood plasma," *Food and Chemical Toxicology*, vol. 43, no. 4, pp. 515–520, 2005.

[13] A. L. Dawidowicz and M. Olszowy, "Does antioxidant properties of the main component of essential oil reflect its antioxidant properties? The comparison of antioxidant properties of essential oils and their main components," *Natural Product Research*, vol. 28, no. 22, pp. 1952–1963, 2014.

[14] D.-Y. Kim, K.-J. Won, D. I. Hwan, S. M. Park, B. Kim, and H. M. Lee, "Chemical composition, antioxidant and anti-melanogenic activities of essential oils from *Chrysanthemum boreale* Makino at different harvesting stages," *Chemistry & Biodiversity*, vol. 15, no. 2, article e1700506, 2018.

[15] X. Han and T. L. Parker, "Anti-inflammatory activity of clove (*Eugenia caryophyllata*) essential oil in human dermal fibroblasts," *Pharmaceutical Biology*, vol. 55, no. 1, pp. 1619–1622, 2017.

[16] L. Ferrero-Miliani, O. H. Nielsen, P. S. Andersen, and S. E. Girardin, "Chronic inflammation: importance of NOD2 and NALP3 in interleukin-1β generation," *Clinical and Experimental Immunology*, vol. 147, no. 2, pp. 227–235, 2007.

[17] R. de Cássia da Silveira e Sá, L. N. Andrade, and D. P. de Sousa, "A review on anti-inflammatory activity of monoterpenes," *Molecules*, vol. 18, no. 1, pp. 1227–1254, 2013.

[18] R. Cássia da Silveira e Sá, L. N. Andrade, and D. P. de Sousa, "Anti-inflammation activities of essential oil and its constituents from indigenous cinnamon (*Cinnamomum osmophloeum*) twigs," *Bioresource Technology*, vol. 99, no. 9, pp. 3908–3913, 2008.

[19] M. J. Stone, "Regulation of chemokine–receptor interactions and functions," *International Journal of Molecular Sciences*, vol. 18, no. 11, article 2415, 2017.

[20] I. T. Nizamutdinova, G. F. Dusio, O. Y. Gasheva et al., "Mast cells and histamine are triggering the NF-κB-mediated reactions of adult and aged perilymphatic mesenteric tissues to acute inflammation," *Aging*, vol. 8, no. 11, article 3065, 3090 pages, 2016.

[21] J. Wang, Y. T. Liu, L. Xiao, L. Zhu, Q. Wang, and T. Yan, "Anti-inflammatory effects of apigenin in lipopolysaccharide-induced inflammatory in acute lung injury by suppressing COX-2 and NF-kB pathway," *Inflammation*, vol. 37, no. 6, pp. 2085–2090, 2014.

[22] F. Polesso, M. Sarker, A. Anderson, D. C. Parker, and S. E. Murray, "Constitutive expression of NF-κB inducing kinase in regulatory T cells impairs suppressive function and promotes instability and pro-inflammatory cytokine production," *Scientific Reports*, vol. 7, no. 1, article 14779, 2017.

[23] S. S. Islam, I. Al-Sharif, A. Sultan, A. Al-Mazrou, A. Remmal, and A. Aboussekhra, "Eugenol potentiates cisplatin anti-cancer activity through inhibition of ALDH-positive breast

cancer stem cells and the NF-κB signaling pathway," *Molecular Carcinogenesis*, vol. 57, no. 3, pp. 333–346, 2018.

[24] B. L. Bermas, "Non-steroidal anti inflammatory drugs, glucocorticoids and disease modifying anti-rheumatic drugs for the management of rheumatoid arthritis before and during pregnancy," *Current Opinion in Rheumatology*, vol. 26, no. 3, pp. 334–340, 2014.

[25] J. D. Rajput, S. D. Bagul, U. D. Pete, C. M. Zade, S. B. Padhye, and R. S. Bendre, "Perspectives on medicinal properties of natural phenolic monoterpenoids and their hybrids," *Molecular Diversity*, vol. 22, no. 1, pp. 225–245, 2018.

[26] D. P. Sousa, *Medicinal Essential Oils: Chemical, Pharmacological and Therapeutic Aspects*, Nova Science Publishers, 2012.

[27] R. de Cássia da Silveira e Sá, L. N. Andrade, R. dos Reis Barreto de Oliveira, and D. P. de Sousa, "A review on anti-inflammatory activity of phenylpropanoids found in essential oils," *Molecules*, vol. 19, no. 2, pp. 1459–1480, 2014.

[28] S. S. Kim, O. J. Oh, H. Y. Min et al., "Eugenol suppresses cyclooxygenase-2 expression in lipopolysaccharide-stimulated mouse macrophage RAW264. 7 cells," *Life Sciences*, vol. 73, no. 3, pp. 337–348, 2003.

[29] E. Dervis, A. Yurt Kilcar, E. I. Medine et al., "*In vitro* incorporation of radioiodinated eugenol on adenocarcinoma cell lines (Caco2, MCF7, and PC3)," *Cancer Biotherapy & Radiopharmaceuticals*, vol. 32, no. 3, pp. 75–81, 2017.

[30] S. F. Hamed, Z. Sadek, and A. Edris, "Antioxidant and antimicrobial activities of clove bud essential oil and eugenol nanoparticles in alcohol-free microemulsion," *Journal of Oleo Science*, vol. 61, no. 11, pp. 641–648, 2012.

[31] E. Darvishi, M. Omidi, A. A. S. Bushehri, A. Golshani, and M. L. Smith, "The antifungal eugenol perturbs dual aromatic and branched-chain amino acid permeases in the cytoplasmic membrane of yeast," *PLoS One*, vol. 8, no. 10, p. e76028, 2013.

[32] J.-P. Dai, X. F. Zhao, J. Zeng et al., "Drug screening for autophagy inhibitors based on the dissociation of Beclin1-Bcl2 complex using BiFC technique and mechanism of eugenol on anti-influenza A virus activity," *PLoS One*, vol. 8, no. 4, article e61026, 2013.

[33] Y. A. Taher, A. M. Samud, F. E. El-Taher et al., "Experimental evaluation of anti-inflammatory, antinociceptive and antipyretic activities of clove oil in mice," *Libyan Journal of Medicine*, vol. 10, no. 1, article 28685, 2015.

[34] H. Tsuchiya, "Anesthetic agents of plant origin: a review of phytochemicals with anesthetic activity," *Molecules*, vol. 22, no. 8, p. 1369, 2017.

[35] B. Baldisserotto, T. V. Parodi, and E. D. Stevens, "Lack of post-exposure analgesic efficacy of low concentrations of eugenol in zebrafish," *Veterinary Anaesthesia and Analgesia*, vol. 45, no. 1, pp. 48–56, 2018.

[36] R. Perez-Roses, E. Risco, R. Vila, P. Penalver, and S. Canigueral, "Biological and nonbiological antioxidant activity of some essential oils," *Journal of Agricultural and Food Chemistry*, vol. 64, no. 23, pp. 4716–4724, 2016.

[37] L. L. Zhang, L. F. Zhang, J. G. Xu, and Q. P. Hu, "Comparison study on antioxidant, DNA damage protective and antibacterial activities of eugenol and isoeugenol against several food-borne pathogens," *Food & Nutrition Research*, vol. 61, no. 1, article 1353356, 2017.

[38] U. K. Sharma, A. K. Sharma, and A. K. Pandey, "Medicinal attributes of major phenylpropanoids present in cinnamon," *BMC Complementary and Alternative Medicine*, vol. 16, no. 1, p. 156, 2016.

[39] B. Yogalakshmi, P. Viswanathan, and C. V. Anuradha, "Investigation of antioxidant, anti-inflammatory and DNA-protective properties of eugenol in thioacetamide-induced liver injury in rats," *Toxicology*, vol. 268, no. 3, pp. 204–212, 2010.

[40] G. Kaur, M. Athar, and M. S. Alam, "Eugenol precludes cutaneous chemical carcinogenesis in mouse by preventing oxidative stress and inflammation and by inducing apoptosis," *Molecular Carcinogenesis*, vol. 49, no. 3, pp. 290–301, 2010.

[41] X. Huang, Y. Liu, Y. Lu, and C. Ma, "Anti-inflammatory effects of eugenol on lipopolysaccharide-induced inflammatory reaction in acute lung injury via regulating inflammation and redox status," *International Immunopharmacology*, vol. 26, no. 1, pp. 265–271, 2015.

[42] P. Patlevič, J. Vašková, P. Švorc Jr, L. Vaško, and P. Švorc, "Reactive oxygen species and antioxidant defense in human gastrointestinal diseases," *Integrative Medicine Research*, vol. 5, no. 4, pp. 250–258, 2016.

[43] A. Ayala, M. F. Muñoz, and S. Argüelles, "Lipid peroxidation: production, metabolism, and signaling mechanisms of malondialdehyde and 4-hydroxy-2-nonenal," *Oxidative Medicine and Cellular Longevity*, vol. 2014, Article ID 360438, 31 pages, 2014.

[44] N. García, C. Zazueta, and L. Aguilera-Aguirre, "Oxidative stress and inflammation in cardiovascular disease," *Oxidative Medicine and Cellular Longevity*, vol. 2017, Article ID 5853238, 2 pages, 2017.

[45] S. K. Biswas, J. B. Lopes De Faria, S. K. Biswas, and J. B. Lopes De Faria, "Which comes first: renal inflammation or oxidative stress in spontaneously hypertensive rats?," *Free Radical Research*, vol. 41, no. 2, pp. 216–224, 2007.

[46] A. Ambade and P. Mandrekar, "Oxidative stress and inflammation: essential partners in alcoholic liver disease," *International Journal of Hepatology*, vol. 2012, Article ID 853175, 9 pages, 2012.

[47] S. Reuter, S. C. Gupta, M. M. Chaturvedi, and B. B. Aggarwal, "Oxidative stress, inflammation, and cancer: how are they linked?," *Free Radical Biology and Medicine*, vol. 49, no. 11, pp. 1603–1616, 2010.

[48] T. Hussain, B. Tan, Y. Yin, F. Blachier, M. C. B. Tossou, and N. Rahu, "Oxidative stress and inflammation: what polyphenols can do for us?," *Oxidative Medicine and Cellular Longevity*, vol. 2016, Article ID 7432797, 9 pages, 2016.

[49] H. U. von Andrian, J. D. Chambers, L. M. McEvoy, R. F. Bargatze, K. E. Arfors, and E. C. Butcher, "Two-step model of leukocyte-endothelial cell interaction in inflammation: distinct roles for LECAM-1 and the leukocyte beta 2 integrins in vivo," *Proceedings of the National Academy of Sciences*, vol. 88, no. 17, pp. 7538–7542, 1991.

[50] C. F. Estevão-Silva, R. Kummer, F. C. Fachini-Queiroz et al., "Anethole and eugenol reduce in vitro and in vivo leukocyte migration induced by fMLP, LTB$_4$, and carrageenan," *Journal of Natural Medicines*, vol. 68, no. 3, pp. 567–575, 2014.

[51] C. Pan and Z. Dong, "Antiasthmatic effects of eugenol in a mouse model of allergic asthma by regulation of vitamin D$_3$ upregulated protein 1/NF-κB pathway," *Inflammation*, vol. 38, no. 4, pp. 1385–1393, 2015.

[52] C. B. Magalhães, D. R. Riva, L. J. DePaula et al., "In vivo anti-inflammatory action of eugenol on lipopolysaccharide-

induced lung injury," *Journal of Applied Physiology*, vol. 108, no. 4, pp. 845–851, 2010.

[53] W. A. Zin, A. G. L. S. Silva, C. B. Magalhães et al., "Eugenol attenuates pulmonary damage induced by diesel exhaust particles," *Journal of Applied Physiology*, vol. 112, no. 5, pp. 911–917, 2012.

[54] D. M. Abd el Motteleb, S. A. Selim, and A. M. Mohamed, "Differential effects of eugenol against hepatic inflammation and overall damage induced by ischemia/re-perfusion injury," *Journal of Immunotoxicology*, vol. 11, no. 3, pp. 238–245, 2014.

[55] K. Mnafgui, R. Hajji, F. Derbali et al., "Anti-inflammatory, antithrombotic and cardiac remodeling preventive effects of eugenol in isoproterenol-induced myocardial infarction in Wistar rat," *Cardiovascular Toxicology*, vol. 16, no. 4, pp. 336–344, 2016.

[56] G. Arango Duque and A. Descoteaux, "Macrophage cytokines: involvement in immunity and infectious diseases," *Frontiers in Immunology*, vol. 5, p. 491, 2014.

[57] J. L. Yeh, J. H. Hsu, Y. S. Hong et al., "Eugenolol and glyceryl-isoeugenol suppress LPS-induced iNOS expression by down-regulating NF-κB AND AP-1 through inhibition of MAPKS and AKT/IκBα signaling pathways in macrophages," *International Journal of Immunopathology and Pharmacology*, vol. 24, no. 2, pp. 345–356, 2011.

[58] M. de Paula Porto, G. N. Da Silva, B. C. O. Luperini et al., "Citral and eugenol modulate DNA damage and pro-inflammatory mediator genes in murine peritoneal macrophages," *Molecular Biology Reports*, vol. 41, no. 11, pp. 7043–7051, 2014.

[59] V. Deepak, A. Kasonga, M. C. Kruger, and M. Coetzee, "Inhibitory effects of eugenol on RANKL-induced osteoclast formation via attenuation of NF-κB and MAPK pathways," *Connective Tissue Research*, vol. 56, no. 3, pp. 195–203, 2015.

[60] H. M. Abuohashish, D. A. Khairy, M. M. Abdelsalam, A. Alsayyah, M. M. Ahmed, and S. S. Al-Rejaie, "In-vivo assessment of the osteo-protective effects of eugenol in alveolar bone tissues," *Biomedicine & Pharmacotherapy*, vol. 97, pp. 1303–1310, 2018.

[61] S. Faizel, S. Thomas, V. Yuvaraj, S. Prabhu, and G. Tripathi, "Comparision between neocone, alvogyl and zinc oxide eugenol packing for the treatment of dry socket: a double blind randomised control trial," *Journal of Maxillofacial and Oral Surgery*, vol. 14, no. 2, pp. 312–320, 2015.

[62] A. Martínez-Herrera, A. Pozos-Guillén, S. Ruiz-Rodríguez, A. Garrocho-Rangel, A. Vértiz-Hernández, and D. M. Escobar-García, "Effect of 4-allyl-1-hydroxy-2-methoxybenzene (eugenol) on inflammatory and apoptosis processes in dental pulp fibroblasts," *Mediators of Inflammation*, vol. 2016, Article ID 9371403, 7 pages, 2016.

[63] A. Hussain, K. Brahmbhatt, A. Priyani, M. Ahmed, T. A. Rizvi, and C. Sharma, "Eugenol enhances the chemotherapeutic potential of gemcitabine and induces anticarcinogenic and anti-inflammatory activity in human cervical cancer cells," *Cancer Biotherapy and Radiopharmaceuticals*, vol. 26, no. 5, pp. 519–527, 2011.

[64] F. Esmaeili, S. Rajabnejhad, A. R. Partoazar et al., "Anti-inflammatory effects of eugenol nanoemulsion as a topical delivery system," *Pharmaceutical Development and Technology*, vol. 21, no. 7, pp. 887–893, 2016.

[65] J. S. Jesudasan, P. U. A. Wahab, and M. R. M. Sekhar, "Effectiveness of 0.2% chlorhexidine gel and a eugenol-based paste on postoperative alveolar osteitis in patients having third

molars extracted: a randomised controlled clinical trial," *British Journal of Oral and Maxillofacial Surgery*, vol. 53, no. 9, pp. 826–830, 2015.

[66] Y. H. Shih, D. J. Lin, K. W. Chang et al., "Evaluation physical characteristics and comparison antimicrobial and anti-inflammation potentials of dental root canal sealers containing hinokitiol *in vitro*," *PLoS One*, vol. 9, no. 6, article e94941, 2014.

[67] M. Escobar-García, K. Rodríguez-Contreras, S. Ruiz-Rodríguez, M. Pierdant-Pérez, B. Cerda-Cristerna, and A. Pozos-Guillén, "Eugenol toxicity in human dental pulp fibroblasts of primary teeth," *Journal of Clinical Pediatric Dentistry*, vol. 40, no. 4, pp. 312–318, 2016.

12

ALDH2 Activity Reduces Mitochondrial Oxygen Reserve Capacity in Endothelial Cells and Induces Senescence Properties

G. Nannelli,[1] E. Terzuoli,[1] V. Giorgio ⓘ,[2,3] S. Donnini ⓘ,[1] P. Lupetti,[1] A. Giachetti,[1] P. Bernardi,[2,3] and M. Ziche ⓘ[1]

[1]Department of Life Sciences, University of Siena, Siena, Italy
[2]Department of Biomedical Sciences, University of Padua, Padua, Italy
[3]Consiglio Nazionale delle Ricerche, Neuroscience Institute, Padua, Italy

Correspondence should be addressed to M. Ziche; marina.ziche@unisi.it

Academic Editor: Márcio Carocho

Endothelial cells (ECs) are dynamic cells that turn from growth into senescence, the latter being associated with cellular dysfunction, altered metabolism, and age-related cardiovascular diseases. Aldehyde dehydrogenase 2 (ALDH2) is a mitochondrial enzyme metabolizing acetaldehyde and other toxic aldehydes, such as 4-hydroxynonenal (4-HNE). In conditions in which lipid peroxidation products and reactive oxygen species (ROS) are accumulated, ECs become dysfunctional and significantly contribute to the progression of vascular-dependent diseases. The aim of the present study has been to investigate whether inhibition of ALDH2 alters endothelial functions together with the impairment of bioenergetic functions, accelerating the acquisition of a senescent phenotype. HUVECs transfected with siRNA targeting ALDH2 or treated with daidzin, an ALDH2 inhibitor, were used in this study. We observed an alteration in cell morphology associated with endothelial dysfunctions. Loss of ALDH2 reduced cell proliferation and migration and increased paracellular permeability. To assess bioenergetic function in intact ECs, extracellular flux analysis was carried out to establish oxygen consumption rates (OCR). We observed a decrease in mitochondrial respiration and reserve capacity that coincided with SA-β-Gal accumulation and an increase in p21 and p53 expression in siALDH2 or daidzin-treated HUVECs. Treatment with N-acetyl-L-cysteine (NAC) reduced endothelial dysfunctions mediated by siALDH2, indicating that oxidative stress downstream to siALDH2 plays an instrumental role. Our results highlight that ALDH2 impairment accelerates the acquisition of a premature senescent phenotype, a change likely to be associated with the observed reduction of mitochondrial respiration and reserve capacity.

1. Introduction

The aging process reflects the age-dependent functional decline of body tissues and organs [1]. The progressive decline also affects the vascular endothelium, resulting in an impairment of its important functions such as the capacity to supply nutrients and growth factors to organs, the barrier function, and the capacity to form new vessels or angiogenesis [2, 3]. Vascular cell senescence is widely considered one of the causative factors of peripheral and central nervous system pathologies [4], as it promotes reactive oxygen species (ROS) production and the ensuing vascular inflammatory responses [5]. For instance, frequent stroke episodes in patients affected by cerebral amyloid angiopathy (CAA) are related to the

perivascular deposition of amyloid beta peptides (Aβ), which promote ROS production and, in turn, reduce endothelial cell (EC) responsiveness. Similarly, in MELAS, a disease characterized by encephalomyopathy, high ROS levels, derived from dysfunctional mitochondria, compromise EC-mediated vasodilatation, which explains the susceptibility of these patients to stroke-like episodes [6–8]. Besides increased ROS production, nine hallmarks have been proposed to contribute to the aging phenotype, including the phenomenon of cellular senescence as a stable arrest of cell cycle coupled with phenotypic changes, mitochondrial dysfunction, and activation of the p53 pathway [1].

Even though ECs appear to meet most of their energy needs anaerobically, they have an extensive mitochondrial network and consume oxygen. Their mitochondria are essential to endothelial functions [9–11]. It is broadly accepted that, as cells are exposed to stressors, mitochondria are able to rely on a "reserve capacity," referred to as the difference between the maximum respiratory capacity and the basal respiratory capacity. This reserve capacity is suitable to provide the increased energy demands to preserve cellular functions and repair or detoxification of reactive species [11, 12].

In this study, we sought to gain insights into the role of endothelial mitochondria in the senescence process, taking advantage of the recent progress gathered on the role of aldehyde dehydrogenases (ALDHs), particularly ALDH2 isozyme (one of 19 enzymes belonging to the same superfamily). The ALDH2 isozyme is located in the mitochondrial matrix and is predominantly responsible for the acetaldehyde detoxification in alcohol metabolism. It is also a key to detoxification of endogenous aldehydes, such as 4-hydroxy-2-nonenal (4-HNE), which arise from lipid peroxidation under oxidative stress, and of exogenous aldehyde products, such as acrolein from tobacco smoke and car exhausts [13, 14]. Increasing evidence has revealed a cardioprotective and neuroprotective role of ALDH2 in myocardial ischemia-reperfusion injury and Aβ-induced damage, respectively. Studies from our laboratory have provided evidence on the contribution of ALDH2 to Aβ-induced endothelial dysfunction and on the possibility of preserving the endothelial function in some pathological conditions by activating the ALDH2 enzyme [15]. In this study, we focused on ALDH2 and its role as a critical metabolic checkpoint for endothelial function. The aim of the study was to move beyond correlative analyses between ALDH2 and hallmarks of aging, providing causal evidence of the implication of ALDH2 in endothelial senescence.

2. Materials and Methods

2.1. Cell Cultures. Human umbilical vein endothelial cells (HUVECs) (Lonza, Basel, Switzerland) were used. Cells were cultured on gelatin-coated dishes with endothelial growth medium (EGM-2) (Lonza) supplemented with antibiotics (100 U/ml penicillin and 100 μg/ml streptomycin, Euroclone, Milan, Italy), glutamine (2 mM, Euroclone), and 10% fetal bovine serum (FBS, Hyclone, GE Healthcare, Little Chalfont, UK). Progressively passaged HUVECs were utilized up to senescence as already described [16]. The formula PD = (ln n_{ch} – ln n_{cs})/ln 2 was used to calculate the number of cumulative population doublings (PD), where n_{ch} is the number of cells harvested and n_{cs} is the number of cells seeded.

2.2. Small Interfering RNA Transfection. Transient knockdown experiments were performed using control and specific siRNAs (OriGene, Rockville, MD, USA). Subconfluent cells were seeded in 60 mm or 100 mm or 6-well plate dishes in EGM-2 plus 10% FBS. After 24 h, cells were transfected in endothelial basal medium (EBM-2) without serum and antibiotics using Lipofectamine® 3000 (Invitrogen, Carlsbad, CA, USA) and 20 nM targeting siRNA (siALDH2) or scrambled control siRNA (siCTR) diluted in Opti-MEM (Gibco, Thermo Fisher Scientific, Waltham, MA, USA). Serum was

added 6–8 h posttransfection. Where indicated, cells were harvested 24 h posttransfection. Cells were assayed 2–6 days posttransfection. The transfection was repeated every 72 h. We evaluated the knockdown efficiency using immunoblotting or quantitative RT-PCR (qRT-PCR) analysis at the indicated time.

2.3. Immunoblot Analysis. Subconfluent cells were plated in 60 mm or 100 mm or 6-well plate gelatin-coated dishes and transfected as above or treated with 10 μM daidzin, for 48 h. Daidzin was dissolved in DMSO (Sigma-Aldrich). The treatment with daidzin was repeated every day. Where indicated, siCTR and siALDH2 HUVECs have been pretreated with 5 mM N-acetyl-L-cysteine (NAC), as reported [17]. Next, cells were washed and lysed, and an equal amount of proteins was used for immunoblot analysis, as described [15]. The blotted membranes were incubated with anti-ALDH2 (OriGene), anti-p21, anti-Egr-1, anti-c-Myc (Cell Signaling Technology, Danvers, MA, USA), anti-tubulin, anti-p53 (Santa Cruz, Heidelberg, Germany), anti-β-actin (Sigma-Aldrich), anti-4-HNE (Abcam, Cambridge, United Kingdom), and OXPHOS antibody cocktail kit (Abcam) antibodies. Super-Signal West Pico Chemiluminescent Substrate (Thermo Fisher Scientific) was used to develop signals, which were detected and quantified by the ChemiDoc system and Quantity One software (Bio-Rad, Hercules, CA, USA). For all experiments using whole-cell lysate, β-actin or β-tubulin was used as loading controls.

2.4. Real-Time PCR. The RNeasy Plus Kit (Qiagen, Hilden, Germany) was used according to the manufacturer's instructions to extract and prepare total RNA. A total amount of 1 μg RNA was transcribed, and quantitative RT-PCR was performed as reported [18]. The fold change expression was determined using the comparative Ct method ($\Delta\Delta$Ct) normalized to 60S ribosomal protein L19 expression. Data are reported as fold change relative to siCTR (control), which was set to 1.

2.5. ALDH Enzymatic Activity. The conversion of acetaldehyde to acetic acid was determined in order to evaluate ALDH enzyme activity, as reported [15]. Briefly, 1×10^6 of seeded cells were transfected as described above, and after 48 h, cells were scraped into 100 μl of CelLytic™ MT Cell Lysis (Sigma-Aldrich) supplied with protease inhibitors (Sigma-Aldrich) and sodium orthovanadate (Sigma-Aldrich). Then, lysates were centrifuged for 20 min at 4°C at 14000 × g. The protein content in the supernatant was quantified in a Bradford assay. ALDH2 activity was measured in an assay mix (0.8 ml) containing 100 mM sodium pyrophosphate (Sigma-Aldrich) at pH 9 and 10 mM NAD+ (Sigma-Aldrich) and 300 μg of sample protein. Then, acetaldehyde (10 mM, Sigma-Aldrich) was added to the cuvette to start the reaction. NADH formation from NAD+ was monitored at 25°C in a spectrophotometer Infinite F200 Pro at 340 nm (Tecan Life Sciences, Switzerland). Where indicated, supernatants of HUVECs were challenged with daidzin for 10 min before the acetaldehyde was added; the compound was tested at 1 and 10 μM to monitor the extent of ALDH inhibition in these cell lysates. Enzyme-specific activity was expressed as % nmol NADH/minute/mg protein.

2.6. Cell Survival and Area.

Cells were transfected with siRNA for ALDH2 as described above. Then, cells were harvested and seeded (1.5×10^3/well) in triplicate in 96-multiwell plates. Adherent cells were exposed to EBM-2 with 2% FBS for 2 and 5 days. Where indicated, HUVECs were treated with 5 mM NAC (Sigma-Aldrich) before the administration of 2% FBS. This treatment was repeated every three days. Further, HUVECs were also pretreated for 30 min with 10 μM daidzin in EBM-2 before the administration of 2% FBS for 2 or 5 days. Then, cells were fixed and stained with the PanReac kit (Darmstadt, Germany), and five fields per well were counted. Data are analyzed in triplicate, and results are expressed as the cell number counted/well. To calculate the area of cells, three fields in which cells were at 60% confluence for each condition were measured using ImageJ software and results are expressed as square pixel.

2.7. Senescence-Associated β-Galactosidase (SA-β-Gal) Activity Assay.

Cells were seeded in 6-well multiplates (8×10^4 or 1.5×10^5 cells/well). Adherent cells were treated with 10 μM daidzin for 2 days or transfected with siRNA as described above. Where indicated, 24 h posttransfection, a preincubation of 30 min with 5 mM NAC was carried out before the administration of 2% FBS. This treatment was repeated every three days. At 2 and 6 days, SA-β-Gal activity was assessed by using the Senescence β-Galactosidase Staining Kit (Cell Signaling) following the manufacturer's manual. Data are reported as a fold increase vs. siCTR of positive cells for SA-β-Gal activity.

2.8. BrdU Incorporation Assay.

Cell proliferative capacity was evaluated using a chemiluminescence ELISA (Roche Diagnostic S.p.A, Monza, Italy) which assesses the 5-bromo-2′-deoxy-uridine (BrdU) incorporation. 3×10^3 cells were seeded in a 96-well plate in triplicate 24 h posttransfection. Adherent cells were exposed to EBM-2 in the presence or absence of serum (2% and 0.1% FBS, respectively) for 48 h. 8 hours before the end of incubation, BrdU was added in each well. Then, the assay was carried out as reported [18].

2.9. Wound Healing Assay.

siRNA transfection of adherent cells was conducted as described above, and after 24 h, cells were harvested. siCTR, siALDH2, and wild-type HUVECs were seeded (1×10^5 cells/well) into 24-well plates and incubated until they were grown into a confluent monolayer (24–30 h). Then, a sterile 100–1000 μl micropipette tip was used to scrape the confluent monolayer and create a wound $\pm$ 500 μm. The cells were washed twice with PBS and exposed to fresh EBM-2 medium supplemented with 0.1 or 2% FBS and ARA-C (2.5 mg/ml, Sigma-Aldrich) to suppress cell proliferation. Where indicated, confluent HUVECs were pretreated for 30 min with daidzin and then treated with 2% FBS. Images of the wound in each well were acquired from 0 to 18 h under a phase contrast microscope at 10x magnification. Then, cells were fixed and stained with the PanReac kit. Results were quantified using ImageJ software, and data are reported as % of scratch closure.

2.10. Immunofluorescence Microscopy Analysis.

Cells were transfected with siRNA as described above, and 24 h posttransfection, ECs were harvested and seeded (8×10^4 cells) on 8 mm ∅ glass coverslips in triplicate. After 24 h, cells were exposed to EBM-2 with 0.1% FBS for 8 h. 4% paraformaldehyde/PBS with Ca^{2+} and Mg^{2+} and 3% bovine serum albumin (BSA) were used to fix cells and block unspecific binding sites, respectively. Then, cells were incubated with a monoclonal rabbit anti-VE-cadherin diluted to 1 : 400 (Cell Signaling Technology) and a polyclonal rabbit anti-ZO-1 (Life Technologies, Carlsbad, CA, USA) diluted to 1 : 50 in 0.5% BSA in PBS for 18 h at 4°C. After incubation with the secondary antibody, Alexa Fluor© 488-labeled anti-rabbit (1 : 200, 1 h, Invitrogen) and Alexa Fluor© 555-labeled anti-rabbit (1 : 200, 1 h) were used for 1 h at room temperature, and then the protocol was completed according to Terzuoli et al. [19]. Leica SP5 confocal microscopy (63x objective) was used to capture images of stained cells.

2.11. Paracellular Permeability Assay.

Cells were seeded (8×10^4 cells/well) 24 h post-ALDH2 silencing on gelatin-coated insert membranes (0.4 μm diameter pores, Corning, New York, USA), and the inserts were placed in 24-multiwell plates and incubated for 24 h. Next, cells were exposed to EBM-2 with 0.1% FBS for 8 h. The assay was carried out as described [20]. Briefly, the fluorescent permeability tracer (3 kDa FITC-Dextran, 10 μM) was added, and the fluorescence was measured after 7 min in the medium present in the bottom of the well, in a multiplate reader (Infinite 200 Pro, SpectraFluor, Tecan), at 485/535 nm (excitation/emission). Results are reported as relative fluorescence units (RFU) [20].

2.12. ROS Measurement.

siCTR and siALDH2 cells (24 h posttransfection) were seeded (1.5×10^3 cells/well) in triplicate in a 96-well plate, and after adherence (6–8 h), the medium was replaced with EBM-2 with 0.1% FBS in the presence or absence of 5 mM NAC for 24 h. DCFH2-DA (2,-7-dichlorodihydrofluorescein diacetate, Invitrogen) was used, and intracellular ROS were measured as previously described [20]. The results are reported as fold change vs. siCTR of relative fluorescence units (RFU) corrected for the cell number counted [20].

2.13. Measurement of the Oxygen Consumption Rate.

The measurement of oxygen consumption rates (OCR) was carried out using the Seahorse XF24 extracellular flux analyzer as described previously [21, 22]. siCTR and siALDH2 ECs were harvested and seeded 24 h posttransfection in XF24 cell culture plates at 3×10^4 cells/well density in 200 μl of EGM-2 supplemented with 10% FBS and incubated at 37°C in 5% CO_2 for 6–8 h. Then, adherent cells were exposed to EBM-2 supplemented with 2% FBS for 24 h. Assays were performed as reported [22]. Independent titration was routinely carried out to determine the optimal concentration of FCCP (carbonylcyanide-p-trifluoromethoxyphenyl hydrazone), which was ranged between 0.2 and 0.4 μM. Initially, a stable OCR baseline was determined, and then, oligomycin, FCCP, rotenone, and antimycin A were supplied as reported in the figure legend.

2.14. Transmission Electron Microscopy. 1×10^4 cells transfected with siRNA as above were harvested and seeded 24 h posttransfection in a small chamber prepared with cylinder part of BEEM® (Ted Pella Inc., Redding, CA, USA) capsule glued to the coverslip as previously described [23]. After 6–8 h of incubation needed for adhesion, cells were exposed to EBM-2 with 2% FBS for 24 h. The medium was replaced with 2.5% glutaraldehyde (Ted Pella, Redding, CA, USA) in 0.1 M phosphate buffer (pH 7.2) for 2 h at RT and postfixed with buffered 1% OsO_4 (EMS, Hatfield, PA, USA) for 1 h and processed by standard dehydration through a graded series of ethanol (50°–100°). Specimens were then embedded in pure Epon (EMS, Hatfield, PA, USA) resin. Polymerization was done in an oven at 60°C for 48 h. Then, slides were dropped into liquid nitrogen to detach the resin from coverslips. 60–70 nm thick sections were cut with an Ultracut E (Reichert-Jung, Wien, AT) ultramicrotome, stained with uranyl acetate and lead citrate, and examined in a TEM Jeol 1010 (Peabody, MA, USA) transmission electron microscope.

2.15. Statistical Analysis. Results are expressed as means ± SD or SEM. Statistical analysis was generated by GraphPad software (San Diego, CA, USA). Statistical analysis was performed by Student's *t*-test and two-way ANOVA. $p < 0.05$ was considered statistically significant.

3. Results

3.1. ALDH2 Silencing or Inhibition Impairs Endothelial Cell Functions. To examine the role of ALDH2 in endothelial function, HUVECs were treated with 1 and 10 μM daidzin, an inhibitor of ALDH2 activity [14], or transiently knocked down for ALDH2 (siALDH2) and compared with wild-type cells transfected with an empty vector (siCTR), throughout this work. 10 μM daidzin was the higher concentration without a significant effect of its solvent on HUVEC survival.

Whereas in siCTR cells ALDH2 protein expression was easily detected by Western blot, the enzyme expression was drastically reduced in siALDH2 (Figure 1(a)). Silencing of ALDH2 also reduced the mRNA levels and activity of the enzyme (Figures 1(b) and 1(c)) and promoted a significant change in HUVEC morphology, characterized by the irregular elongated shape instead of the regular polygonal shape of siCTR cells (Figure 1(d)). As expected, 10 μM daidzin significantly reduced ALDH2 activity, while at 1 μM, it did not affect the enzyme activity (Figure 1(e)).

Next, we determined the involvement of ALDH2 activity on cell viability, proliferation, and migration, as well as on cell permeability, key features of endothelial cell functions. The proliferation of siALDH2 ECs, assessed by the BrdU incorporation assay, was significantly reduced relative to siCTR ECs and not recovered in the presence of serum (Figure 2(a)). Accordingly, both deficiency and pharmacological inhibition of ALDH2 in HUVECs resulted in a consistent reduction of cell viability, particularly visible after 5 days

(Figures 2(b) and 2(c)). Moreover, cell migration, evaluated by the scratch assay, was significantly inhibited in both daidzin-treated and siALDH2 ECs (Figure 2(d)). ALDH2 ablation also affected the adherence and tight junctions of HUVECs altering their barrier function. Indeed, in confluent siCTR, the expression of VE-cadherin and ZO-1, examined by immunofluorescence, was mainly localized at cell-cell contacts and disappeared in cells whose ALDH2 was silenced (Figure 2(e)).

To corroborate the immunofluorescence analysis, we evaluated the paracellular flux in a confluent monolayer of siCTR and siALDH2 ECs. Consistent with the above data, we observed an increase in permeability in siALDH2 when compared to siCTR ECs, as shown by increased paracellular flux of fluorescence-conjugated dextran (Figure 2(f)).

Of note, silencing the ALDH2 triggered the accumulation of 4-HNE-induced covalent adducts, as well as ROS products [24] in ECs (Figures 3(a) and 3(b)), suggesting that the intracellular abundance of these toxic products might contribute to the impairment of the endothelium and trigger the premature senescence process seen below.

To get insight into the role of ROS in the dysfunction of ECs whose ALDH2 was silenced, 5 mM NAC, a ROS scavenger, was used. In particular, as shown in Figures 3(b)–3(e), NAC treatment in siALDH2 ECs affected the pattern of 4-HNE protein adducts and reduced their expression, significantly inhibited the production of total ROS levels, and improved viability at 5 days. Taken together, these results indicate that ALDH2 silencing affects the healthy phenotype of HUVECs by increasing the accumulation of 4-HNE-induced adducts and ROS products, leading to changes in morphology and disassembling of intercellular junctions, and impairs endothelial cell barrier function and mobilization capacity.

3.2. ALDH2 Silencing or Inhibition Promotes the Onset of Senescence in Endothelial Cells. In light of the above findings, showing a pervasive dysfunction of endothelial cells upon ALDH2 silencing, we wondered whether this impaired state might be associated with the acquisition of premature senescence. Morphological modifications characterize usually senescent cells in *in vitro* culture: cells become large, flat, vacuolated, and occasionally multinucleated [25]. Therefore, we quantified the size of the cells and reported it as the area of the cells expressed as square pixel. siALDH2 cells presented a larger cell area in comparison to siCTR cells (Figures 4(a) and 4(b)). We next measured the cumulative population doubling (PD) in long-term cultured endothelial cells at predetermined set points, an experimental protocol we devised to study senescence [16]. We performed measurements of PD and of several senescence markers at PD 5 and PD 21, corresponding to the time-dependent progress from premature to moderate-full senescent cells, respectively. Senescent cells vary from other nonproliferating cells by several markers. Besides the expression of signals belonging to the two major senescence-inducing pathways (p53/p21, c-Myc, Egr-1), we also evaluated beta-galactosidase (SA-β-Gal) activity. As shown in Figures 4(c), 4(d), and 4(g), HUVECs at PD 21 overexpressed SA-β-Gal activity and senescence markers

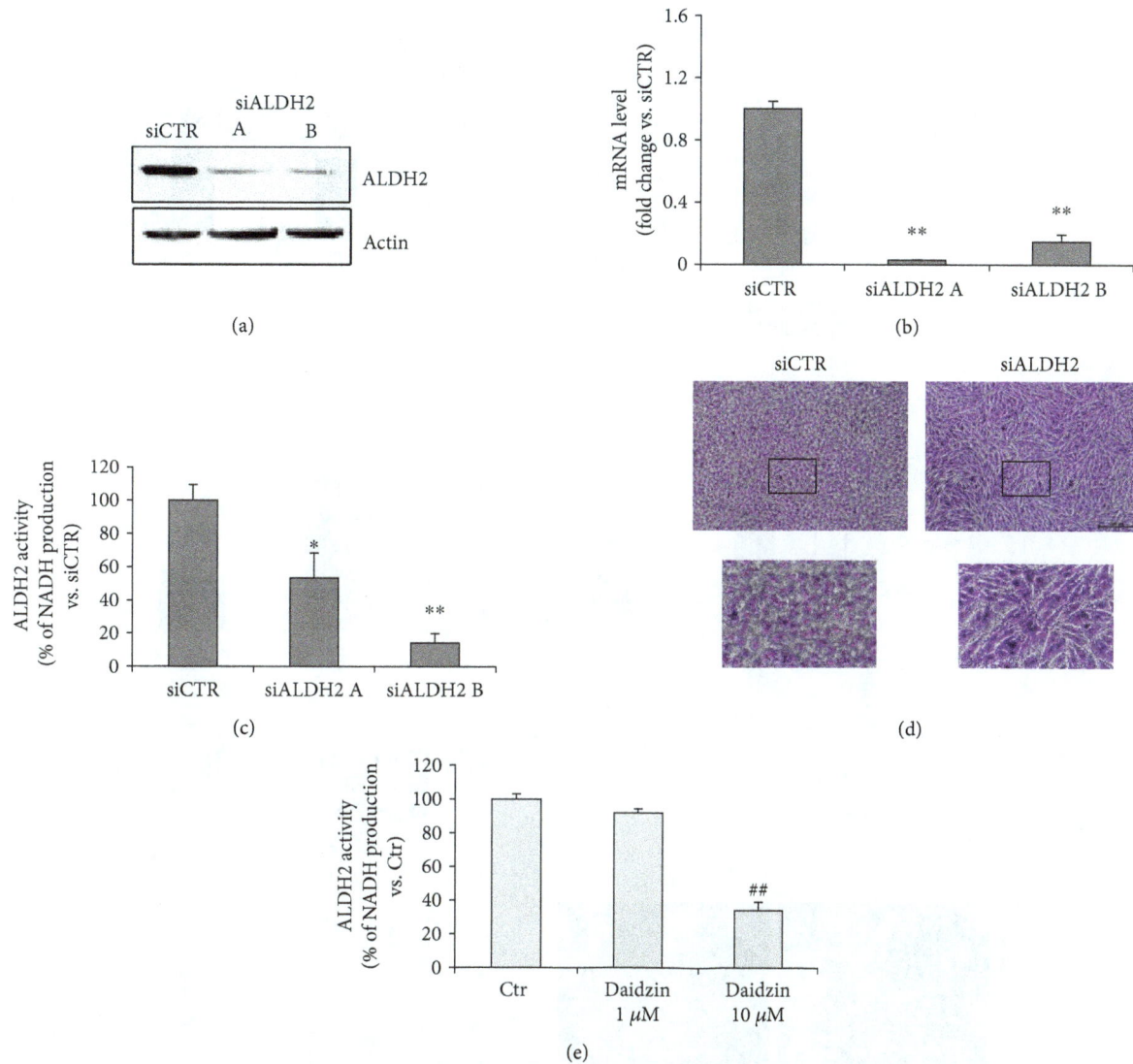

FIGURE 1: Characterization of siALDH2 and daidzin-treated HUVECs. (a) Immunoblotting and (b) qPCR analysis of ALDH2 silencing (siALDH2) in ECs, 48 h posttransfection. Representative blots of at least 3 with similar results are shown. qPCR data are expressed as the mean of fold change ± SD vs. siCTR cells, which were assigned to 1. $^{**}p < 0.01$ vs. siCTR. (c) ALDH2 activity measured in siALDH2 EC lysates (48 h posttransfection). Data are presented as the mean ± SD of % NADH production vs. siCTR. $^{*}p < 0.05$ and $^{**}p < 0.01$ vs. siCTR. (d) Morphology of confluent monolayers of siCTR and siALDH2 B ECs fixed and stained 48 h posttransfection. A representative image for each condition is shown. Scale bar: 100 μm. (e) ALDH2 activity measured in ECs in the presence or absence of daidzin (1–10 μM). D10: 10 μM daidzin. Data are presented as the mean ± SD of % NADH production vs. Ctr. $^{\#\#}p < 0.01$ vs. Ctr.

compared to HUVECs at PD 5. Of note, in HUVECs at PD 5 whose ALDH2 was silenced, we observed the overexpression of p53 and p21, c-Myc, and Egr-1 (Figures 4(e), 4(f), and 4(h)).

In addition, evaluation of SA-β-Gal revealed significant differences in its expression between siCTR PD 5 cells and those of siALDH2 groups and PD 21 groups (see Figure 4(i)). A time-related increase in SA-β-Gal expression (3- to 5-fold difference) was evident in siALDH2 but not in siCTR cells (Figure 4(j)). Similarly, treatment with 10 μM daidzin significantly increased senescence markers in PD 5 ECs (Figures 4(k) and 4(l)). Of note, 5 mM NAC partially reversed SA-β-Gal expression in siALDH2 ECs (Figure 4(m)), corroborating the instrumental role played by ROS in the impairment of the endothelium whose ALDH2 was silenced.

These data clearly indicate that ALDH2 silencing and inhibition are associated with the onset of early signs of a senescent phenotype.

3.3. ALDH2 Silencing Alters Bioenergetic Functions in Endothelial Cells.
Adjusting metabolism to a quiescent state is central to normal vessel function [9, 10]. As we observed that ablation of ALDH2 causes an impairment of permeability leading to a senescent phenotype in HUVECs, we investigated whether ALDH2 would affect cell oxidative metabolism. We evaluated oxygen consumption rates (OCR) in siCTR compared to siALDH2 at baseline and in response to oligomycin (Oligo), fluoro-carbonyl cyanide phenylhydrazone (FCCP), or antimycin A (AA) and rotenone (R). We found that ALDH2 silencing reduced basal

(a)

(b)

(c)

(d)

(e)

(f)

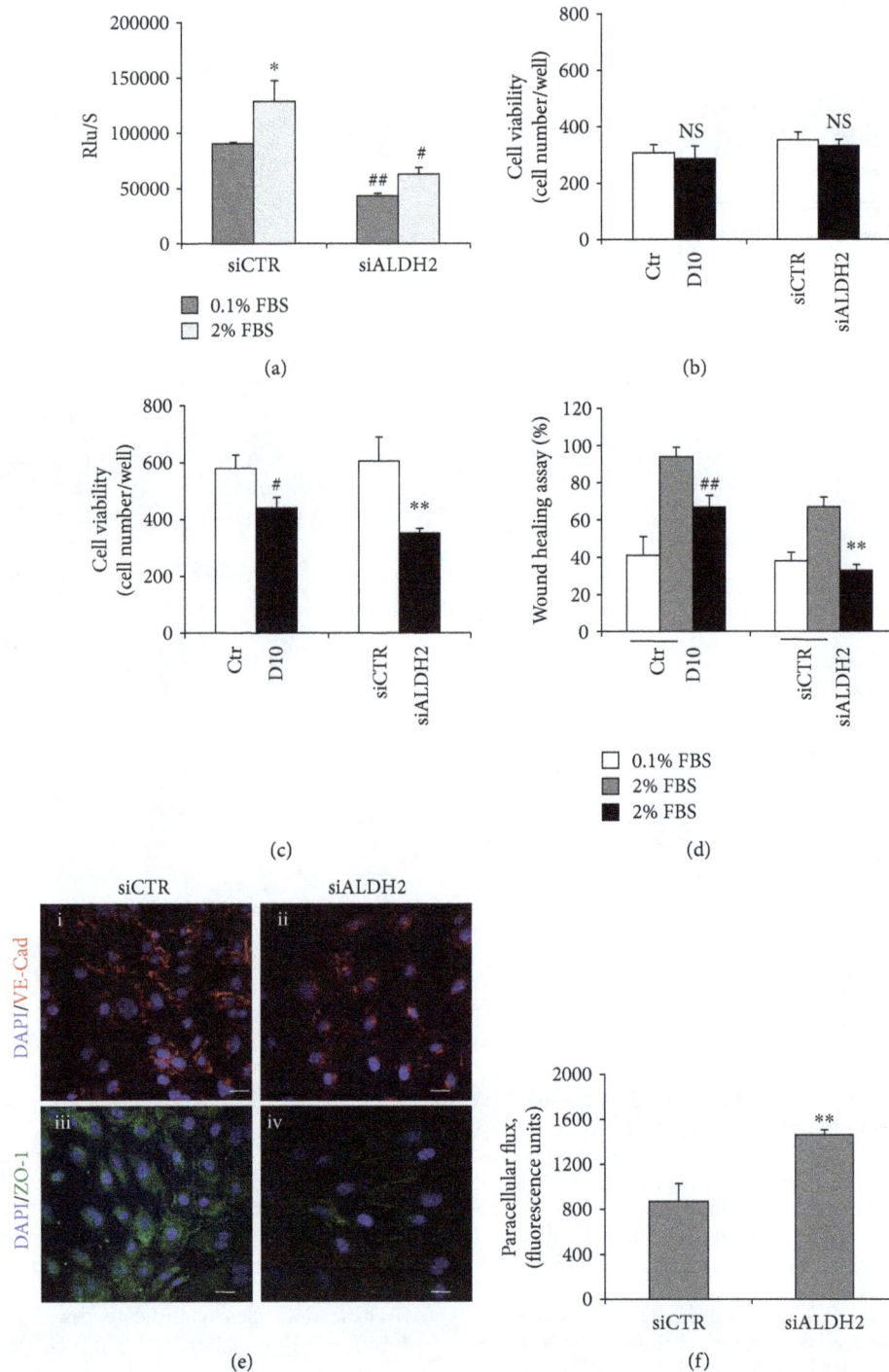

Figure 2: ALDH2 silencing or inhibition impairs endothelial functions. (a) BrdU incorporation in ECs transfected with siRNA for 24 h. Proliferative capacity was assessed after 48 h treatment with 0.1%–2% FBS. Data are reported as mean ± SD. $^*p < 0.05$ vs. siCTR with 0.1% FBS; $^{\#}p < 0.05$ and $^{\#\#}p < 0.01$ vs. siCTR. (b) Cell survival in 10 μM daidzin-treated ECs or siCTR and siALDH2 ECs exposed to 2% FBS for 2 and (c) 5 days. Data are expressed as means ± SD of the cell number counted/well. Dimethyl sulfoxide (DMSO) is used as a solvent to dissolve daidzin. No significant effect of DMSO was observed in HUVEC survival (DMSO-treated cell numbers/well: 329 ± 30). NS: not statistically significant; $^{\#}p < 0.05$ vs. Ctr; $^{**}p < 0.01$ vs. siCTR. D10: 10 μM daidzin. (d) Scratch assay in 10 μM daidzin-treated ECs or in siCTR and siALDH2 ECs cultured in 0.1% or 2% FBS for 18 h. Means ± SD of % of scratch closure ($^{\#\#}p < 0.01$ vs. Ctr; $^{**}p < 0.01$ vs. siCTR). (e) Confocal analysis of VE-cadherin and ZO-1 patterns in control (i–iii) and siALDH2 ECs (ii–iv) after exposure to EBM-2 with 0.1% FBS for 8 h. Representative images of three experiments at 63x magnification are shown. Scale bar: 20 μm. (f) Permeability in siCTR and siALDH2 ECs detected as fluorescence-conjugated FITC-dextran diffusion through the confluent monolayers after exposure to EBM-2 with 0.1% FBS for 8 h. $^{**}p < 0.01$ vs. siCTR. Images are representative of results obtained with siALDH2 B.

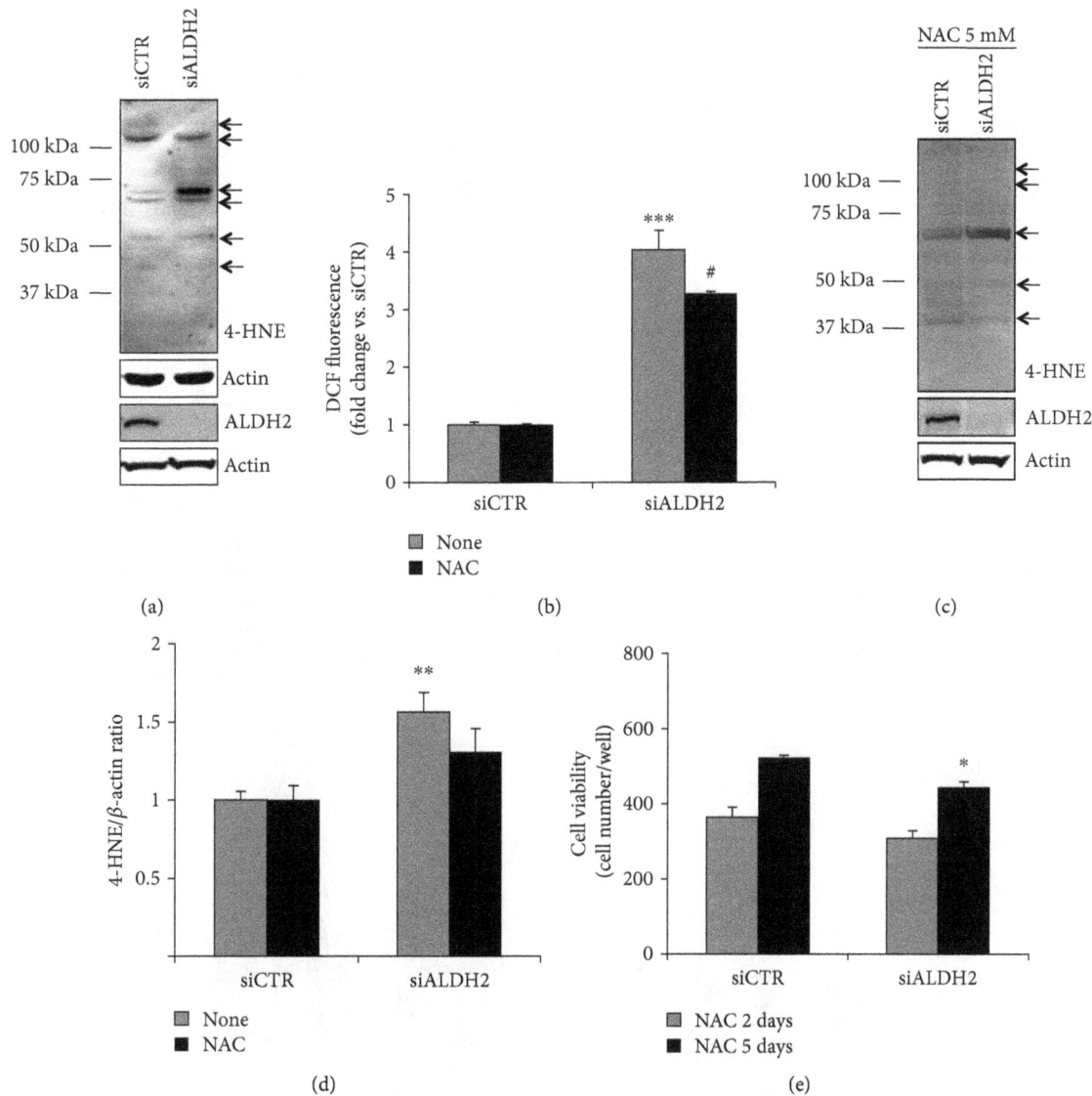

FIGURE 3: ALDH2 silencing increases 4-HNE protein adducts and ROS levels. (a) Western blot analysis of 4-HNE protein adducts in siCTR and siALDH2 ECs cultured in 2% FBS for 24 h. Knockdown efficiency was checked using immunoblotting with an ALDH2 antibody. The arrows indicate bands quantified in (d). Representative blots of at least 3 with similar results are shown. (b) ROS production in siCTR and siALDH2 ECs cultured in 0.1% FBS for 24 h in the presence/absence of NAC (5 mM). Cells were pretreated for 30 min with NAC before FBS treatment. Data, normalized for the cell number, are expressed as the mean of fold change ± SD vs. siCTR of DCF fluorescence. $***p < 0.01$ vs. siCTR; $^{\#}p < 0.05$ vs. untreated siALDH2 ECs. (c) Western blot analysis of 4-HNE protein adducts in siCTR and siALDH2 ECs cultured in 2% FBS for 24 h with or without pretreatment (30 min) with NAC (5 mM). Knockdown efficiency was checked using immunoblotting with an ALDH2 antibody. The arrows indicate bands quantified in (d). Representative blots of 3 with similar results are shown. (d) Quantification of major bands (indicated with arrows), normalized to actin, is reported as a fold increase ± SD of ADU vs. siCTR. $**p < 0.01$ vs. siCTR. (e) Cell survival in siCTR and siALDH2 ECs exposed to 2% FBS in the presence/absence of NAC (5 mM) for 2 (grey bars) or 5 (black bars) days. Data are expressed as means ± SD of the cell number counted/well. $*p < 0.05$ vs. siCTR. Images are representative of results obtained with siALDH2 B.

and maximal respiration and decreased the respiratory reserve capacity (Figures 5(a) and 5(b)). Importantly, Western blot analysis of constitutive respiratory complexes including CII, CIII, and CIV, known to be sensible to the ROS increase in mitochondria, indicated that ALDH2 did not alter the abundance of these respiratory complexes (Figure 5(c)).

Given the significant changes of the metabolic function reported, we assessed whether they were associated with morphological modification of cellular components. TEM images showed minor morphological changes in mitochondria of siALDH2 cells (Figure 6). In particular, smaller mitochondria in Figure 6(b) were observed when compared to those in Figure 6(a), and cristae in the centre of mitochondria in Figure 6(d) appear to be deleted.

In conclusion, bioenergetic analysis revealed that ALDH2 deficiency specifically reduced both mitochondrial respiration

(a)

(b)

(c)

(d)

(e)

(f)

(g)

(h)

(i)

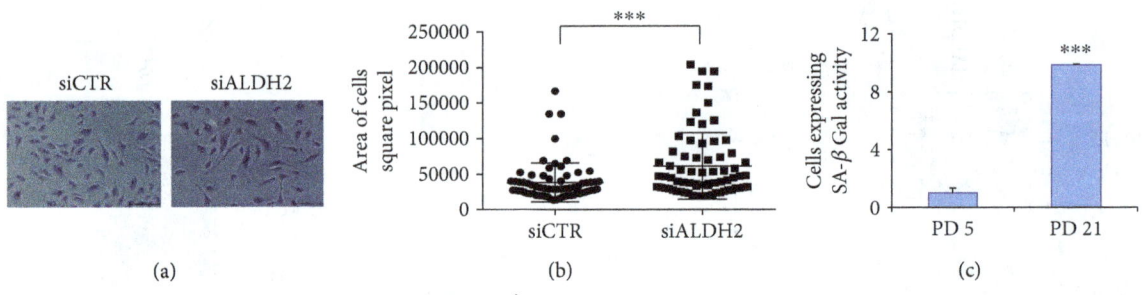

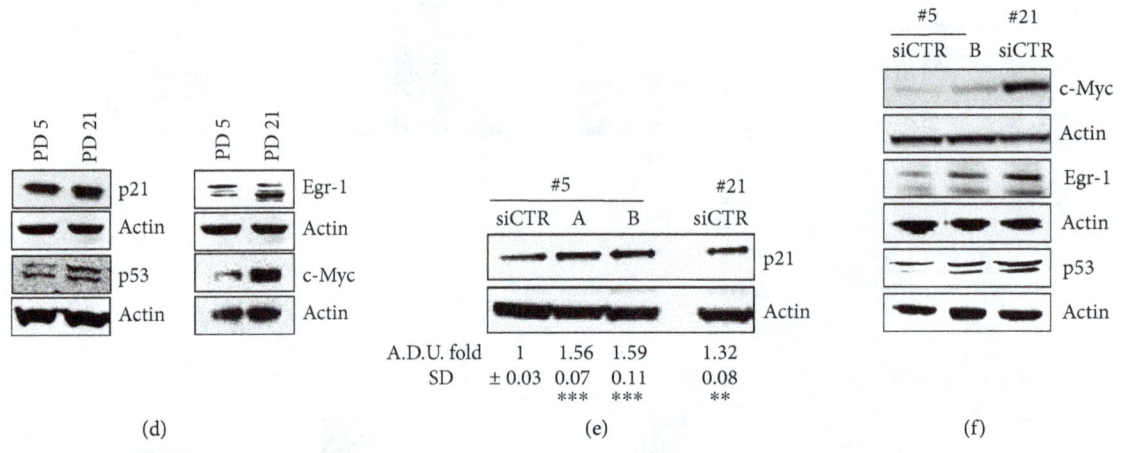

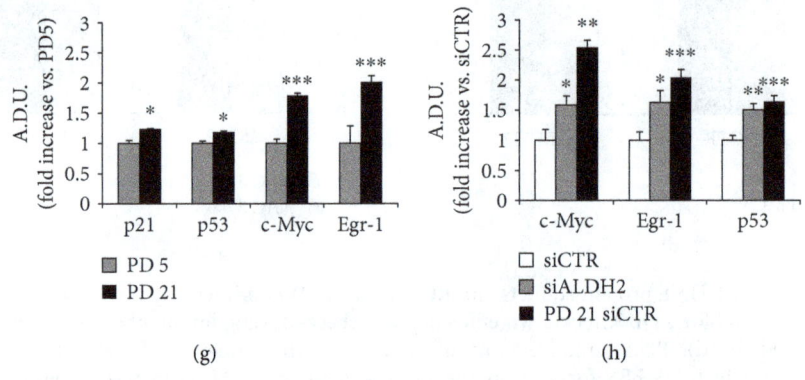

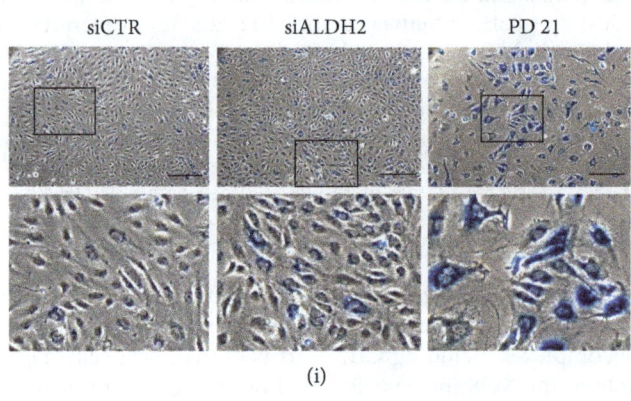

FIGURE 4: Continued.

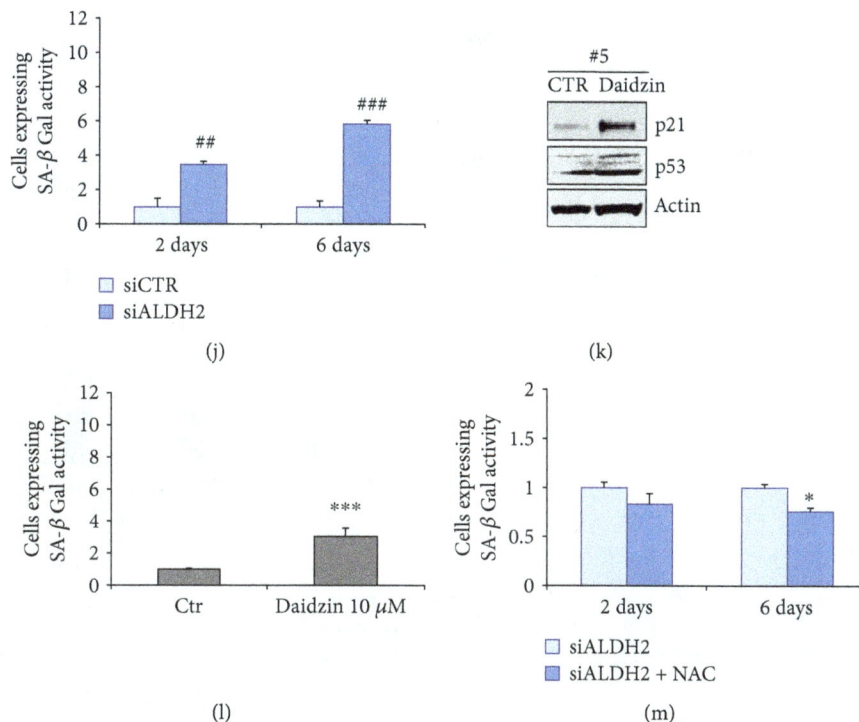

FIGURE 4: ALDH2 silencing or inhibition induces the expression of senescence markers in HUVECs. (a, b) Images and area of cells in siCTR and siALDH2 ECs cultured in EBM-2 supplemented with 2% FBS for 48 h. Data are expressed as a square pixel of cells analyzed using ImageJ. Quantification of 70 cell areas for each condition is reported. ***$p < 0.001$ vs. siCTR. Two-way ANOVA was used. (c) SA-β-Gal quantification, expressed as a fold increase in positive cells for SA-β-Gal activity ± SD vs. PD 5. ***$p < 0.001$ vs. PD 5. (d, e, f) Western blot analysis of a pattern of senescent markers (d, left: p21 and p53 or right: Egr-1 and c-Myc) in HUVECs at PD 5 (#5, PD 5) and PD 21 (#21, PD 21) or (e, p21 or f c-Myc, Egr-1, and p53) in siCTR and siALDH2 HUVECs, 48 h posttransfection (#5, PD 5; #21, PD 21). Representative blots of 3 with similar results are shown (e, g, h). Quantification of immunoblot in (d), (e), and (f). Data are reported as an ADU fold increase vs. siCTR (e, h) or vs. PD 5 (g). (e) ***$p < 0.001$ and **$p < 0.01$ vs. siCTR. (g) ***$p < 0.001$ and *$p < 0.05$ vs. PD5. (h) ***$p < 0.001$, **$p < 0.01$, and *$p < 0.05$ vs. siCTR. (i) Images of SA-β-Gal staining of siCTR and siALDH2 ECs and PD 21 groups obtained with a Leica DMI4000 microscope. Images of HUVECs at PD 21 were reported as a positive control. Scale bar: 250 μm. The insets show boxed areas in detail. (j) Cells were transfected with siRNA for 2 or 6 days. The transfection was repeated every 72 h. SA-β-Gal quantification, expressed as a fold increase ± SD vs. siCTR of positive cells for SA-β-Gal activity. ##$p < 0.01$ and ###$p < 0.001$. (k) Western blot analysis of senescent markers in HUVECs at PD 5 in the presence/absence of daidzin (10 μM) for 48 h (#5, PD 5). Representative blots of 3 with similar results are shown. (l) SA-β-Gal quantification in ECs treated or not with daidzin (10 μM) for 48 h, expressed as a fold increase in positive cells for SA-β-Gal activity ± SD vs. untreated cells. ***$p < 0.001$ vs. untreated cells. (m) Cells were transfected with siRNA for 2 or 6 days in the presence/absence of NAC (5 mM). The transfection was repeated every 72 h. Cells were pretreated for 30 min with NAC, before the treatment with 2% of FBS. The pretreatment with NAC and the treatment with 2% FBS were repeated every 3 days. SA-β-Gal quantification, expressed as a fold decrease ± SD vs. untreated cells positive for SA-β-Gal activity. *$p < 0.05$. Images are representative of results obtained with siALDH2 B.

and reserve capacity, which presumably contribute to the reduction of the endothelial responsiveness.

4. Discussion

ALDH2, a mitochondrial enzyme, is known for its detoxifying properties, which provide living organisms with a protective shield against endogenous and exogenous toxic agents [26], such as acetaldehyde (alcohol metabolism) and products originating from lipid peroxidation (4-HNE) and ROS. The relevance of ALDH2 in providing strong protection toward toxic insults has been described in numerous reports, demonstrating its efficacy in various models of human diseases such as ischemia-reperfusion and ischemic stroke characterized by overwhelming oxidative stress [27]. Note that

the above pathologies have the vascular endothelium as an underlying component whose function might be compromised by ROS and aldehyde surge.

Previous data from our group documented that alteration in endothelial function induced by Aβ was restored by the activation of mitochondrial ALDH2 in the endothelium [15]. However, the contribution of ALDH2 to endothelial senescence remains unresolved.

Here, we have described the role of ALDH2 in endothelial growth and function, using HUVECs as a model, whose ALDH2 was silenced through transfection of targeting siRNA or exposure to the pharmacological inhibitor of ALDH2, daidzin. The resulted cellular models displayed a number of morphological and functional changes. Morphologically, we observed a subverted phenotype of silenced cells,

(a)

(b)

(c)

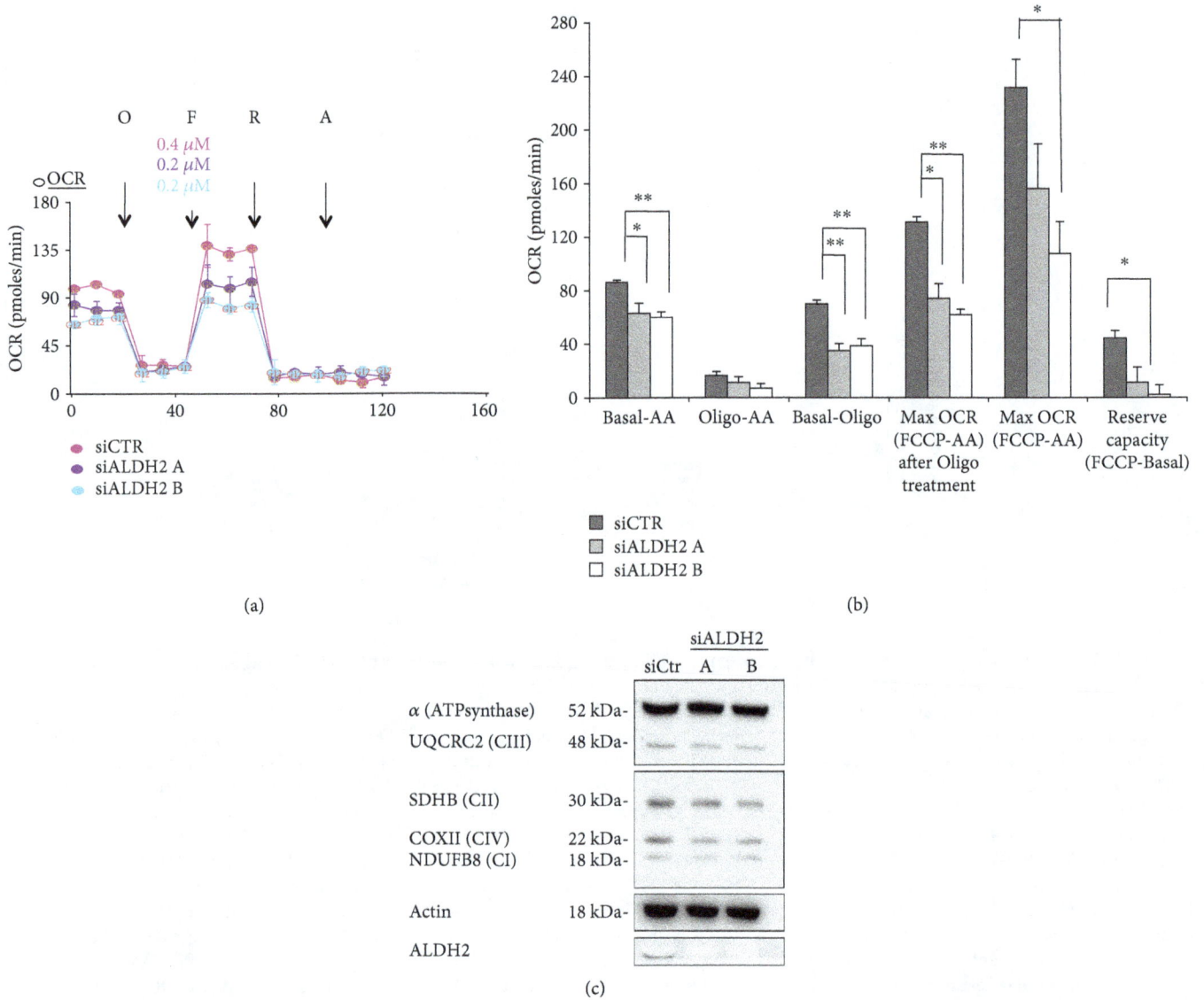

FIGURE 5: ALDH2 silencing is associated with mitochondrial dysfunction. (a) OCR was assessed by a Seahorse XF24 cell culture microplate in siCTR and siALDH2 ECs that were harvested and seeded 24 h posttransfection in XF24 cell culture plates at a density of 3×10^4 cells/well. Where indicated (arrows), oligomycin (O) (1 μg $\times$ ml^{-1}), FCCP (F) (0.2–0.4 μM), rotenone (R) (1 μM), and antimycin A (AA) (1 μM) were added. Data are representative of three experiments. (b) Basal OCR, proton leak, ATP-linked OCR, maximal OCR, and reserve capacity in siALDH2 ECs exposed to 2% FBS for 24 h. The means $\pm$ SEM of each parameter are shown. $^{**}p < 0.01$ and $^*p < 0.05$ vs. siCTR. (c) Western blot analysis of OXPHOS representative complexes detected by the OXPHOS antibody cocktail kit in siALDH2 (two clones A and B) or siCTR cultured in 2% FBS for 24 h. Knockdown efficiency was verified with an ALDH2 antibody. Actin was used as a loading control. Blots are representative of 3 with similar results.

characterized by an enlarged and elongated cell shape, in sharp contrast to the polygonal one of wild-type endothelial cells. Functionally, the ALDH2 loss yielded a reduced mobility and augmented permeability, a finding consistent with the marked decline of VE-cadherin and ZO-1 expression at cell-cell contacts and with the changes in cell morphology. We also observed a reduction of cell proliferation that results in a reduction of the cell number. Predictably, ALDH2 silencing produced intracellular accumulation of 4-HNE adducts and ROS production, which appears to be the primary cause of the observed impairment of endothelial cell

functions and morphological changes, as corroborated by using the scavenger NAC.

The study of mitochondrial respiration provided further insight into the mechanism underlying endothelial dysfunction, as mitochondria possess a considerable respiratory reserve, which is important in the response to oxidative stress [11, 12]. Indeed, we found that ALDH2 silencing diminished the inherent oxidative metabolism, as indicated by a decline in the oxygen consumption rate. Specifically, siALDH2 cells showed a reduction in basal and maximal respiration measured under basal conditions

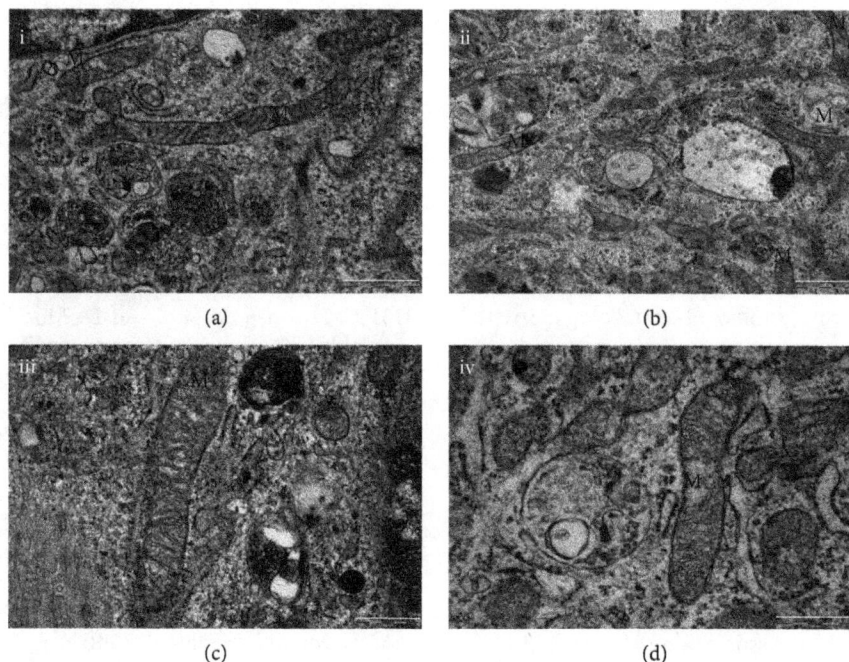

FIGURE 6: ALDH2 silencing affects the HUVEC mitochondrial ultrastructure. Cells were transfected with siRNA as described above. Then, they were harvested and seeded 24 h posttransfection and treated as described in Materials and Methods. TEM representative images of siCTR or siALDH2: (a, c) siCTR and (b, d) siALDH2. M: mitochondria. Scale bar: (a, b) 1 μm and (c, d) 500 nm. Images are representative of results obtained with siALDH2 B.

and in response to FCCP, with a clear decrease in the reserve capacity. While mitochondrial respiration decreased, the analysis of the expression of all respiratory complexes does not change upon ALDH2 downregulation, indicating that the protein level of all respiratory complexes is not the leading cause of reduced respiration in siALDH2 cells. We therefore suggested that the decrease in basal OCR and spare reserve capacity might be due to some posttranslational modifications.

Furthermore, TEM images suggest alterations in mitochondrial morphology of siALDH2 cells. Thus, the endothelial dysfunction, noted in siALDH2 cells and in ECs exposed to daidzin, may be attributed to the effects of accumulated toxic products and to subtle defects of mitochondrial respiration.

Investigation on endothelial cell senescence was initiated in view of the observed morphological similarities between siALDH2 and those typical of senescent cells, i.e., the flat morphology and enlarged cell size. Evidence sustaining the hypothesis of an incipient senescent state was gleaned from the analysis of SA-β-Gal activity and specific intracellular signals measured in siALDH2 cells and in daidzin-treated cells subjected to stress-induced senescence experiments in which population doublings (PD) were recorded. Indeed, cellular senescence ensued as early as at PD 5 progressing steadily up to PD 21. In fact, increases in signals, e.g., SA-β-Gal, p21/p53, Egr1, and c-Myc, were noted when comparing signalling patterns at PD 5 vs. PD 21. The onset of senescence in siALDH2 cells as well as in ECs exposed to daidzin is considerably faster than what was observed in the earlier work on HUVECs exposed to exogenous amyloid peptides (PD 5 vs. PD 21) [16]. This underscores the

protective role of ALDH2 exerted toward the endothelium to an extent not appreciated before.

5. Conclusions

Our results demonstrate that in the vascular endothelium, loss of ALDH2 accelerates the acquisition of a premature senescence phenotype leading to endothelial dysfunction. These events are associated with an increase in ROS levels, accumulation of 4-HNE protein adducts, and impairment of mitochondrial bioenergetic functions. The senescence phenotype of the endothelium, with exhaustion of the regenerative capacity, may represent a defensive response from the damage caused by an accumulation of toxic aldehydes and can lead to the expansion of the senescent cell population further aggravating the loss of function in the vasculature.

Abbreviations

AA:	Antimycin A
ALDH2:	Aldehyde dehydrogenase 2
DAPI:	4′,6-diamidino-2-phenylindole
EGM-2:	Endothelial growth medium
EBM-2:	Endothelial basal medium
ECs:	Endothelial cells
FCCP:	Carbonylcyanide-p-trifluoromethoxyphenyl hydrazone

NAC: N-Acetyl-L-cysteine
PD: Cumulative population doubling
siALDH2:   siRNA targeting ALDH2
siCTR: Scrambled control siRNA.

Disclosure

Some results showed in the manuscript have been presented in the 1st Meeting in Translational Pharmacology: Invited Societies SPF-SIF-EEI.

Acknowledgments

We thank Daria Mochly-Rosen (Stanford University) for stimulating discussions during the course of this work. We are grateful to Eugenio Paccagnini (University of Siena) for the technical support with electron microscopy analysis. This work was supported by Associazione Ricerca sul Cancro (AIRC) (IG 15443) and MIUR-PRIN (20152HKF3Z) through MZ.

References

[1] C. López-Otin, M. Blasco, L. Partridge, M. Serrano, and G. Kroeme, "The hallmarks of aging," *Cell*, vol. 153, no. 6, pp. 1194–1217, 2013.

[2] J. D. Erusalimsky, "Vascular endothelial senescence: from mechanisms to pathophysiology," *J Appl Physiol. 1985.*, vol. 106, no. 1, pp. 326–332, 2009.

[3] X. L. Tian and Y. Li, "Endothelial cell senescence and age-related vascular diseases," *Journal of Genetics and Genomics*, vol. 41, no. 9, pp. 485–495, 2014.

[4] F. Paneni, C. Diaz Cañestro, P. Libby, T. F. Lüscher, and G. G. Camici, "The aging cardiovascular system: understanding it at the cellular and clinical levels," *Journal of the American College of Cardiology*, vol. 69, no. 15, pp. 1952–1967, 2017.

[5] M. Mittal, M. R. Siddiqui, K. Tran, S. P. Reddy, and A. B. Malik, "Reactive oxygen species in inflammation and tissue injury," *Antioxidants & Redox Signaling*, vol. 20, no. 7, pp. 1126–1167, 2014.

[6] A. Quaegebeur, C. Lange, and P. Carmeliet, "The neurovascular link in health and disease: molecular mechanisms and therapeutic implications," *Neuron*, vol. 71, no. 3, pp. 406–424, 2011.

[7] Y. Koga, Y. Akita, N. Junko et al., "Endothelial dysfunction in MELAS improved by l-arginine supplementation," *Neurology*, vol. 66, no. 11, pp. 1766–1769, 2006.

[8] L. H. Rodan, G. D. Wells, L. Banks, S. Thompson, J. E. Schneiderman, and I. Tein, "L-Arginine affects aerobic capacity and muscle metabolism in MELAS (mitochondrial encephalomyopathy, lactic acidosis and stroke-like episodes) syndrome," *PLoS One*, vol. 10, no. 5, article e0127066, 2015.

[9] M. Potente and P. Carmeliet, "The link between angiogenesis and endothelial metabolism," *Annual Review of Physiology*, vol. 79, no. 1, pp. 43–66, 2017.

[10] P. Fraisl, M. Mazzone, T. Schmidt, and P. Carmeliet, "Regulation of angiogenesis by oxygen and metabolism," *Developmental Cell*, vol. 16, no. 2, pp. 167–179, 2009.

[11] M. A. Kluge, J. L. Fetterman, and J. A. Vita, "Mitochondria and endothelial function," *Circulation Research*, vol. 112, no. 8, pp. 1171–1188, 2013.

[12] B. P. Dranka, B. G. Hill, and V. M. Darley-Usmar, "Mitochondrial reserve capacity in endothelial cells: the impact of nitric oxide and reactive oxygen species," *Free Radical Biology & Medicine*, vol. 48, no. 7, pp. 905–914, 2010.

[13] C. H. Chen, L. Sun, and D. Mochly-Rosen, "Mitochondrial aldehyde dehydrogenase and cardiac diseases," *Cardiovascular Research*, vol. 88, no. 1, pp. 51–57, 2010.

[14] C. Chen, C. B. Julio Ferreira, E. Gross, and D. Mochly-Rosen, "Targeting aldehyde dehydrogenase 2: new therapeutic opportunities," *Physiological Reviews*, vol. 94, no. 1, pp. 1–34, 2014.

[15] R. Solito, F. Corti, C. Chen et al., "Mitochondrial aldehyde dehydrogenase-2 activation prevents β-amyloid-induced endothelial cell dysfunction and restores angiogenesis," *Journal of Cell Science*, vol. 126, no. 9, pp. 1952–1961, 2013.

[16] S. Donnini, R. Solito, E. Cetti et al., "Aβ peptides accelerate the senescence of endothelial cells in vitro and in vivo, impairing angiogenesis," *The FASEB Journal*, vol. 24, no. 7, pp. 2385–2395, 2010.

[17] M. Monti, I. Hyseni, A. Pacini, E. Monzani, L. Casella, and L. Morbidelli, "Cross-talk between endogenous H$_2$S and NO accounts for vascular protective activity of the metal-nonoate Zn(PipNONO)Cl," *Biochemical Pharmacology*, vol. 152, pp. 143–152, 2018.

[18] L. Bazzani, S. Donnini, A. Giachetti, G. Christofori, and M. Ziche, "PGE2 mediates EGFR internalization and nuclear translocation," *Oncotarget*, vol. 9, no. 19, pp. 14939–14958, 2018.

[19] E. Terzuoli, G. Nannelli, M. Frosini, A. Giachetti, M. Ziche, and S. Donnini, "Inhibition of cell cycle progression by the hydroxytyrosol-cetuximab combination yields enhanced chemotherapeutic efficacy in colon cancer cells," *Oncotarget*, vol. 8, no. 47, pp. 83207–83224, 2017.

[20] V. Ciccone, M. Monti, G. Antonini et al., "Efficacy of Adipo-Dren® in reducing interleukin-1-induced lymphatic endothelial hyperpermeability," *Journal of Vascular Research*, vol. 53, no. 5-6, pp. 255–268, 2016.

[21] V. Giorgio, V. Petronilli, A. Ghelli et al., "The effects of idebenone on mitochondrial bioenergetics," *Biochimica et Biophysica Acta*, vol. 1817, no. 2, pp. 363–369, 2012.

[22] M. Schiavone, A. Zulian, S. Menazza et al., "Alisporivir rescues defective mitochondrial respiration in Duchenne muscular dystrophy," *Pharmacological Research*, vol. 125, Part B, pp. 122–131, 2017.

[23] L. Stepanek and G. Pigino, "Millisecond time resolution correlative light and electron microscopy for dynamic cellular processes," *Methods in Cell Biology*, vol. 140, pp. 1–20, 2017.

[24] O. I1, K. Nishimaki, C. Yasuda, K. Kamino, and S. Ohta, "Deficiency in a mitochondrial aldehyde dehydrogenase increases vulnerability to oxidative stress in PC12 cells," *Journal of Neurochemistry*, vol. 84, no. 5, pp. 1110–1117, 2003.

[25] D. Muñoz-Espín and M. Serrano, "Cellular senescence: from physiology to pathology," *Nature Reviews Molecular Cell Biology*, vol. 15, no. 7, pp. 482–496, 2014.

[26] V. Vasiliou and D. W. Nebert, "Analysis and update of the human aldehyde dehydrogenase (ALDH) gene family," *Human Genomics*, vol. 2, no. 2, pp. 138–143, 2005.

[27] C. H. Chen, G. R. Budas, E. N. Churchill, M. H. Disatnik, T. D. Hurley, and D. Mochly-Rosen, "Activation of aldehyde dehydrogenase-2 reduces ischemic damage to the heart," *Science*, vol. 321, no. 5895, pp. 1493–1495, 2008.

13

Extracts from the Mediterranean Food Plants *Carthamus lanatus, Cichorium intybus,* and *Cichorium spinosum* Enhanced GSH Levels and Increased Nrf2 Expression in Human Endothelial Cells

Dimitrios Stagos ⓘ,[1] **Dimitrios Balabanos,**[1] **Salomi Savva,**[1] **Zoi Skaperda,**[1] **Alexandros Priftis,**[1] **Efthalia Kerasioti,**[1] **Eleni V. Mikropoulou,**[2] **Konstantina Vougogiannopoulou,**[2] **Sofia Mitakou,**[2] **Maria Halabalaki,**[2] **and Demetrios Kouretas ⓘ**[1]

[1]*Department of Biochemistry and Biotechnology, University of Thessaly, Viopolis, Larissa 41500, Greece*
[2]*Division of Pharmacognosy and Natural Product Chemistry, Department of Pharmacy, University of Athens, Panepistimiopolis, Athens 15771, Greece*

Correspondence should be addressed to Dimitrios Stagos; stagkos@med.uth.gr

Guest Editor: Pavel Pospisil

The Mediterranean diet is considered to prevent several diseases. In the present study, the antioxidant properties of six extracts from Mediterranean plant foods were assessed. The extracts' chemical composition analysis showed that the total polyphenolic content ranged from 56 to 408 GAE mg/g dw of extract. The major polyphenols identified in the extracts were quercetin, luteolin, caftaric acid, caffeoylquinic acid isomers, and cichoric acid. The extracts showed *in vitro* high scavenging potency against $ABTS^{\bullet+}$ and $O_2^{\bullet-}$ radicals and reducing power activity. Also, the extracts inhibited peroxyl radical-induced cleavage of DNA plasmids. The three most potent extracts, *Cichorium intybus, Carthamus lanatus,* and *Cichorium spinosum,* inhibited $OH^{\bullet}$-induced mutations in *Salmonella typhimurium* TA102 cells. Moreover, *C. intybus, C. lanatus,* and *C. spinosum* extracts increased the antioxidant molecule glutathione (GSH) by 33.4, 21.5, and 10.5% at 50 μg/ml, respectively, in human endothelial EA.hy926 cells. *C. intybus* extract was also shown to induce in endothelial cells the transcriptional expression of Nrf2 (the major transcription factor of antioxidant genes), as well as of antioxidant genes GCLC, GSR, NQO1, and HMOX1. In conclusion, the results suggested that extracts from edible plants may prevent diseases associated especially with endothelium damage.

1. Introduction

Reactive oxygen species (ROS) are generated within living organisms by different physiological processes such as metabolism and inflammation [1, 2]. Although basic levels of ROS are needed for cellular homeostasis, they can be harmful when they are overproduced, a condition called oxidative stress [1, 2]. An excessive production of ROS intracellularly may induce oxidative damage to important biological macromolecules [3]. Thus, oxidative stress may be the aetiological factor for a number of pathological conditions, such as cancer, neurodegenerative diseases, diabetes, and cardiovascular diseases [4, 5].

Especially, oxidative stress-induced damage of the vascular endothelium is considered a major cause of cardiovascular ailments [6–8]. For instance, oxidative stress may induce acute and chronic phases of leukocyte adhesion to the endothelium [6, 9]. Moreover, the interplay between ROS and nitric oxide induces a vicious circle that may cause further endothelial activation and inflammation [6, 7]. Furthermore, ROS like hydrogen peroxide (H_2O_2) may enter into endothelial cells and interact with cysteine groups in proteins to alter their function [6, 10]. Consequently, oxidative stress may induce different abnormalities to endothelial cells such as progress to senescence loss of integrity and detach into the circulation [11].

Living organisms produce antioxidant molecules, enzymatic and nonenzymatic, for protection against oxidative stress [1, 3]. Moreover, an organism may also obtain antioxidant compounds through diet, especially from plant foods [12, 13]. The antioxidant properties of plant foods are mainly attributed to polyphenols, a large group of secondary metabolites acting as free radical scavengers and metal chelators and affecting the activity of antioxidant enzymes [14]. Consumption of plant products is of great importance in the Mediterranean diet known for its benefits on human health [15]. For example, wild and semidomesticated edible plants containing high polyphenolic content and exhibiting strong antioxidant activity form a major part of the Mediterranean diet [16–20]. Specifically, in Greece, the term "chórta" means wild or semidomesticated edible herbaceous plants, which are cooked or consumed as raw salads as part of the Mediterranean-style Greek diet [16, 17, 21–23]. Currently, there have been few studies on the antioxidant activity of wild edible greens of Greece and especially on the molecular mechanisms accounting for this activity. In a recent preliminary study, we have found that extracts from "chórta" species possessed anticarcinogenic and antioxidant potential [24].

Therefore, the aim of the present study was a further investigation of the antioxidant properties of extracts derived from six wild edible greens (i.e., *Carthamus lanatus*, *Crepis sancta*, *Cichorium intybus*, *Cichorium spinosum*, *Amaranthus blitum*, and *Sonchus asper*) from Greece. Thus, the extracts were examined for their free radical scavenging activity against the ABTS$^{\bullet+}$ radical and superoxide anion radical (O2$^{\bullet-}$), for their reducing power activity and for their antimutagenic activity against ROS-induced mutagenicity. Moreover, the extracts' possible enhancement of antioxidant defense in endothelial cells and the molecular mechanisms accounting for these effects was investigated.

2. Materials and Methods

2.1. Plant Material and Isolation of Extracts. Six plant species, *C. lanatus* (gkourounáki), *C. intybus* (kavouráki), *C. sancta* (ladáki), *S. asper* (zochós), *C. spinosum* (stamnagkáthi), and *A. blitum* (vlíto), were obtained from local markets in Athens (Greece; spring of 2015). Five of them were from the family of Asteraceae and one from the family of Amaranthaceae (i.e., *A. blitum*). The samples were botanically characterized at the Laboratory of Pharmacognosy and Natural Products Chemistry. As described previously [24], the leaves and stems were boiled with water (500 g of plant material/1 l of water), for 20 minutes. After cooling at room temperature, the decoctions were filtered through paper and evaporated to dryness. Moreover, three of the extracts and more specifically those of *C. lanatus*, *C. sancta*, and *C. intybus* were enriched by using XAD7 HP Amberlite® adsorption resin. All of the dry extracts were submitted to HPLC-PDA chemical analysis.

2.2. HPLC-PDA Analysis. For the HPLC analysis of the extracts, a Thermo Finnigan® HPLC-PDA System (P4000 Pump, AS3000 Autosampler, PDA Detector UV8000,

ChromQuest™ 4.2 Software) and a Supelco® RP18 Discovery HS-C18 (250 mm, 4.6 mm, and 5 μm) column were employed. 20 μl of water extracts at 1.5 mg/ml was injected. The mobile phase was 0.1% formic acid in water (A) and MeOH (B). Elution started with 2% (B), reaching 100% (B) in 60 minutes. These conditions were kept for 4 minutes before getting back to initial conditions in 2 min for a 4 min reequilibration. The flow rate was maintained at 1 ml/min and the column temperature at 25°C. Relative quantification of the main secondary metabolites was performed at 280 nm absorbance.

2.3. Evaluation of the Total Polyphenolic Content (TPC) of the Extracts. The evaluation of the TPC of the plant extracts was assessed spectrophotometrically at 765 nm by using the Folin-Ciocalteu reagent as described previously [25]. TPC was determined by a standard curve of absorbance values in correlation with standard concentrations (50–1500 μg/ml) of gallic acid. The TPC was expressed as mg of gallic acid equivalents (GAE) per g of dry weight (dw) of extract.

2.4. ABTS$^{\bullet+}$ Radical Scavenging Assay. ABTS$^{\bullet+}$ radical scavenging capacity of the extracts was performed as described previously [26]. Briefly, ABTS$^{\bullet+}$ radical was generated by mixing 2 mM ABTS with 30 μM H$_2$O$_2$ and 6 μM horseradish peroxidase (HRP) enzyme in 1 ml of distilled water. The mixture was vortexed vigorously and left at room temperature in the dark for 45 min. Subsequently, 10 μl of extract at different concentrations was added in the reaction solution and the absorbance at 730 nm was read. In each experiment, a blank was used consisting of the tested sample in distilled water, ABTS$^{\bullet+}$, and H$_2$O$_2$. The ABTS$^{\bullet+}$ radical solution with 10 μl H$_2$O was used as control. After measuring the absorbance, the percentage of radical scavenging capacity (RSC) of the tested extracts was calculated. In addition, for comparison of the extracts' radical scavenging efficiency, IC$_{50}$ value indicating the concentration that caused 50% scavenging of ABTS$^{\bullet+}$ radical was calculated from the graph-plotted RSC percentage against extract concentration. At least two independent experiments in triplicate were performed for each tested compound.

2.5. Superoxide Radical Scavenging Assay. The superoxide anion radical (O$_2$$^{\bullet-}$) scavenging activity of the extracts was evaluated as described previously [27]. In brief, O$_2$$^{\bullet}$ is produced by the PMS-NADH system through oxidation of NADH and is measured spectrophotometrically at 560 nm by the reduction of nitroblue tetrazolium (NBT). Antioxidants may scavenge O$_2$$^{\bullet-}$ and consequently reduce absorbance. The RSC and the IC$_{50}$ values for O$_2$$^{\bullet-}$ were evaluated as mentioned above for ABTS$^{\bullet+}$ radical. At least two independent experiments in triplicate were performed for each tested compound.

2.6. Reducing Power Assay. Reducing power was determined spectrophotometrically as described previously [28]. RP$_{0.5AU}$ value showing the extract concentration-caused absorbance of 0.5 at 700 nm was calculated from the graph-plotted absorbance against extract concentration. At least two independent experiments in triplicate were performed for each tested compound.

2.7. Peroxyl Radical-Induced DNA Plasmid Strand Cleavage.

The assay was performed as described previously [29]. In brief, peroxyl radicals (ROO•) were produced from thermal decomposition of 2,2′-azobis (2-amidinopropane hydrochloride) (AAPH). The reaction mixture (10 μl) containing 1 μg pBluescript-SK+ plasmid DNA, 2.5 mM AAPH in phosphate-buffered saline (PBS), and the tested extract at different concentrations was incubated in the dark for 45 min at 37°C. Then the reaction was stopped by the addition of 3 μl loading buffer (0.25% bromophenol blue and 30% glycerol). After analyzing the DNA samples by agarose gel electrophoresis, they were photographed and analyzed using the Alpha Innotech Multi Image (Protein-Simple, California, USA). In addition, plasmid DNA was treated with each extract alone at the highest concentration used in the assay in order to test their effects on plasmid DNA conformation. The percentage of the protective activity of the tested extracts from ROO•-induced DNA strand breakage was calculated using the following formula:

$$\%\text{inhibition} = \left[\frac{(S - S_0)}{(S_{\text{control}} - S_0)} \right] \times 100, \quad (1)$$

where S_{control} is the percentage of supercoiled DNA in the negative control sample (plasmid DNA alone), S_0 is the percentage of supercoiled plasmid DNA in the positive control sample (without tested extracts but in the presence of the radical initiating factor), and S is the percentage of supercoiled plasmid DNA in the sample with the tested extracts and the radical initiating factor. Moreover, IC$_{50}$ values showing the concentration that inhibited the AAPH-induced relaxation by 50% were calculated from the graph-plotted percentage inhibition against extract concentration. At least two independent experiments in triplicate were performed for each tested compound.

2.8. Bacterial Strain.

Seven hundred microliters of the stock culture of *Salmonella typhimurium* TA102 strain (MOLTOX,

Boone, NC) was used to inoculate 30 ml of Oxoid nutrient broth no. 2. The inoculated cultures were placed on a shaker (100 rpm) and incubated in the dark at 37°C until the cells reached a density of 1-2 × 10^9 colony forming units (CFU/ml, OD$_{540}$ between 0.1 and 0.2).

2.9. The Antimutagenicity Test.

Two of the extracts (i.e., *C. lanatus* and *C. intybus*) enriched with polyphenols that exhibited the highest protective activity against ROO•-induced DNA plasmid damage were also examined for their inhibitory activity against ROS-induced mutagenicity in *S. typhimurium* TA102 bacterial cells. Similarly, *C. spinosum* extract, the most potent among nonenriched extracts, was also examined for its antimutagenic activity in *S. typhimurium* TA102 bacterial cells.

For the antimutagenicity examination, the standard plate incorporation procedure was used as described previously [27, 30, 31]. *Tert*-butyl hydroperoxide (*t*-BOOH) was used as mutagenic agent. Specifically, the following substances were added in screwed sterile tubes maintained at 45°C ± 2°C: 2 ml top agar, 100 μl bacterial culture of *S. typhimurium* TA102 strain, 50 μl *t*-BOOH solution (0.4 mM final concentration), and 50 μl extract at various concentrations. The contents of the tubes were mixed and poured onto the surface of glucose minimal agar plates. Then the plates were inverted and placed in an incubator, at 37°C ± 2°C for 48 h. Afterwards, the histidine revertant colonies (His$^+$) were counted. Before counting, the agar plates were microscopically checked for toxicity [31]. Each assay included both positive (oxidizing agent alone) and negative (plates without oxidizing agent or tested extract) controls. Also, each antioxidant was checked at the two highest concentrations used in the antimutagenicity assay, for possible induction of mutations.

For evaluation of the percent inhibition of mutagenicity, the number of induced revertants was obtained by subtracting the number of spontaneous revertants from the number of revertants on the plates containing the mutagen and/or antioxidant. The percentage inhibition of mutagenicity was calculated as follows:

$$\text{Inhibition} = \left[1 - \frac{\text{number of colonies/plate with oxidant + test compound}}{\text{number of colonies/plate with oxidant alone}} \right] \times 100. \quad (2)$$

At least two independent experiments in triplicate were performed for each tested compound.

2.10. Cell Culture Conditions.

As described previously [32], human endothelial EA.hy926 cells were cultured in normal Dulbecco's modified Eagle's medium (DMEM) in plastic disposable tissue culture flasks at 37°C in 5% carbon dioxide.

2.11. XTT Assay.

To examine the extracts' antioxidant activity in endothelial cells, noncytotoxic concentrations

were used. For selection of these concentrations, extracts' cytotoxicity in endothelial cells was checked using the cell viability XTT assay kit (Roche, Switzerland) as described previously [28]. Briefly, EA.hy926 cells were seeded into a 96-well plate with 1 × 10^4 cells per well in DMEM medium. After 24 h incubation, the cells were treated with different concentrations of the extracts in serum-free DMEM medium for 24 h. Then 50 μl of XTT test solution was added to each well. After 4 h of incubation, absorbance was measured at 450 nm and also at 630 nm as a reference wavelength in

TABLE 1: The sequence of primers used for the assessment of mRNA levels of *NFE2L2, GCLC, GSR, GPX1, HMOX1, CAT, NQO1, SOD1*, and *TXN* genes in EA.hy926 cells by qRT-PCR.

Gene	Access no.	Primer (5'-3')
CAT	847	Forward: CCAGAAGAAAGCGGTCAAGAA
		Reverse: TGGATGTGGCTCCCGTAGTC
SOD1	6647	Forward: AGGGCATCA TCAATTTCGAG
		Reverse: GGGCCTCAGACTACATCCAA
TXN	7295	Forward: TTTCCATCGGTCCTTACAGC
		Reverse: TTGGCTCCAGAAAATTCACC
HMOX1	3162	Forward: GGCCTGGCCTTCTTCACCTT
		Reverse: GAGGGGCTCTGGTCCTTGGT
NFE2L2	4780	Forward: *ATTGCCTGTAAGTCCTGGTCA*
		Reverse: *ACTGCTCTTTGGACATCATTTCG*
NQO1	1728	Forward: GGGCAAGTCCATCCCAACTG
		Reverse: GCAAGTCAGGGAAGCCTGGA
GCLC	2729	Forward: GAAGAAGATATTTTTCCTGTCATTGAT
		Reverse: CCATTCATGTATTGAAGAGTGAATTT
GSR	2936	Forward: CCAGCTTAGGAATAACCAGCGATGG
		Reverse: GTCTTTTTAACCTCCTTGACCTGGGAGAAC
GPX1	2876	Forward: CGCTTCCAGACCATTGACATC
		Reverse: CGAGGTGGTATTTTCTGTAAGATCA
GAPDH	2597	Forward: *TGCACCACCAACTGCTTAG*
		Reverse: *GATGCAGGGATGATGTTC*

a Biotek ELx800 microplate reader (Winooski, Vermont, USA). Negative control was DMEM serum-free medium. The absorbance values of the control and samples were used for calculation of the percentage inhibition of cell growth caused by the extract treatment. All experiments were carried out in triplicate and on two separate occasions.

2.12. Treatment of EA.hy926 Cells with the Extracts.

C. lanatus and *C. intybus* extracts which exhibited the highest free radical scavenging potency among extracts enriched with polyphenols were examined for their antioxidant capacity in endothelial EA.hy926 cells. *C. spinosum* extract, the most potent of nonenriched with polyphenols extracts, was also examined in endothelial cells. The cells were cultured in flasks for 24 h. Afterwards, the medium was replaced with serum-free medium containing the tested extracts at noncytotoxic concentrations. The cells were treated with the extracts for 24 h, and then they were trypsinized, collected, and centrifuged twice at 300 × g for 10 min at 5°C. At the end of the first centrifugation, the supernatant fluid was discarded and the cellular pellet was resuspended in PBS. After the second centrifugation, the cell pellet was collected and used to measure the glutathione (GSH) and ROS levels and the mRNA levels of antioxidant genes.

2.13. Assessment of GSH and ROS Levels by Flow Cytometry Analysis in Endothelial Cells.

The GSH and ROS levels in EA.hy926 cells were assessed using mercury orange and DCF-DA, respectively, as described previously [33, 34]. In brief, for assessment of the GSH and ROS levels, the cells were resuspended in PBS at 1×10^6 cells/ml and incubated in the presence of mercury orange ($10 \mu M$) and DCF-DA ($40 \mu M$), respectively, in the dark at 37°C for 30 min. Then the cells were washed, resuspended in PBS, and submitted to flow cytometric analysis using a FACSCalibur flow cytometer (Becton Dickinson, New Jersey, USA) with excitation and emission wavelengths at 488 and 530 nm for ROS and at 488 and 580 nm for GSH. Data were analyzed using "BD CellQuest" software (Becton Dickinson). Each experiment was repeated at least three times.

2.14. Quantitative Real-Time PCR (qRT-PCR) of Antioxidant Genes.

The extract that exhibited the highest antioxidant potency in endothelial cells (i.e., *C. intybus*) was examined for its effects on the transcriptional expression of major antioxidant genes, as described previously [35]. Specifically, EA.hy926 cells were treated with *C. intybus* extract at $50 \mu g/ml$ for 3, 12, and 24 h. Then RNA was extracted from cell pellet (see Section 2.11) using an RNA isolation kit (PureLink™ RNA kit, Invitrogen, USA). The extracted RNA ($\sim 10 \mu g$) was treated with DNase (RQ1 RNase-Free DNase, $1 U/\mu l$, Promega, USA). DNA-free RNA was then reverse transcribed to obtain cDNA (SuperScript II Reverse Transcriptase, Invitrogen, USA) using oligo (dT) 12-18 primers (Invitrogen, USA). Amplification of cDNAs for the *NFE2L2, GCLC, GSR, GPX1, HMOX1, CAT, SOD1, NQO1, TXN,* and *GAPDH* genes was carried out in $10 \mu l$ reactions containing SYBR® Select Master Mix 2X (Applied Biosystems, CA, USA), $0.25 \mu M$ of each primer, 50 nM ROX Low, and 25 ng cDNA for the amplification of all genes. The utilized primers are shown in Table 1. The thermocycling conditions used for the amplification of the aforementioned genes were the

TABLE 2: Total phenolic content, free radical scavenging activity against $ABTS^{\bullet+}$ and $O_2^{\bullet-}$ radicals, protective activity against peroxyl (ROO•) radical-induced DNA damage, and reducing power of the extracts.

Plant variety	TPC[a] (mg GAE/gr dw)	IC_{50} ($\mu g/ml$)[e]			Reducing power[e] $(RP_{0.5AU})$[d]
		$ABTS^{\bullet+}$	$O_2^{\bullet-}$	ROO•	
Carthamus lanatus	408	7.9 ± 0.9[b]	6.3 ± 0.4[b]	110.0 ± 8.2[c]	5.0 ± 0.3[b]
Cichorium intybus	320	9.1 ± 0.6	8.2 ± 0.7	105.0 ± 7.6	6.0 ± 0.2
Cichorium spinosum	117	28.0 ± 3.1	21.0 ± 1.4	300.0 ± 17.3	8.0 ± 0.6
Crepis sancta	288	12.0 ± 1.5	7.5 ± 0.6	132.0 ± 9.8	10.5 ± 0.9
Sonchus asper	56	66.0 ± 7.2	56.0 ± 3.8	970.0 ± 53.4	47.0 ± 3.3
Amaranthus blitum	63	72.0 ± 9.6	21.0 ± 1.2	443.0 ± 19.5	65.0 ± 4.6

[a]TPC: total polyphenolic content. [b]Values are the mean ± SD of at least two separate triplicate experiments. [c]Values are the mean ± SD from three independent experiments. [d]$RP_{0.5AU}$: extract concentration ($\mu g/ml$) caused absorbance of 0.5 at 700 nm. [e]Values are statistically significant, $p < 0.05$.

following: 3 min at 95°C, 45 cycles of 15 sec at 95°C, and 30 sec at 53°C followed by 30 sec at 72°C. Finally, a melting curve was carried out from 53°C to 95°C to check the specificity of the products. All qRT-PCR were performed on a μx3005P system (Stratagene, UK). Amplification efficiencies were >86% with r^2 values > 0.981 for all genes.

2.15. Statistical Analysis. All results were expressed as mean ± SD. Differences were considered significant at $p < 0.05$. One-way ANOVA was performed followed by Tukey's test for multiple pair-wise comparisons using the SPSS 20.0 software.

3. Results and Discussion

3.1. Polyphenolic Composition of Extracts. The range of the TPC in the tested extracts was from 56 to 408 mg GAE/gr dw (Table 2). As expected, *C. lanatus*, *C. intybus*, and *C. sancta* exhibited the higher TPC values (408, 320, and 288 mg GAE/gr dw of extract, respectively), since they were enriched with polyphenols by using absorption resin (Table 2). All the extracts from the Asteraceae family were rich in phenolic compounds and particularly hydroxycinnamic acids and flavonoid derivatives. All the members of the Cichoriae tribe (i.e., *C. spinosum*, *C. intybus*, *C. sancta*, and *S. asper*) presented a similar chemical profile (Figure 1) with variations to the relative percentages of specific secondary metabolites in each extract (supplementary material (available here)). Based on the literature [36] and previous LC-MS analyses (data not shown) of the extracts, we estimated that two caffeoyl tartaric acid derivatives, namely, caftaric acid and cichoric acid, constituted the predominant compounds of these extracts and could be responsible for the decoctions' biological activities. *C. lanatus*-enriched decoction appeared to possess extremely high amounts of phenolic substances, most probably glycosides of the flavonoids quercetin and luteolin, while its profile was complimented by the presence of caffeoylquinic acid isomers and dimers. On the other hand, the *A. blitum* extract was quite poor in phenolic compounds with only a few, minor peaks observed in the medium polarity area of its chromatogram. However, as expected from a member of the Amaranthaceae family, the presence of the nonpolar triterpene saponins was evident.

3.2. Free Radical Scavenging Activity and Reducing Power of Extracts. The IC_{50} values against $ABTS^{\bullet+}$ and $O_2^{\bullet-}$ radicals are shown in Table 2. Low IC_{50} values mean strong antioxidant potency. In the $ABTS^{\bullet+}$ method, the IC_{50} extended from 7.9 (*C. lanatus*) to 72.0 $\mu g/ml$ (*A. blitum*), and in $O_2^{\bullet-}$ radical assay, it was from 6.3 (*C. lanatus*) to 56.0 $\mu g/ml$ (*S. asper*) (Table 2). It was remarkable that *C. lanatus* extract had the highest potency in $ABTS^{\bullet+}$ and $O_2^{\bullet-}$ radical assays and exhibited activity at too low concentrations. As mentioned, *C. lanatus* had also the highest TPC, and so, its rich polyphenolic content may explain the high antioxidant activity. Moreover, the polyphenols (i.e., quercetin, luteolin, and caffeoylquinic acid derivatives) found in *C. lanatus* have been known as strong free radical scavengers [37, 38]. In general, the three extracts (i.e., *C. lanatus*, *C. intybus*, and *C. sancta*) enriched with polyphenols due to use of absorption resin exhibited IC_{50} values which were at least 2-fold lower than those of the other extracts (Table 2). Although $ABTS^{\bullet+}$ radical is one of the most used for examining compounds' antioxidant activity, it is a synthetic radical. However, $O_2^{\bullet-}$ is one of the most common and reactive radicals found in living organisms [3]. Superoxide radical may be produced *in vivo* by the reactions of the electron transport chains in mitochondria (1–3% of electrons forming $O_2^{\bullet-}$), activated phagocytic cells, enzymatic activity (e.g., P450 enzymes and xanthine oxidase), and autooxidation reactions of biomolecules (e.g., adrenalin and $FADH_2$) [2]. Superoxide radical may cause damage to DNA, proteins, and lipids, and these effects seem to increase with aging [3]. Thus, it is important for prevention of oxidative stress-induced diseases to find out compounds which effectively scavenge $O_2^{\bullet-}$.

In the reducing power assay, $RP_{0.5AU}$ values ranged from 5.0 (*C. lanatus*) to 65.0 (*A. blitum*) (Table 2). Like IC_{50} values, the lower the $RP_{0.5AU}$ value is, the higher is the reducing power activity. The reducing power of a compound is an indication of its antioxidant activity, because it shows its ability to act as an electron donor and consequently to neutralize free radicals [39]. Again, *C. lanatus* extract was the most potent in this assay, while the other two extracts (i.e., *C. intybus* and *C. sancta*) that were enriched with polyphenols had also high reducing activity (Table 2). However, in this assay, *C. spinosum* extract also exhibited high reducing potency ($RP_{0.5AU}$: 8.0), although it was not processed with absorption resins (Table 2). This *C. spinosum* extract's high

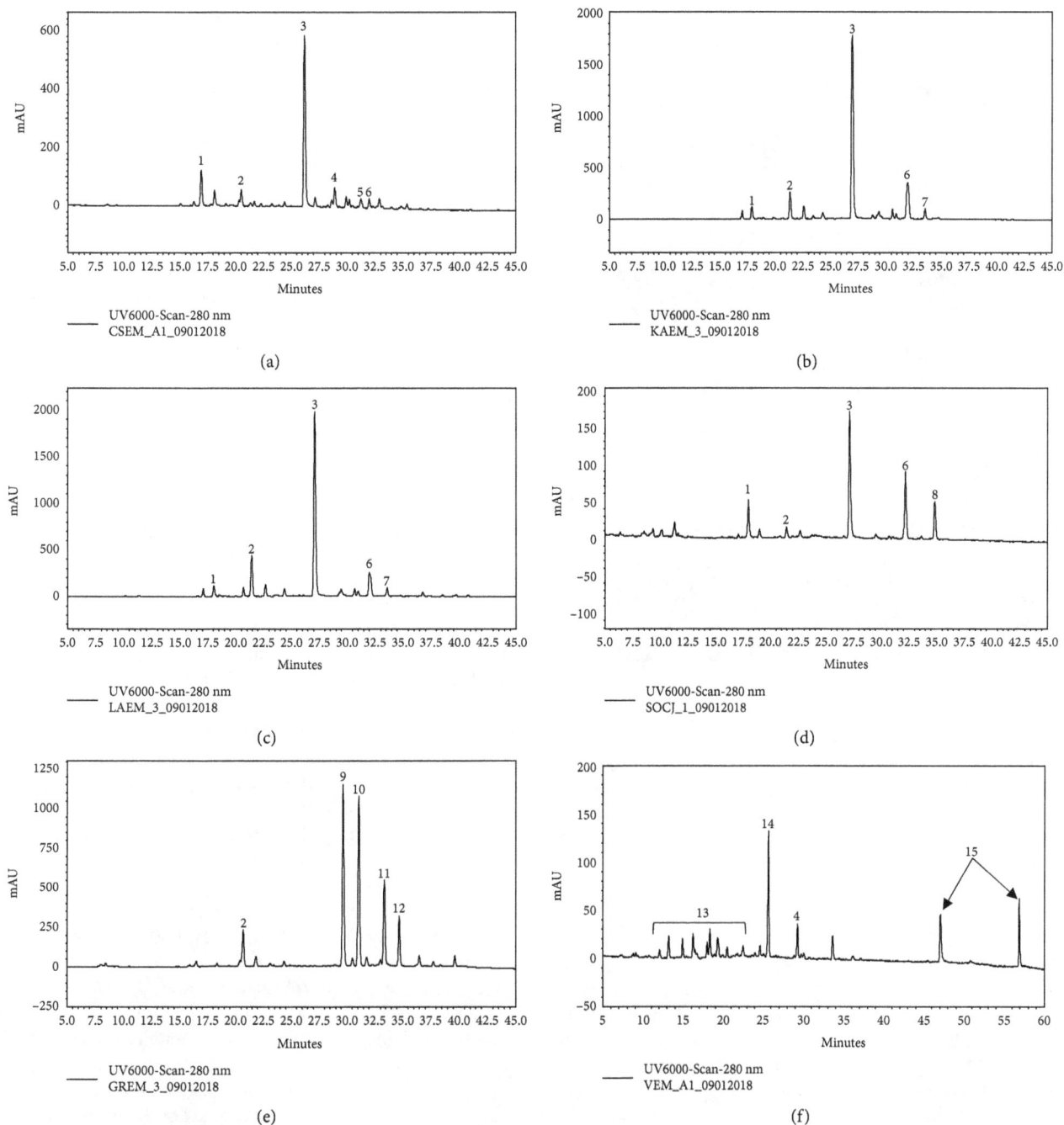

FIGURE 1: HPLC-PDA profiles of plant decoctions: (a) *Cichorium spinosum,* (b) *Cichorium intybus,* (c) *Crepis sancta,* (d) *Sonchus asper,* (e) *Carthamus lanatus,* (f) *Amaranthus blitum,* and their main metabolites: 1: caftaric acid; 2: caffeoylquinic acid isomer; 3: cichoric acid; 4: luteolin diglycoside; 5: quercetin glucuronide; 6: luteolin glucuronide; 7: dicaffeoylquinic acid isomer; 8: apigenin glucuronide; 9: quercetin glucoside; 10: luteolin glucoside; 11: quercetin acetyl glucoside; 12: luteolin acetyl glucoside; 13: hydroxycinnamates; 14: rutin; 15: triterpene saponins.

activity may be explained by the type of its polyphenols or by the presence of other chemical compounds which may be very effective as hydrogen donors.

3.3. Antimutagenic Activity of Extracts against ROS-Induced DNA Damage.
All the tested extracts inhibited ROO•-induced DNA plasmid breakage, with IC_{50} values ranging from 105 to 970 μg/ml (Table 2 and Figure 2). The potency

order was *C. lanatus = C. intybus > C. sancta > C. spinosum > A. blitum > S. asper* (Table 2). Similar to antioxidant assays, the three extracts enriched with polyphenols by passage through resin column exhibited at least 2-fold higher protective activity compared to other extracts. The ROO• radicals that caused the DNA damage in this assay are produced within cells after the addition of O_2 to carbon-centered radicals [40]. Subsequently, ROO• can oxidize

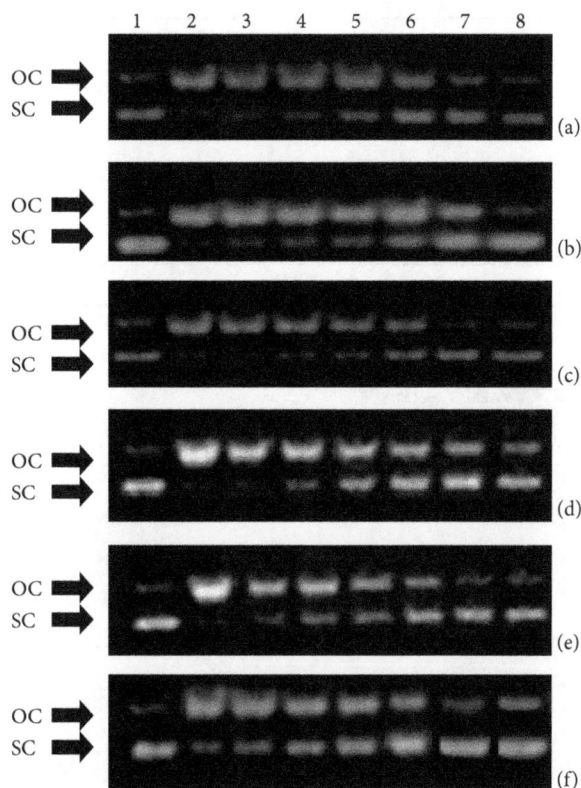

FIGURE 2: Protective activity of extracts from (a) *Crepis sancta*, (b) *Cichorium intybus*, (c) *Carthamus lanatus*, (d) *Amaranthus blitum*, (e) *Cichorium spinosum*, and (f) *Sonchus asper* plants against ROO• radicals: 1: pBluescript-SK+ plasmid DNA without any treatment; 2: plasmid DNA exposed to ROO• radicals alone; 3, 4, 5, 6, and 7: plasmid DNA exposed to ROO• radicals in the presence of extract concentrations: 0.015, 0.030, 0.060, 0.120, and 0.240 mg/mL, respectively (a–c) and 0.030, 0.060, 0.120, 0.240, and 0.480 mg/ml, respectively (e) and 0.120, 0.240, 0.480, 0.960, and 1.920 mg/ml, respectively (d, f); 8: plasmid DNA exposed to the maximum tested concentration of each extract alone. OC: open circular; SC: supercoiled.

DNA bases to their hydroxyl derivatives resulting in mutations and manifestation of diseases [41]. These detrimental effects may be prevented by the use of the tested extracts through diet as the present findings suggested. Interestingly, quercetin, luteolin, and caffeoylquinic acid found in *C. lanatus* extract have been demonstrated to scavenge ROO• [42, 43].

The two most potent extracts enriched with polyphenols due to passage through resin (i.e., *C. lanatus* and *C. intybus*) and the most potent (i.e., *C. spinosum*) among nonenriched extracts were also tested for their inhibitory potency against ROS-induced mutagenicity in *S. typhimurium* TA102 bacterial cells. The results from this assay supported those from DNA plasmid cleavage assay, since all three extracts inhibited dose-dependent *t*-BOOH-induced mutagenicity (Figure 3). Specifically, *C. lanatus* extract inhibited significantly *t*-BOOH-induced mutations by 12.3, 17.9, 31.7, 48.7, and 66.9% at 5, 10, 25, 50, and 100 μg/plate, respectively, *C. intybus* extract by 17.0, 19.6, 30.0, 38.0, and 56.9% at 5, 10, 25, 50, and 100 μg/plate, respectively, and *C. spinosum*

extract by 12.2, 24.7, and 48.1% at 100, 200, and 400 μg/plate, respectively (Figure 3). The two extracts enriched with polyphenols had higher inhibitory activity than the nonenriched extract, indicating that the polyphenols accounted mainly for the observed protection from mutagenicity. The *t*-BOOH reacts with Fe^{2+} in cells and generates HO• causing DNA damage [3]. The OH• radicals are the major ROS to react with either DNA bases or deoxyribose resulting in DNA damage and mutations [3]. Thus, it was important that the tested extracts protected from OH•-induced DNA mutations. *C. lanatus* extract was again the most potent due, at least in part, to its identified polyphenols, since previous studies have shown that quercetin and luteolin inhibited *t*-BOOH-induced mutagenicity in TA102 cells [44]. Moreover, Jho et al. [45] have reported that a caffeoylquinic derivative inhibited *t*-BOOH-induced DNA damage in human liver HepG2 cells.

3.4. Effects of Extracts on the Antioxidant Status of Endothelial Cells. *C. lanatus* and *C. intybus* extracts, the two most potent extracts enriched with polyphenols, and *C. spinosum* extract, the most potent among nonenriched extracts, were examined for their antioxidant activity in human endothelial EA.hy926 cells. Firstly, the extracts' cytotoxicity was evaluated, so as noncytotoxic concentrations to be used for the assessment of the antioxidant activity. The results from XTT assay showed that *C. intybus*, *C. lanatus*, and *C. spinosum* extracts exhibited significant cytotoxicity above 100, 200, and 600 μg/ml, respectively (Figure 4). Thus, the selected concentrations of the *C. intybus*, *C. lanatus*, and *C. spinosum* extracts in the following assays were up to 50, 100, and 400 μg/ml, respectively.

The assessment of the extracts' effects on the antioxidant capacity of endothelial cells was based on the measurement of GSH and ROS levels by flow cytometry. The results showed that *C. intybus* increased significantly GSH levels by 10.8, 15.2, and 33.4% at 10, 25, and 50 μg/ml, respectively, compared to control, *C. lanatus* by 15.9, 21.5, and 24.7% at 25, 50, and 100 μg/ml, respectively, and *C. spinosum* by 10.5 and 21.6% at 50 and 100 μg/ml, respectively (Figure 5). The increase in GSH after extract treatment is important, since GSH is considered as a significant endogenous antioxidant molecule in cells [46]. GSH may scavenge directly free radicals by donating one hydrogen atom from its sulfhydryl group or is used as substrate by antioxidant enzymes such as glutathione transferase (GST) and glutathione peroxidase (GPx) [46]. Especially for endothelial cells, GSH is important not only as antioxidant but also as a crucial regulator of cell signaling [47, 48]. Although the effects of *C. intybus* and *C. lanatus* on GSH were dose dependent, the *C. spinosum* extract did not affect GSH at higher concentrations than 100 μg/ml (Figure 5). This intriguing observation may be explained by the fact that *C. spinosum* at 200 and 400 μg/ml exhibited a tension to decrease cell viability (Figure 4). That is, for *C. spinosum*, 100 μg/ml seemed to be a crucial concentration, above which cytotoxicity was caused. In turn, this cytotoxicity was encountered by GSH consumption. It is known that polyphenols sometimes have a biphasic effect, namely, at low concentrations, they act as antioxidants and

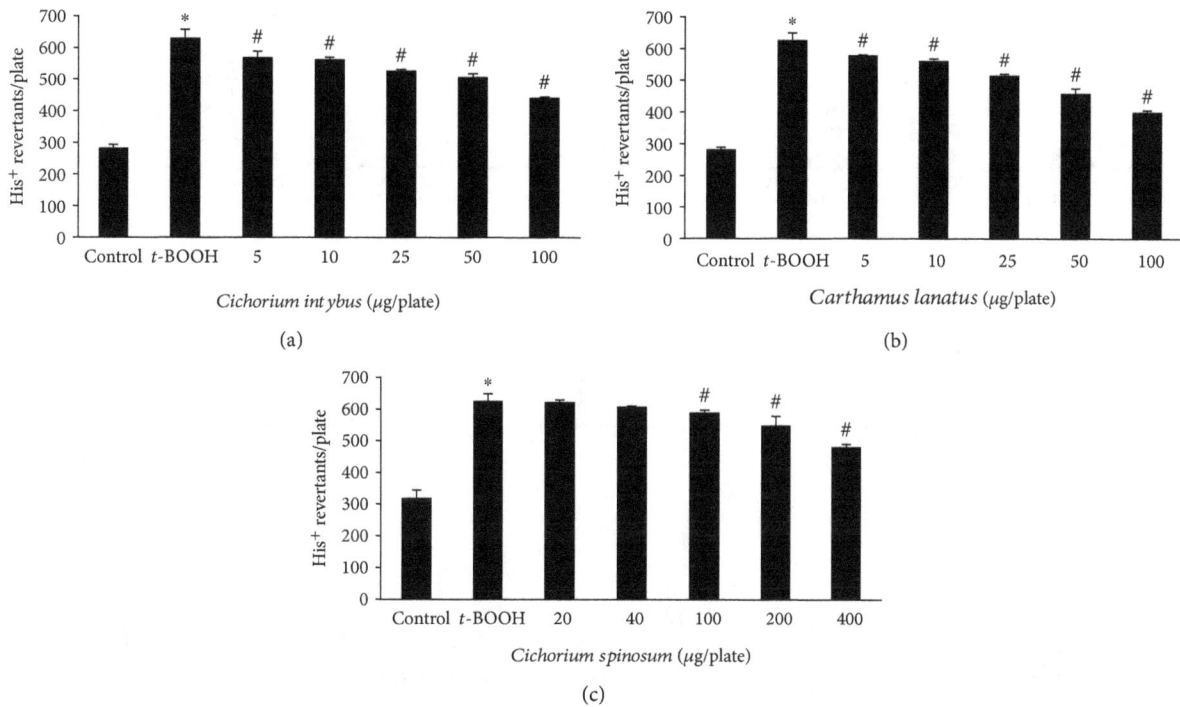

FIGURE 3: Antimutagenic effects of *C. intybus*, *C. lanatus*, and *C. spinosum* extracts on *t*-BOOH-induced mutagenicity in *S. typhimurium* TA102 cells. Values are the mean $\pm$ SD number of histidine revertants of three independent experiments carried out in triplicate. The concentration of *t*-BOOH was 0.4 mM/plate. $^*p < 0.05$ when compared with control. $^\#p < 0.05$ when compared with the *t*-BOOH alone sample.

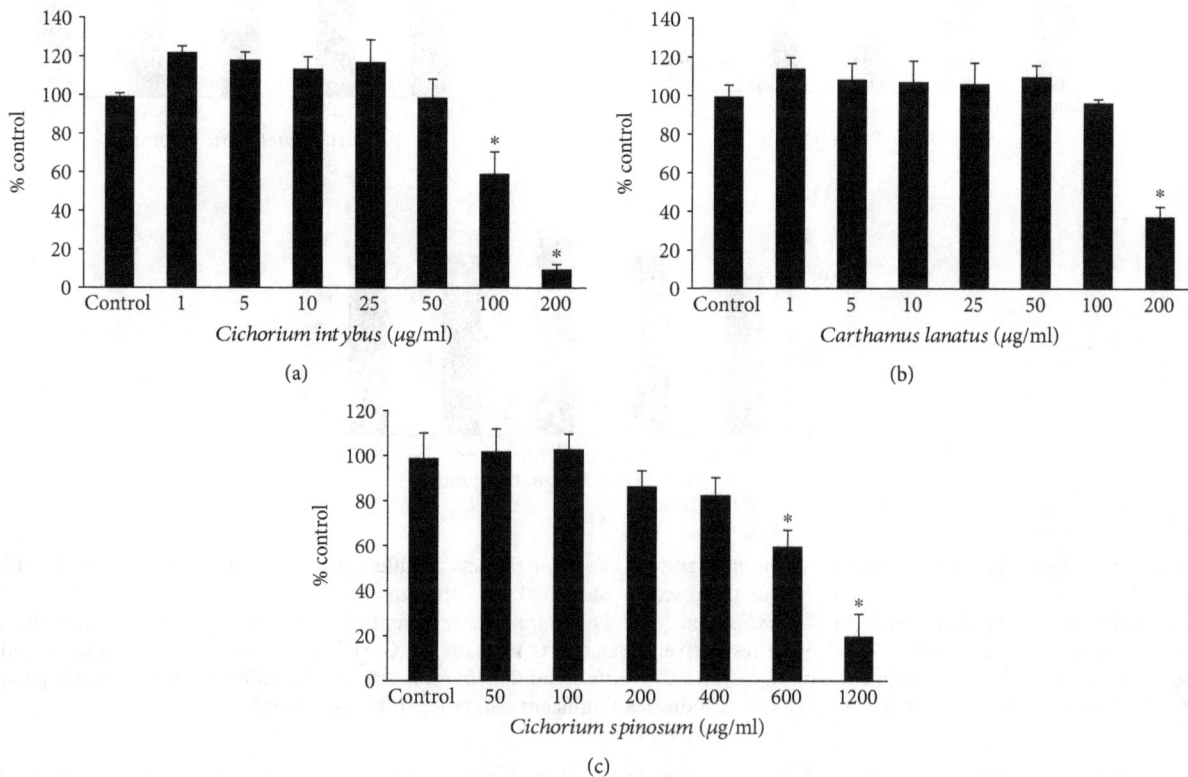

FIGURE 4: Cell viability following treatment with *C. intybus*, *C. lanatus*, and *C. spinosum* extracts in EA.hy926 cells. The results are presented as the means $\pm$ SEM of three independent experiments carried out in triplicate. $^*p < 0.05$ indicates significant difference from the control value.

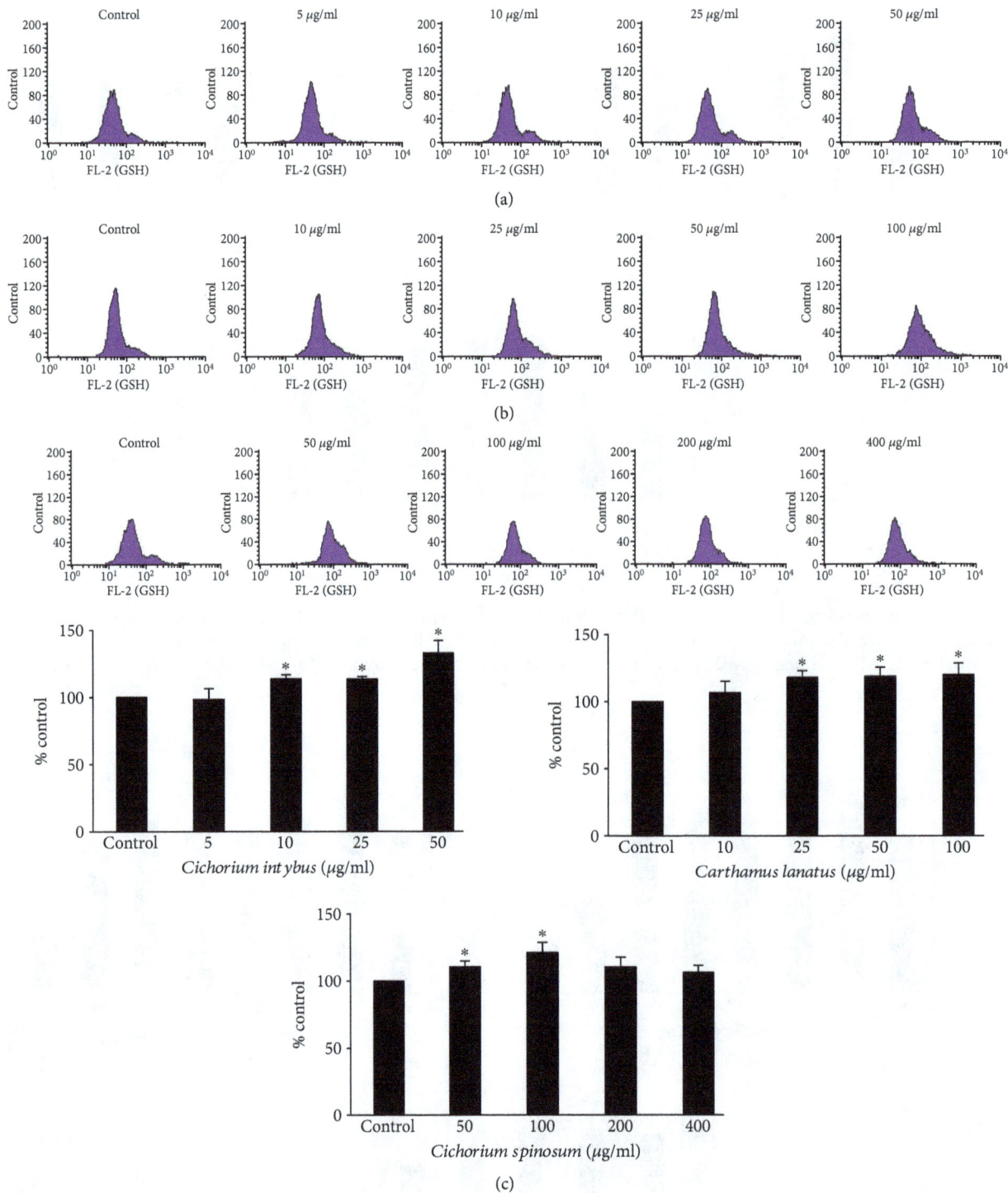

FIGURE 5: Effects of treatment with *C. intybus*, *C. lanatus*, and *C. spinosum* extracts at different concentrations for 24 h on GSH levels in EA.hy926 cells. The histograms of cell counts versus fluorescence of 10,000 cells analyzed by flow cytometry for the detection of GSH levels after treatment with (a) *C. intybus*, (b) *C. lanatus*, and (c) *C. spinosum*. FL2 represents the detection of fluorescence using 488 and 580 nm as the excitation and emission wavelength, respectively. Bar charts indicate the GSH levels as % of control as estimated by the histograms in EA.hy926 cells after treatment with *C. intybus*, *C. lanatus*, and *C. spinosum* extracts. All values of bar charts are presented as the mean ± SEM of 3 independent experiments. $^*p < 0.05$ indicates significant difference from the control.

at high concentrations, they act as prooxidants resulting in cytotoxicity [49]. It is also worth mentioning that polyphenols identified in the tested extracts have been reported to increase GSH levels. For example, quercetin has been demonstrated recently to enhance GSH levels in human aortic endothelial cells (HAEC) through increased expression of glutamate-cysteine ligase (GCL), one of the major enzymes involved in GSH synthesis [50]. Moreover, luteolin has been

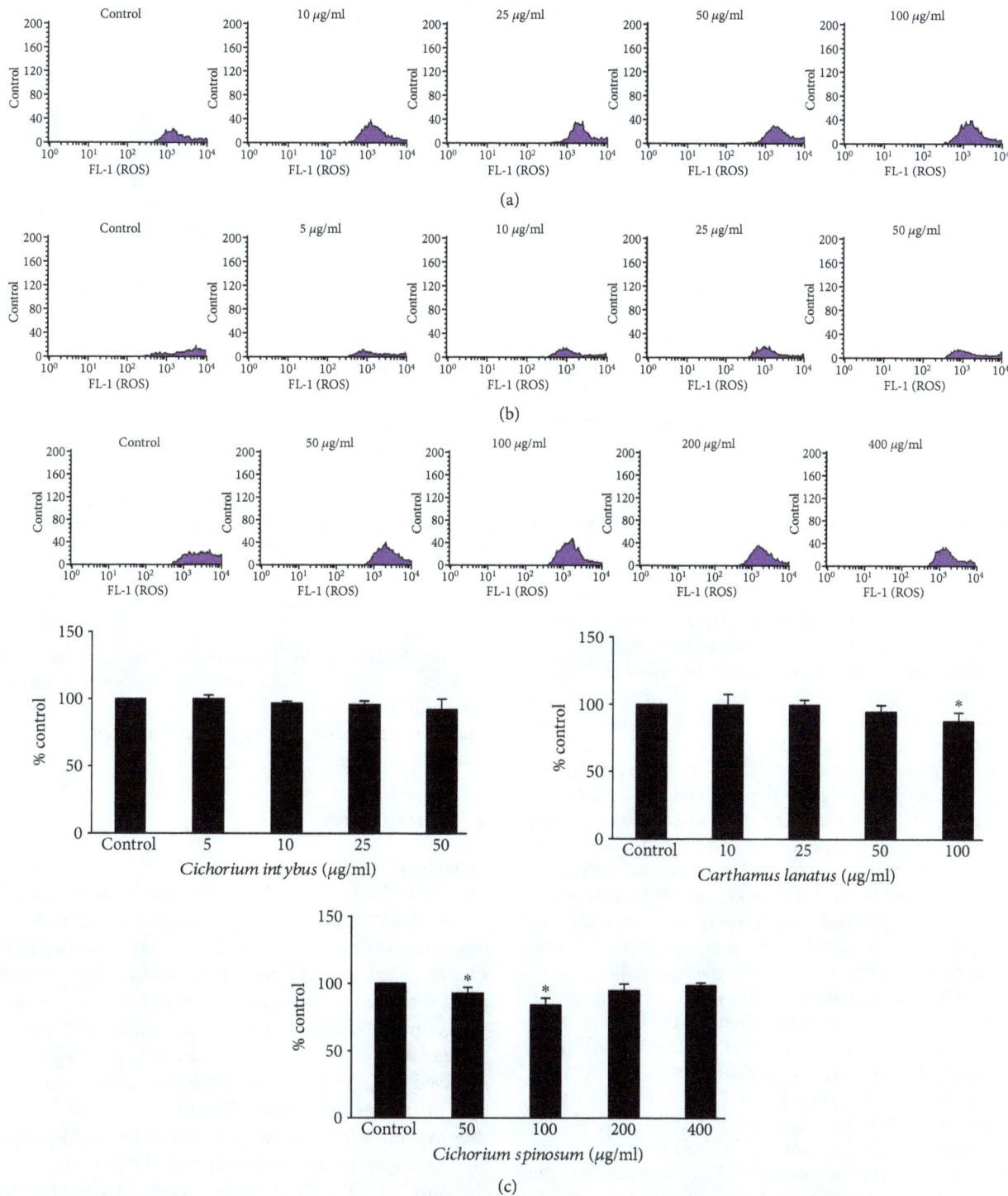

FIGURE 6: Effects of treatment with *C. intybus*, *C. lanatus*, and *C. spinosum* extracts at different concentrations for 24 h on ROS levels in EA.hy926 cells. The histograms of cell counts versus fluorescence of 10,000 cells analyzed by flow cytometry for the detection of ROS levels after treatment with (a) *C. intybus*, (b) *C. lanatus*, and (c) *C. spinosum*. FL2 represents the detection of fluorescence using 488 and 530 nm as the excitation and emission wavelength, respectively. Bar charts indicate the ROS levels as % of control as estimated by the histograms in EA.hy926 cells after treatment with *C. intybus*, *C. lanatus*, and *C. spinosum* extracts. All values of bar charts are presented as the mean ± SEM of 3 independent experiments. $^*p < 0.05$ indicates significant difference from the control.

demonstrated to decrease oxidative stress in the mouse lung through, among other mechanisms, increase of GSH [51]. Additionally, administration of caftaric acid to rats inhibited lead-induced decrease in GSH in the kidney [52].

Unlike GSH, extract treatment did not affect ROS levels too intensively (Figure 6). Only *C. lanatus* extract reduced significantly ROS by 12.1% and *C. spinosum* extract by 6.8 and 15.6% at 50 and 100 μg/ml, respectively, compared to control (Figure 6). The weak extracts' effect on ROS levels may be attributed to the fact that their impact was examined on the baseline ROS levels, that is, there was not an oxidant stimulus to cells. Nevertheless, the observed decrease in ROS, even only at the higher extract concentrations, was in accordance with and might be attributed to the corresponding increase in the antioxidant molecule of GSH by the extracts (Figure 5). Interestingly, *C. spinosum* at concentrations higher than 100 μg/ml did not decrease further ROS levels (Figure 6). This finding supported our hypothesis mentioned above, that is, *C. spinosum* at concentrations above 100 μg/ml may exhibit prooxidant effect and cytotoxicity.

Since *C. intybus* extract induced the highest increase in antioxidant mechanism (i.e., GSH) in endothelial cells, its effects on the expression at a transcriptional level of antioxidant genes were assessed (Figure 7). Specifically, it was examined if the extract affected the expression of the nuclear factor (erythroid-derived 2)-like 2 (Nrf2), the most important transcription factor regulating antioxidant genes [53]. The results from the qRT-PCR showed that *C. intybus* treatment upregulated significantly the expression of *NFE2L2* gene encoding for Nrf2 by 7.3-fold and 8.5-fold at 12 and 24 h, respectively, compared to control (Figure 7). This finding was significant, because it indicated that the extract's compounds exerted antioxidant activity not only as direct free radical scavengers but also as modulators of molecular mechanisms. Interestingly, chicoric acid found in *C. intybus* extract has been reported to increase Nrf2 expression in mouse muscle [54]. The increase in Nrf2 expression was supported by the extract treatment-induced increase in expression of genes regulated by Nrf2. Namely, extract treatment upregulated significantly the expression of *GCLC* by 6.2-fold, 6.3-fold, and 3.4-fold at 3, 12, and 24 h, respectively, *GSR* by 9.8-fold, 8.0-fold, and 5.0-fold at 3, 12, and 24 h, respectively, *NQO1* by 8.4-fold, 12.1-fold, and 6.7-fold at 3, 12, and 24 h, respectively, and *HMOX1* by 4.0-fold, 4.5-fold, and 2.7-fold at 3, 12, and 24 h, respectively, compared to control (Figure 7). Especially, the increase in *GCLC* and *GSR* expression was important, since it accounted for the *C. intybus* extract-induced increase in GSH levels (Figure 5). *GCLC* gene encodes the catalytic subunit of the GCL protein, the main enzyme involved in GSH synthesis [40]. *GSR* encodes for glutathione reductase (GR) enzyme regenerating GSH from the oxidized glutathione (GSSG) [40]. *HMOX1* and *NQO1*, the other two upregulating genes, encode for heme oxygenase 1 (HO-1) and NAD (P)H:quinone oxidoreductase 1 (NQO1), respectively. The increase in the expression of these enzymes supported further the ability of the *C. intybus* extract to enhance endothelial cells' antioxidant capacity, since HO-1 and NQO1 are important antioxidant enzymes participating in iron sequestration and quinone detoxification, respectively [55, 56]. *C. intybus* treatment did not affect the expression of *CAT*, *SOD1*, and *GPX1* genes, while it downregulated significantly *TXN* gene expression by 35.7-fold, 10.3-fold, and 10.0-fold at 3, 12, and 24 h, respectively (Figure 7). The lack of effect on *CAT*, *SOD1*, and *GPX1* and the downregulation of *TXN* gene were intriguing, since Nrf2 activates their expression [53]. This contradiction may be explained by the high complexity of

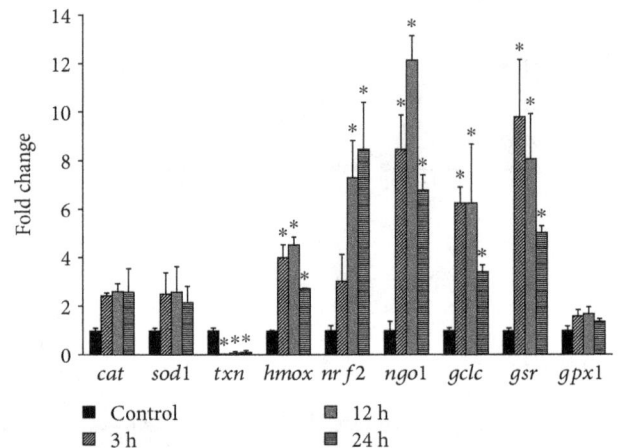

FIGURE 7: Gene expression profiles of *NFE2L2*, *GCLC*, *GSR*, *GPX1*, *HMOX1*, *NQO1*, *CAT*, *SOD1*, and *TXN* genes in EA.hy926 cells after treatment with *C. intybus* extract at 50 μg/ml for 3, 12, and 24 h. mRNA levels were determined by qRT-PCR, and relative levels were expressed as fold of control (untreated cells) after normalization to GAPDH. The results are expressed as mean ± SD of three independent experiments. $*p < 0.05$ indicates significant difference from the control.

the regulation of the antioxidant mechanisms and the interaction between them, namely, when some antioxidant mechanisms are enhanced, some others remain inactive as a compensation adaptive response of the cell [57].

4. Conclusions

In conclusion, the present findings demonstrated for the first time that extracts from the edible plants *C. lanatus*, *C. intybus*, and *C. spinosum* enhanced antioxidant defense mechanism such as GSH in endothelial cells. Especially, *C. spinosum* extract was shown to mediate this antioxidant effect through increased expression of Nrf2, the most crucial transcription factor of antioxidant genes, and subsequent upregulation of important antioxidant genes including those involved in GSH synthesis. Since, these plants constitute a part of the Mediterranean diet, their observed bioactivities may explain, at least in part, the prevention of this type of diet against diseases associated with endothelial function such as the cardiovascular disease [58]. Moreover, the results suggested that these extracts may be used for the development of food supplements or biofunctional foods that would protect from diseases caused by oxidative stress-induced endothelium damage.

Authors' Contributions

Dimitrios Balabanos, Salomi Savva, and Zoi Skaperda contributed equally to the present study.

Acknowledgments

The work was funded by the "Toxicology" MSc program in the Department of Biochemistry and Biotechnology at the University of Thessaly. The current work was also supported by the EU and project MediHealth-H2020-MSCA-RISE-2015—"Novel natural products for healthy ageing from Mediterranean diet and food plants of other global sources" (Proposal number: 691158) under the Horizon 2020 framework.

References

[1] P. D. Ray, B. W. Huang, and Y. Tsuji, "Reactive oxygen species (ROS) homeostasis and redox regulation in cellular signaling," *Cellular Signalling*, vol. 24, no. 5, pp. 981–990, 2012.

[2] A. Priftis, D. Stagos, K. Konstantinopoulos et al., "Comparison of antioxidant activity between green and roasted coffee beans using molecular methods," *Molecular Medicine Reports*, vol. 12, no. 5, pp. 7293–7302, 2015.

[3] B. Halliwell, *Free Radicals and Other Reactive Species in Disease*, John Wiley & Sons, Ltd, eLS, 2005.

[4] V. Sosa, T. Moliné, R. Somoza, R. Paciucci, H. Kondoh, and M. E. LLeonart, "Oxidative stress and cancer: an overview," *Ageing Research Reviews*, vol. 12, no. 1, pp. 376–390, 2013.

[5] L. Rochette, M. Zeller, Y. Cottin, and C. Vergely, "Diabetes, oxidative stress and therapeutic strategies," *Biochimica et Biophysica Acta (BBA) - General Subjects*, vol. 1840, no. 9, pp. 2709–2729, 2014.

[6] P. Kouka, A. Priftis, D. Stagos et al., "Assessment of the antioxidant activity of an olive oil total polyphenolic fraction and hydroxytyrosol from a Greek Olea europea variety in endothelial cells and myoblasts," *International Journal of Molecular Medicine*, vol. 40, no. 3, pp. 703–712, 2017.

[7] J. E. Deanfield, J. P. Halcox, and T. J. Rabelink, "Endothelial function and dysfunction: testing and clinical relevance," *Circulation*, vol. 115, no. 10, pp. 1285–1295, 2007.

[8] V. M. Victor, M. Rocha, E. Solá, C. Bañuls, K. Garcia-Malpartida, and A. Hernández-Mijares, "Oxidative stress, endothelial dysfunction and atherosclerosis," *Current Pharmaceutical Design*, vol. 15, no. 26, pp. 2988–3002, 2009.

[9] S. Kokura, R. E. Wolf, T. Yoshikawa, D. N. Granger, and T. Y. Aw, "Molecular mechanisms of neutrophil-endothelial cell adhesion induced by redox imbalance," *Circulation Research*, vol. 84, no. 5, pp. 516–524, 1999.

[10] S. G. Rhee, "Cell signaling. H2O2, a necessary evil for cell signaling," *Science*, vol. 312, no. 5782, pp. 1882-1883, 2006.

[11] A. Woywodt, F. H. Bahlmann, K. De Groot, H. Haller, and M. Haubitz, "Circulating endothelial cells: life, death, detachment and repair of the endothelial cell layer," *Nephrology, Dialysis, Transplantation*, vol. 17, no. 10, pp. 1728–1730, 2002.

[12] J. M. Landete, "Dietary intake of natural antioxidants: vitamins and polyphenols," *Critical Reviews in Food Science and Nutrition*, vol. 53, no. 7, pp. 706–721, 2013.

[13] Y. Z. Fang, S. Yang, and G. Wu, "Free radicals, antioxidants, and nutrition," *Nutrition*, vol. 18, no. 10, pp. 872–879, 2002.

[14] J. M. Landete, "Updated knowledge about polyphenols: functions, bioavailability, metabolism, and health," *Critical Reviews in Food Science and Nutrition*, vol. 52, no. 10, pp. 936–948, 2012.

[15] M. Battino and B. Mezzetti, "Update on fruit antioxidant capacity: a key tool for Mediterranean diet," *Public Health Nutrition*, vol. 9, no. 8A, pp. 1099–1103, 2006.

[16] M. Leonti, S. Nebel, D. Rivera, M. Heinrich, and M. Leonti, "Wild gathered food plants in the European Mediterranean: a comparative analysis," *Economic Botany*, vol. 60, no. 2, pp. 130–142, 2006.

[17] A. C. H. Hadjichambis, D. Paraskeva-Hadjichambi, A. Della et al., "Wild and semi-domesticated food plant consumption in seven circum-Mediterranean areas," *International Journal of Food Sciences and Nutrition*, vol. 59, no. 5, pp. 383–414, 2008.

[18] E. Vasilopoulou and A. Trichopoulou, "Green pies: the flavonoid rich Greek snack," *Food Chemistry*, vol. 126, no. 3, pp. 855–858, 2011.

[19] E. Vasilopoulou, K. Georga, M. B. Joergensen, A. Naska, and A. Trichopoulou, "The antioxidant properties of Greek foods and the flavonoid content of the Mediterranean menu," *Current Medicinal Chemistry - Immunology, Endocrine & Metabolic Agents*, vol. 5, no. 1, pp. 33–45, 2005.

[20] F. Conforti, S. Sosa, M. Marrelli et al., "The protective ability of Mediterranean dietary plants against the oxidative damage: the role of radical oxygen species in inflammation and the polyphenol, flavonoid and sterol contents," *Food Chemistry*, vol. 112, no. 3, pp. 587–594, 2009.

[21] S. Zeghichi, S. Kallithraka, A. P. Simopoulos, and Z. Kypriotakis, "Nutritional composition of selected wild plants in the diet of Crete," *World Review of Nutrition and Dietetics*, vol. 91, pp. 22–40, 2003.

[22] C. I. Vardavas, D. Majchrzak, K. H. Wagner, I. Elmadfa, and A. Kafatos, "The antioxidant and phylloquinone content of wildly grown greens in Crete," *Food Chemistry*, vol. 99, no. 4, pp. 813–821, 2006.

[23] S. Nebel, A. Pieroni, and M. Heinrich, "Ta chòrta: wild edible greens used in the Graecanic area in Calabria, Southern Italy," *Appetite*, vol. 47, no. 3, pp. 333–342, 2006.

[24] E. V. Mikropoulou, K. Vougogiannopoulou, E. Kalpoutzakis et al., "Phytochemical composition of the decoctions of Greek edible greens (chórta) and evaluation of antioxidant and cytotoxic properties," *Molecules*, vol. 23, no. 7, article 1541, 2018.

[25] S. Makri, I. Kafantaris, S. Savva et al., "Novel feed including olive oil mill wastewater bioactive compounds enhanced the redox status of lambs," *In Vivo*, vol. 32, no. 2, pp. 291–302, 2018.

[26] D. Stagos, N. Soulitsiotis, C. Tsadila et al., "Antibacterial and antioxidant activity of different types of honey derived from Mount Olympus in Greece," *International Journal of Molecular Medicine*, vol. 42, no. 2, pp. 726–734, 2018.

[27] A. Priftis, D. Mitsiou, M. Halabalaki et al., "Roasting has a distinct effect on the antimutagenic activity of coffee varieties," *Mutation Research*, vol. 829-830, pp. 33–42, 2018.

[28] E. Kerasioti, D. Stagos, A. Priftis et al., "Antioxidant effects of whey protein on muscle C2C12 cells," *Food Chemistry*, vol. 155, pp. 271–278, 2014.

[29] C. Spanou, D. Stagos, L. Tousias et al., "Assessment of antioxidant activity of extracts from unique Greek varieties of Leguminosae plants using in vitro assays," *Anticancer Research*, vol. 27, no. 5A, pp. 3403–3410, 2007.

[30] D. M. Maron and B. N. Ames, "Revised methods for the Salmonella mutagenicity test," *Mutation Research*, vol. 113, no. 3-4, pp. 173–215, 1983.

[31] K. Mortelmans and E. Zeiger, "The Ames Salmonella/microsome mutagenicity assay," *Mutation Research*, vol. 455, no. 1-2, pp. 29–60, 2000.

[32] A. Priftis, E. M. Panagiotou, K. Lakis et al., "Roasted and green coffee extracts show antioxidant and cytotoxic activity in myoblast and endothelial cell lines in a cell specific manner," *Food and Chemical Toxicology*, vol. 114, pp. 119–127, 2018.

[33] N. Goutzourelas, D. Stagos, N. Demertzis et al., "Effects of polyphenolic grape extract on the oxidative status of muscle and endothelial cells," *Human & Experimental Toxicology*, vol. 33, no. 11, pp. 1099–1112, 2014.

[34] E. Kerasioti, D. Stagos, V. Georgatzi et al., "Antioxidant effects of sheep whey protein on endothelial cells," *Oxidative Medicine and Cellular Longevity*, vol. 2016, Article ID 6585737, 10 pages, 2016.

[35] A. Priftis, N. Goutzourelas, M. Halabalaki et al., "Effect of polyphenols from coffee and grape on gene expression inmyoblasts," *Mechanisms of Ageing and Development*, vol. 172, pp. 115–122, 2018.

[36] V. Brieudes, A. Angelis, K. Vougogiannopoulou et al., "Phytochemical analysis and antioxidant potential of the phytonutrient-rich decoction of Cichorium spinosum and C. intybus," *Planta Medica*, vol. 82, no. 11-12, pp. 1070–1078, 2016.

[37] A. W. Boots, G. R. Haenen, and A. Bast, "Health effects of quercetin: from antioxidant to nutraceutical," *European Journal of Pharmacology*, vol. 585, no. 2-3, pp. 325–337, 2008.

[38] Y. C. Zhang, F. F. Gan, S. B. Shelar, K. Y. Ng, and E. H. Chew, "Antioxidant and Nrf 2 inducing activities of luteolin, a flavonoid constituent in Ixeris sonchifolia Hance, provide neuroprotective effects against ischemia-induced cellular injury," *Food and Chemical Toxicology*, vol. 59, pp. 272–280, 2013.

[39] S. Chanda and R. Dave, "In vitro models for antioxidant activity evaluation and some medicinal plants possessing antioxidant properties: an overview," *African Journal of Microbiology Research*, vol. 3, pp. 981–996, 2009.

[40] T. A. Dix and J. Aikens, "Mechanisms and biological relevance of lipid peroxidation initiation," *Chemical Research in Toxicology*, vol. 6, no. 1, pp. 2–18, 1993.

[41] T. Simandan, J. Sun, and T. A. Dix, "Oxidation of DNA bases, deoxyribonucleosides and homopolymers by peroxyl radicals," *The Biochemical Journal*, vol. 335, no. 2, pp. 233–240, 1998.

[42] E. Rodrigues, L. R. Mariutti, and A. Z. Mercadante, "Carotenoids and phenolic compounds from *Solanum sessiliflorum*, an unexploited Amazonian fruit, and their scavenging capacities against reactive oxygen and nitrogen species," *Journal of Agricultural and Food Chemistry*, vol. 61, no. 12, pp. 3022–3029, 2013.

[43] M. Terashima, Y. Kakuno, N. Kitano et al., "Antioxidant activity of flavonoids evaluated with myoglobin method," *Plant Cell Reports*, vol. 31, no. 2, pp. 291–298, 2012.

[44] R. Edenharder and D. Grünhage, "Free radical scavenging abilities of flavonoids as mechanism of protection against mutagenicity induced by tert-butyl hydroperoxide or cumene hydroperoxide in Salmonella typhimurium TA102," *Mutation Research*, vol. 540, no. 1, pp. 1–18, 2003.

[45] E. H. Jho, K. Kang, S. Oidovsambuu et al., "Gymnaster koraiensis and its major components, 3,5-di-O-caffeoylquinic acid and gymnasterkoreayne B, reduce oxidative damage induced by tert-butyl hydroperoxide or acetaminophen in HepG2 cells," *BMB Reports*, vol. 46, no. 10, pp. 513–518, 2013.

[46] K. Aquilano, S. Baldelli, and M. R. Ciriolo, "Glutathione: new roles in redox signaling for an old antioxidant," *Frontiers in Pharmacology*, vol. 5, p. 196, 2014.

[47] S. J. Elliott and S. K. Koliwad, "Redox control of ion channel activity in vascular endothelial cells by glutathione," *Microcirculation*, vol. 4, no. 3, pp. 341–347, 1997.

[48] C. Espinosa-Díez, V. Miguel, S. Vallejo et al., "Role of glutathione biosynthesis in endothelial dysfunction and fibrosis," *Redox Biology*, vol. 14, pp. 88–99, 2018.

[49] A. M. Mileo and S. Miccadei, "Polyphenols as modulator of oxidative stress in cancer disease: new therapeutic strategies," *Oxidative Medicine and Cellular Longevity*, vol. 2016, Article ID 6475624, 17 pages, 2016.

[50] C. Li, W. J. Zhang, J. Choi, and B. Frei, "Quercetin affects glutathione levels and redox ratio in human aortic endothelial cells not through oxidation but formation and cellular export of quercetin-glutathione conjugates and upregulation of glutamate-cysteine ligase," *Redox Biology*, vol. 9, pp. 220–228, 2016.

[51] B. Liu, H. Yu, R. Baiyun et al., "Protective effects of dietary luteolin against mercuric chloride-induced lung injury in mice: involvement of AKT/Nrf 2 and NF-κB pathways," *Food and Chemical Toxicology*, vol. 113, pp. 296–302, 2018.

[52] K. M. M. Koriem and M. S. Arbid, "Role of caftaric acid in lead-associated nephrotoxicity in rats via antidiuretic, antioxidant and anti-apoptotic activities," *Journal of Complementary and Integrative Medicine*, vol. 15, no. 2, article 20170024, 2017.

[53] I. Bellezza, I. Giambanco, A. Minelli, and R. Donato, "Nrf2-Keap1 signaling in oxidative and reductive stress," *Biochimica et Biophysica Acta (BBA) - Molecular Cell Research*, vol. 1865, no. 5, pp. 721–733, 2018.

[54] D. Zhu, X. Zhang, Y. Niu et al., "Cichoric acid improved hyperglycaemia and restored muscle injury via activating antioxidant response in MLD-STZ-induced diabetic mice," *Food and Chemical Toxicology*, vol. 107, Part A, pp. 138–149, 2017.

[55] J. F. Ndisang, "Synergistic interaction between heme oxygenase (HO) and nuclear-factor E2- related factor-2 (Nrf 2) against oxidative stress in cardiovascular related diseases," *Current Pharmaceutical Design*, vol. 23, no. 10, pp. 1465–1470, 2017.

[56] A. T. Dinkova-Kostova and P. Talalay, "NAD (P)H:quinone acceptor oxidoreductase 1 (NQO1), a multifunctional antioxidant enzyme and exceptionally versatile cytoprotector," *Archives of Biochemistry and Biophysics*, vol. 501, no. 1, pp. 116–123, 2010.

[57] S. Alvarez and A. Boveris, "Antioxidant adaptive response of human mononuclear cells to UV-B: effect of lipoic acid," *Journal of Photochemistry and Photobiology. B*, vol. 55, no. 2-3, pp. 113–119, 2000.

[58] C. M. Erwin, C. T. McEvoy, S. E. Moore et al., "A qualitative analysis exploring preferred methods of peer support to encourage adherence to a Mediterranean diet in a Northern European population at high risk of cardiovascular disease," *BMC Public Health*, vol. 18, no. 1, p. 213, 2018.

14

Uric Acid Protects against Focal Cerebral Ischemia/Reperfusion-Induced Oxidative Stress via Activating Nrf2 and Regulating Neurotrophic Factor Expression

Bai-liu Ya [ID],[1] Qian Liu,[2] Hong-fang Li,[3] Hong-ju Cheng,[1] Ting Yu,[1] Lin Chen,[4] You Wang,[4] Li-li Yuan,[4] Wen-juan Li,[5] Wen-yan Liu,[1] and Bo Bai[1]

[1]Department of Physiology, Jining Medical University, Shandong 272067, China
[2]School of Clinical Medicine, Jining Medical University, Shandong 272067, China
[3]Department of Neurology, Affiliated Hospital of Jining Medical University, Shandong 272067, China
[4]School of Basic Medicine, Jining Medical University, Shandong 272067, China
[5]School of Forensic and Laboratory Medicine, Jining Medical University, Shandong 272067, China

Correspondence should be addressed to Bai-liu Ya; yabailiu@126.com

Guest Editor: Luciano Saso

The aim of this study was to investigate whether uric acid (UA) might exert neuroprotection via activating the nuclear factor erythroid 2-related factor 2 (Nrf2) pathway and regulating neurotrophic factors in the cerebral cortices after transient focal cerebral ischemia/reperfusion (FCI/R) in rats. UA was intravenously injected through the tail vein (16 mg/kg) 30 min after the onset of reperfusion in rats subjected to middle cerebral artery occlusion for 2 h. Neurological deficit score was performed to analyze neurological function at 24 h after reperfusion. Terminal deoxynucleotidyl transferase-mediated dNTP nick end labeling (TUNEL) staining and hematoxylin and eosin (HE) staining were used to detect histological injury of the cerebral cortex. Malondialdehyde (MDA), the carbonyl groups, and 8-hydroxy-2′-deoxyguanosine (8-OHdG) levels were employed to evaluate oxidative stress. Nrf2 and its downstream antioxidant protein, heme oxygenase- (HO-) 1,were detected by western blot. Nrf2 DNA-binding activity was observed using an ELISA-based measurement. Expressions of BDNF and NGF were analyzed by immunohistochemistry. Our results showed that UA treatment significantly suppressed FCI/R-induced oxidative stress, accompanied by attenuating neuronal damage, which subsequently decreased the infarct volume and neurological deficit. Further, the treatment of UA activated Nrf2 signaling pathway and upregulated BDNF and NGF expression levels. Interestingly, the aforementioned effects of UA were markedly inhibited by administration of brusatol, an inhibitor of Nrf2. Taken together, the antioxidant and neuroprotective effects afforded by UA treatment involved the modulation of Nrf2-mediated oxidative stress and regulation of BDNF and NGF expression levels. Thus, UA treatment could be of interest to prevent FCI/R injury.

1. Introduction

The principal therapy for cerebral ischemia is the restoration of cerebral blood flow as early as possible. Early recanalization with recombinant tissue plasminogen activator (rt-PA) has been developed to treat acute ischemic stroke. However, reperfusion after cerebral ischemia may be injurious and increase the risk of brain hemorrhage, promote the development of cerebral edema, and cause more serious damage to the blood-brain barrier. The potential mechanisms responsible for the additional injuries in the ischemic brain caused by reperfusion itself remain unclear [1]. Acute cerebral ischemia starts with cerebral blood flow interruption that causes severely limited oxygen and glucose supply, eliciting a cascade of pathological events such as excitotoxicity, calcium dysregulation, oxidative stress, and inflammatory that could ultimately result in tissue death. Oxidative stress is linked with a progressive increase in reactive oxygen species (ROS), and it affects the pathogenesis of cerebral ischemia/reperfusion (I/R) injury seriously [2–4]. Oxidative insult after I/R injury increases pathological alteration of lipids, proteins, and DNA, thereby damaging function of the cell, which lastly causes the cell death. Enhanced ROS production after reperfusion increases hemorrhagic infarction, brain edema, and infarction size. So the intervention of oxidative damage using safe and effective therapeutic agents with antioxidant properties provides an encouraging therapeutic strategy.

Phase 2 enzymes have been implicated to be the important means by which neurons protect themselves against intense oxidative stress. The expression of phase 2 enzymes, including heme oxygenase (HO)-1, is regulated by nuclear factor E2-related factor 2 (Nrf2) [5]. Considerable efforts have been made to develop effective strategies and drugs to relieve or prevent cerebral I/R injury. Extensive research has confirmed that Nrf2 activation during I/R is becoming a promising therapeutic target for neuroprotection [6, 7]. We also have recently indicated a key role of Nrf2 activation in prevention of ischemic cerebrovascular disease in our previous studies [8].

Neurotrophic factors are essential regulators in post-stroke recovery [9–11]. Both brain-derived neurotrophic factor (BDNF) and nerve growth factor (NGF) have been reported to be neuroprotective in the middle cerebral artery occlusion (MCAO) rat model of ischemia [12, 13]. Previous experimental studies have demonstrated that these neurotrophic factors confer neuroprotective effects as important candidates for prevention of oxidative stress and subsequent neurotoxicity [14, 15]. The expression levels of neurotrophic factors such as BDNF and NGF, which are causally related to oxidative stress, exert key effects in keeping the balance between oxidation and antioxidation mechanisms. Both BDNF and NGF are Nrf2-target genes [16]. In addition, it has been demonstrated that neurotrophins can activate Nrf2 [17–19]. So our choice of regulator molecules, BDNF and NGF, and the transcription factor, Nrf2, which participate in multiple steps of the active process of oxidative stress, is justified because dysfunction of any of these proteins causes a redox imbalance that leads to oxidative damage.

Uric acid (UA) is a major antioxidant in the blood in humans and is responsible for almost two-thirds of all free radical scavenging capacity with a concentration that surpasses other antioxidants by as much as tenfold in plasma [20]. Since UA has a wide variety of profound antioxidant properties, including quenching superoxide and hydroxyl and peroxynitrite radicals, and may have beneficial effects via reducing lipid peroxidation [21, 22]; it should have protective effects against ischemic brain damage. Actually, there are several animal experimental data in which the neuroprotective property of exogenous administration of uric acid is demonstrated [23–27]. Evidence has been presented that UA can exert much of its neuroprotective effect by astrocytic Nrf2/antioxidant response element (ARE) pathway activation indirectly causing increased levels of glutathione concentration [28], which implies that Nrf2 pathway may participate in the neuroprotection of UA. However, it remains unknown whether the Nrf2 pathway activation is involved in the UA-induced neuroprotection against the cerebral I/R injury via neuronal antioxidation approach and

whether neurotrophic factors are involved in the UA's neuroprotection against oxidative damage after stroke. Therefore, we employed the MCAO-induced focal cerebral I/R (FCI/R) rat model to test the hypothesis that UA protects against FCI/R-induced oxidative stress injury by activating Nrf2 pathway and targeting BDNF and NGF expression. Furthermore, this study may help understanding the relationship between Nrf2 signaling activation and the roles of BDNF and NGF in the pathogenesis of the ischemic brain in the neuroprotection induced by UA.

2. Materials and Methods

2.1. FCI/R Rat Model. Male Sprague–Dawley (SD) rats (280–300 g) from Pengyue Experimental Animal Breeding Institute of Jinan, China, were maintained in a room (23-24°C, 50-60% humidity) under 12 h light–dark cycle with free access to water and food. All experimental protocols were conducted according to ARRIVE (Animal Research: Reporting In Vivo Experiments) guidelines. Every effort was made to minimize animal suffering and the number of animals used. The Ethics Committee of Jining Medical University approved all the experimental protocols. All sample analysis was conducted under a strictly blinded manner. 193 rats were used, of which 11 died after transient FCI/R insult and 2 died after left lateral ventricle puncture, and consequently a total of 180 rats were separated randomly into 4 groups which included the sham group ($n = 45$), vehicle-treated I/R group ($n = 45$), 16 mg/kg UA-treated I/R group (UA group, $n = 45$), and UA plus brusatol-treated I/R group (UA + Bru, a specific inhibitor of Nrf2, $n = 45$).

The procedure for transient FCI/R has been described previously [29]. For MCAO, a 4-0 nylon thread with a rounded tip was inserted into the left external carotid artery (CA) and subsequently went into the internal CA approximately 20–21 mm from the carotid bifurcation. Then, the thread was withdrawn to initiate reperfusion after 2 h ischemia. The left CA was isolated with no thread inserted in the sham group. Rectal temperature was monitored and maintained between 37.0 and 37.5°C with a heating pad throughout surgery.

2.2. Drug Treatment and Experimental Design. UA diluted with Locke's buffer (vehicle) was injected intravenously through the tail vein (16 mg/kg) 30 min after reperfusion. An equal volume of vehicle was given to sham and model rats. Rats in the UA + Bru group were treated with UA plus brusatol. The dose of UA was chosen based on previous reports of UA treatment in rats induced by transient FCI/R [24–26]. Left lateral ventricle puncture (anteroposterior, −0.9 mm; lateral, 1.5 mm; depth, 3.6 mm; from bregma) was performed before MCAO. In the UA + Bru group, rats were infused intracerebroventricularly with Nrf2 inhibitor brusatol 30 min prior to ischemia (1 mg/kg, dissolved in 5 μl 1% DMSO) [30]. The other three groups also received equal volume vehicle injection after surgery. After animals underwent neurological evaluation at 24 h of reperfusion, their brains were harvested for the experiments described below.

2.3. Measurement of Cerebral Infarct Area. 2,3,5-Triphenyl-tetrazolium chloride (TTC) staining technique was employed to test the cerebral infarct volume. TTC stains the noninfarcted region with a deep red pigment, while the infarcted brain area appears white. Infarct volume was calculated with correction of edema in the ischemic hemisphere as previously described [29].

2.4. Evaluation of Neurological Deficits. A blinded observer evaluated the neurological status 24 h after FCI/R. A 5-point scale was used as follows [31, 32]: 0, no neurological deficits; 1, failure to fully extend the right forepaw; 2, decreased resistance to a lateral push toward the left side and failure to fully extend the right forepaw; 3, decreased resistance to a lateral push toward the left side, failure to fully extend the right forepaw, and circling to the left side; and 4, inability to walk spontaneously and lack of response to stimulation.

2.5. Determination of Brain Edema. The brains were carefully removed after decapitation. The wet weight was obtained immediately by weighing the ischemic hemispheres. The dry weight was obtained by weighing the samples dried at 60°C for 72 h. The percentage tissue water content was determined as previously described [8].

2.6. Histology and Immunochemistry Analysis. Rats were transcardially perfused with PBS and 4% paraformaldehyde 24 h after transient FCI/R ($n = 3$/group). The brain coronal sections from bregma at 0.3 to −1.8 mm were cut at 20 μm thickness. The sections were stained for hematoxylin and eosin (HE), terminal deoxynucleotidyl transferase- (TdT-) mediated dNTP nick end labeling (TUNEL), the expression of BDNF and NGF, and 8-hydroxy-deoxyguanosine (8-OHdG). Sections were incubated with primary antibody (anti-BDNF, Santa Cruz, USA; anti-NGF, Abcam Inc., Cambridge, MA; anti-8-OHdG, JaICa, Shizuoka, Japan) and then with the biotinylated secondary antibody. Negative controls performed the same staining procedure with the omission of primary antibody. HE staining was performed according to the standard procedure. TUNEL labeling assay kit (Roche Company, Switzerland) was used to measure DNA fragmentation. The number of HE-, TUNEL-, BDNF-, NGF-, and 8-OHdG-positive cells in the penumbra of ischemic ipsilateral parietal cortex in the ischemic area was quantified under a 400x magnification by a blinded investigator.

2.7. Western Blot. The ischemic side cerebral cortex (left side, $n = 4$/group) was dissected to extract total protein using a total protein extraction kit (Applygen Technologies Inc., Beijing). A nuclear-cytosol extraction kit (Applygen Technologies Inc., Beijing) was used to isolate the nuclear and cytosol fractions. We examined the expression levels of Nrf2 in the cytoplasm and nucleus and HO-1 in the cytoplasm. Each sample contained 50 μg protein. The primary antibodies were anti-HO-1 polyclonal antibody (Santa Cruz, USA) and anti-Nrf2 polyclonal antibody (Abcam Inc., Cambridge, MA). Each protein blot was normalized to histone H3 or β-actin to obtain the final result expressed as intensity ratio (% sham-operated control).

2.8. DNA-Binding Activity Assay of Nrf2. A commercially available Active Motif's (Carlsbad, CA, USA) ELISA-based TransAM® Nrf2 kit was used to analyze Nrf2 DNA-binding activity [8]. 10 μg nuclear protein was assayed per the manufacturer's protocol.

2.9. Determination of Protein Oxidation and Lipid Peroxidation. A commercial OxyBlot kit (#S7150; Millipore) was employed to determine the extent of protein oxidation [8]. The protein carbonyl content was used as an index for oxidative protein damage [33]. The cytoplasmic supernatant fluids of tissue samples were reacted with 2,4-dinitrophenyl-hydrazone (DNP) to get the DNP derivatized carbonyl groups. Then western blotting was used to test the DNP-derivatized protein with an anti-DNP antibody.

We analyzed total malondialdehyde (MDA) levels as the indicators of lipid peroxidation with the MDA detection kit (Nanjing Jiancheng, China) [8]. The absorption of the thiobarbituric acid (TBA) reactive substances which were produced by the reaction of TBA with MDA was measured at 532 nm to determine the extent of MDA. Results were presented as nmol/mg protein of wet tissue.

2.10. Statistical Analysis. Neurological deficits were analyzed using the Kruskal-Wallis test followed by Dunn's test, and results are expressed as median ± interquartile range. One-way analysis of variance (ANOVA) with subsequent Duncan's test as post hoc analysis was used for statistical analysis of all the other data, and results are reported as mean ± standard error (SE). A P value < 0.05 was considered to indicate statistical significance.

3. Results

3.1. UA Decreases Cerebral Infarct Size and Improves Neurological Functional Outcome. The infarct size induced by MCAO was determined using TTC staining (Figure 1(a)). No infarct tissue was detected in the sham group, while in the vehicle group, large volumes of infarct tissue were developed. Sections from rats treated with UA had significantly decreased infarct volumes (22.93% ± 3.04%) compared to the vehicle-treated I/R group (40.18% ± 2.30%, $P < 0.01$). In order to evaluate the role of Nrf2 pathway in UA-induced neuroprotection, the effect of brusatol on cerebral infarct volume was also detected. As observed in the UA + Bru group, a larger cerebral infarct volume was presented compared with the UA-treated I/R group (Figures 1(a) and 1(b)). Neurological deficit scores are presented in Figure 1(c). For vehicle-treated I/R animals, the median score was 3.25 (interquartile range (IQR): 2.88 to 3.50), indicative of severe neurological injury. When compared to the vehicle-treated I/R group, treatment with 16 mg/kg UA (median score: 2, IQR: 2 to 2.50) decreased the neurological deficit score significantly. The brain water content decreased significantly in UA-treated rats compared with model rats (83.0 + 1.8% vs. 88.5 + 1.5%, $P < 0.05$), whereas brusatol attenuated the decrease (87.7 + 1.6%, $P < 0.05$, Figure 1(d)).

3.2. UA Attenuated Neuronal Injury. HE staining was an effective way to evaluate neuronal cell death. In the sham

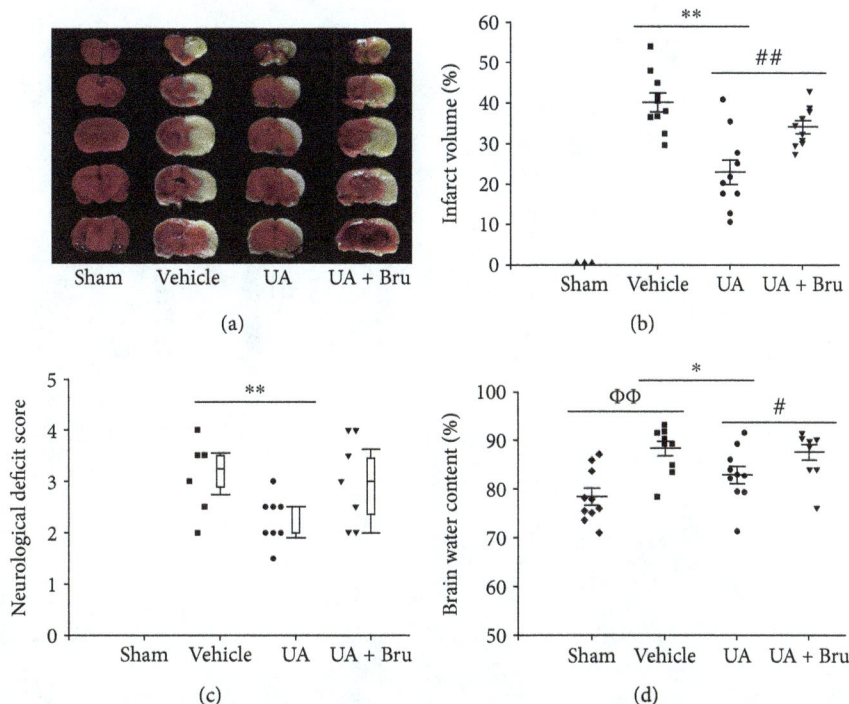

FIGURE 1: Effect of UA on the infarct volume, neurological deficit, and brain water content in rats. (a) Representative TTC-stained coronal sections. (b) Quantification of infarct volume; data are means ± SE ($n = 10$). (c) Neurological deficit scores; data are medians ± interquartile range ($n = 10$). Box plots show the interquartile range (25% to 75%) as the box, median as the horizontal line in the box, and the 95% range as the whiskers. (d) Brain water content; data are means ± SE ($n = 12$). $\Phi\Phi P < 0.01$ vs. the sham group; $^*P < 0.05$, $^{**}P < 0.01$ vs. the vehicle-treated I/R group; $^\#P < 0.05$, $^{\#\#}P < 0.01$ vs. the UA-treated I/R group.

group, no significant neuronal damage or neuronal loss was observed. A significant loss of neuronal cell was observed in model rats compared with sham rats (1150 ± 130 cells/mm^2 vs. 110 ± 23 cells/mm^2, $P < 0.01$). More intact cells in UA-treated rats were observed in comparison with model rats owing to the neuroprotection of UA (890 ± 120 cells/mm^2, $P < 0.01$, Figures 2(a) and 2(b)). Pretreatment with brusatol markedly abolished the protection of UA.

Apoptotic cells were identified by TUNEL staining. The apoptotic cell had round and shrunken shapes and the nuclei were darkly stained. Only few TUNEL-positive cells were observed in sham rats. TUNEL-positive cells increased significantly in model rats compared with sham rats (510 ± 80 cells/mm^2 vs. 60 ± 10 cells/mm^2, $P < 0.01$). TUNEL-positive cells were markedly reduced by UA administration (150 ± 29 cells/mm^2, $P < 0.01$). However, a marked increase of TUNEL-positive cells was observed in the UA + Bru group (390 ± 38 cells/mm^2, $P < 0.01$), suggesting brusatol pretreatment attenuated neuroprotection of UA (Figures 2(c) and 2(d)).

3.3. UA Alleviated Oxidative Injury.

We examined the role of UA in postischemic lipid peroxidation injury by determining the concentration of MDA in ischemic side cerebral cortex. The extent of MDA increased 1.2-fold compared with the sham group. With UA administration, the MDA levels significantly decreased compared with the model group.

However, the decrease was ablated by brusatol pretreatment (Figure 3(a)).

The extent of protein oxidation was measured by the levels of protein carbonylation. The protein carbonylation levels of the model rats significantly increased compared to those of the sham rats, while UA treatment decreased them compared with the model rats ($p < 0.01$, Figures 3(b) and 3(c)). The improving effect of UA on protein carbonylation levels was diminished in the ischemic cortex via pretreatment with brusatol.

Few 8-OHdG-positive cells were observed in sham rats, while a significant amount of 8-OHdG-positive cells was presented in the vehicle group (580 ± 120 cells/mm^2 vs. 240 ± 45 cells/mm^2, $P < 0.01$, Figures 3(d) and 3(e)). UA treatment significantly decreased the amount of 8-OHdG-positive cells. However, preadministration of brusatol significantly increased the levels of 8-OHdG immunoactivity compared with that in the UA-treated group (410 ± 67 cells/mm^2 vs. 240 ± 45 cells/mm^2, $p < 0.01$, Figures 3(d) and 3(e)).

3.4. UA Activated the Nrf2 Pathway.

To find out whether the Nrf2 pathway was involved in the neuroprotection of UA, we detected the expression levels of proteins related to Nrf2 pathway carefully in the cerebral cortices of variously treated animals in the presence of brusatol. UA treatment significantly increased Nrf2 levels in the nucleus, with a corresponding decrease in the cytoplasm, compared with the vehicle group. Further studies showed that cotreatment with

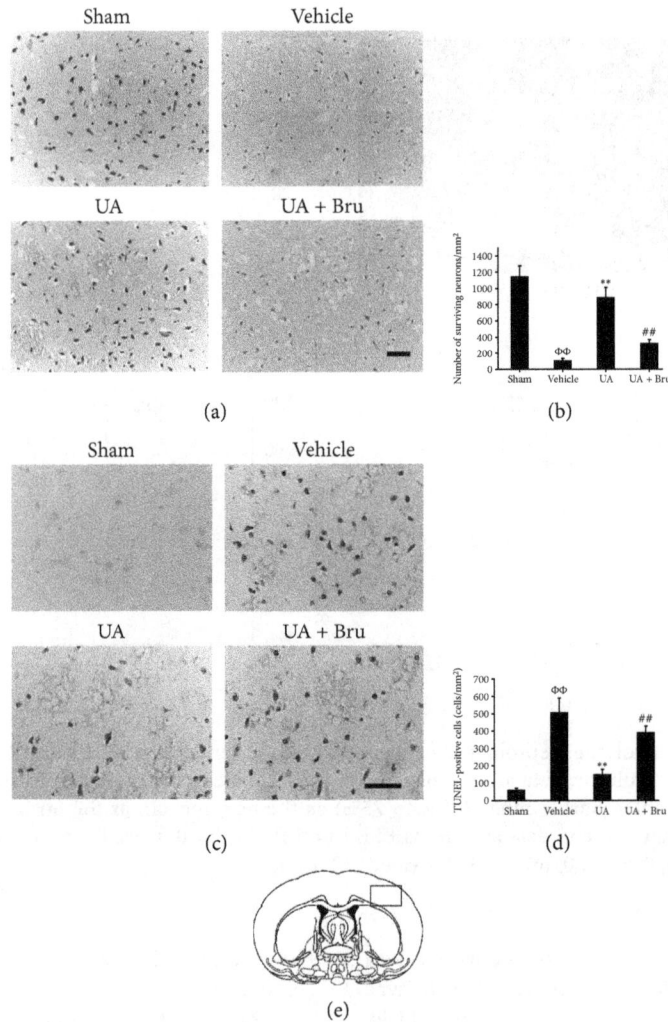

(a)

(b)

(c)

(d)

(e)

FIGURE 2: Effect of UA on neuronal injury in cerebral cortices in rats. (a) Representative photomicrographs of HE staining. Scale bar in all panels = 50 μm. (b) Quantification of surviving neuronal cells. (c) Representative photomicrographs of TUNEL staining. Scale bar in all panels = 50 μm. (d) Quantification of apoptotic cells. (e) Schematic diagram of coronal brain section. Black rectangle in the ischemic ipsilateral parietal cortex of penumbra represents the region selected for histology. Data are means ± SE ($n = 3$). $\Phi\Phi P < 0.01$ vs. the sham group; $^{**}P < 0.01$ vs. the vehicle-treated I/R group; $^{##}P < 0.01$ vs. the UA-treated I/R group.

UA and brusatol significantly attenuated the nuclear translocation of Nrf2 ($P < 0.05$ or $P < 0.01$, Figure 4).

We next examined whether the expression of HO-1 was induced by UA. HO-1 levels were obviously increased by UA treatment, as compared to the vehicle group, an effect that was reversed by pretreatment with brusatol ($P < 0.05$ or $P < 0.01$, Figures 4(c) and 4(e)).

Furthermore, DNA-binding activity of Nrf2 was also analyzed. UA treatment enhanced Nrf2 transcriptional activity; however, brusatol blocked the increased Nrf2 DNA-binding activity of UA significantly ($P < 0.01$, Figure 4(f)).

3.5. UA Upregulated Expression of BDNF and NGF in Ischemic Rat Brain. We examined whether UA had any effect on BDNF and NGF protein expressions using immunohistochemistry. The numbers of BDNF-immunopositive cells and NGF-immunopositive cells significantly decreased in vehicle animals; however, UA treatment successfully restored BDNF and NGF expressions, as indicated by an elevated number of BDNF-immunopositive cells and NGF-immunopositive cells ($P < 0.01$). In addition, cotreatment with UA and brusatol decreased BDNF and NGF expressions comparable to the UA-treated group ($P < 0.05$, Figure 5).

4. Discussion

In this study, where SD rats were exposed to FCI/R, we found that UA treatment (16 mg/kg, i.v.) decreased cerebral infarct volume, neurological deficit core, and degree of brain edema, consistent with the previous studies [23–25]. The neuroprotective properties of UA are related closely to the reduction of oxidative stress known to occur during cerebral I/R. The most novel finding of our study is that UA promoted nuclear translocation of Nrf2 and increased the expression of HO-1, as well as neurotrophic factors such as BDNF and NGF. Furthermore, the neuroprotective effects induced by UA were

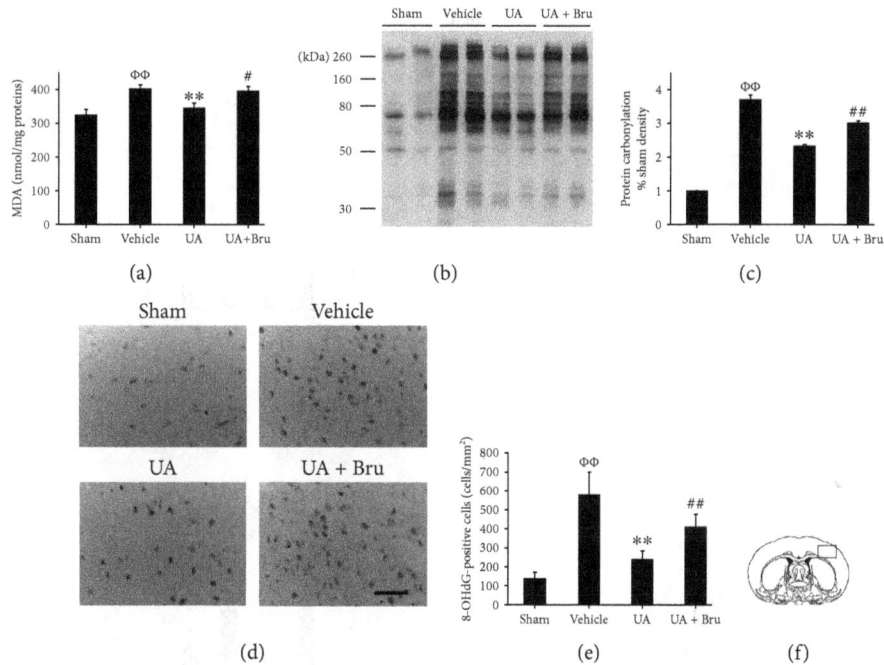

(a)   (b)   (c)

(d)   (e)   (f)

FIGURE 3: Effect of UA on oxidative injury in cerebral cortices in rats. (a) Quantification of MDA; data are means ± SE ($n = 12$). (b, c) Representative blot of protein oxidation. Quantification of carbonyl group bands; data are means ± SE ($n = 4$). (d) Representative photomicrographs of 8-OHdG immunostaining. Scale bar in all panels = 50 μm. (e) Quantification of 8-OHdG-positive cells; data are means ± SE ($n = 3$). (f) Schematic diagram of coronal brain section. The black rectangle in the ischemic ipsilateral parietal cortex of the penumbra represents the region selected for histology. $\Phi\Phi P < 0.01$ vs. the sham group; $^{**}P < 0.01$ vs. the vehicle-treated I/R group; $^{\#}P < 0.05$, $^{\#\#}P < 0.01$ vs. the UA-treated I/R group.

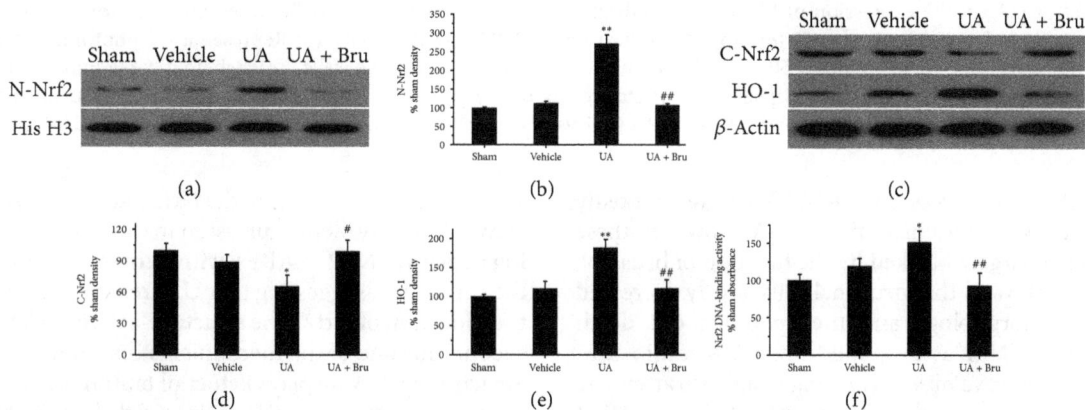

(a)   (b)   (c)

(d)   (e)   (f)

FIGURE 4: Effect of UA on Nrf2 protein distribution, HO-1 protein expression, and Nrf2 DNA-binding activity in cerebral cortices in rats. (a, b) Representative western blot of nuclear Nrf2. Quantification of nuclear Nrf2 normalized with histone H3. (c, d) Representative western blot of cytosolic Nrf2 and HO-1. Quantification of cytosolic Nrf2 and HO-1 normalized with β-actin. (e) Nuclear Nrf2 DNA-binding activity. Data are means ± SE ($n = 4$). $^{*}P < 0.05$, $^{**}P < 0.01$ vs. the vehicle-treated I/R group; $^{\#}P < 0.05$, $^{\#\#}P < 0.01$ vs. the UA-treated I/R group.

prevented by treatment with brusatol, an inhibitor of Nrf2. These results demonstrated that UA protected the brain from I/R injury potently and Nrf2 pathway activation as well as the upregulation of BDNF and NGF expression levels might be involved in this brain protection.

The cellular injury and downstream pathway activation caused by oxidative stress may exacerbate the postischemic brain damage [2]. MDA, protein carbonyls, and 8-OHdG, which are oxidized products of lipid, protein, and DNA,

respectively, are the major oxidative stress biomarkers. We observed a significant amount of MDA, protein carbonyls, and 8-OHdG in I/R rats. UA is a powerful natural antioxidant and radical scavenger that has cytoprotective effects against oxidative stress by scavenging ROS and suppressing lipid peroxidation in cultured hippocampal neurons after exposure to glutamate or cyanide [25]. In addition, UA protects the brain via reducing oxidative/nitrative stress following I/R in rats [24]. In the current study, the concentrations

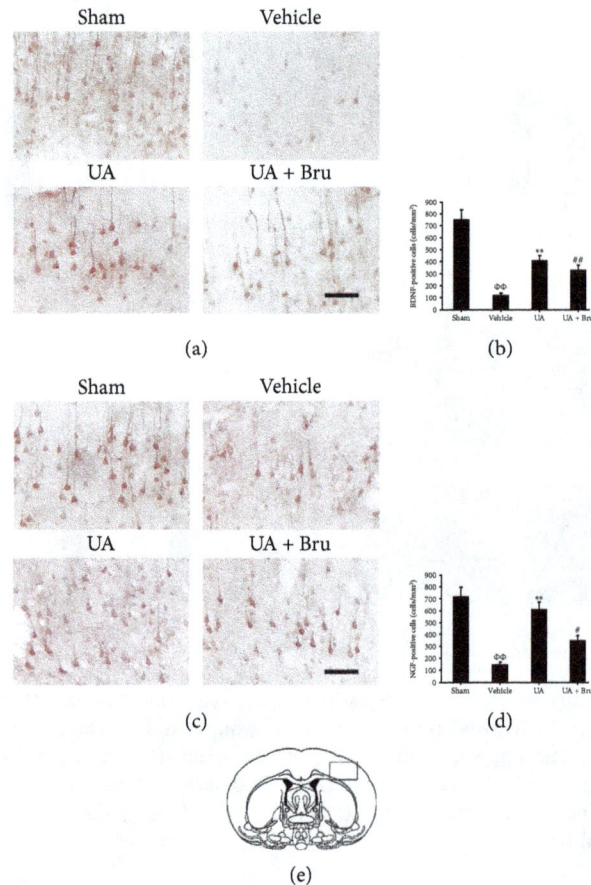

FIGURE 5: Effect of UA on the expression of BDNF and NGF in cerebral cortices in rats. (a) Representative photomicrographs of BDNF immunostaining. Scale bar in all panels = 50 μm. (b) Quantification of BDNF positive cells. (c) Representative photomicrographs of NGF immunostaining. Scale bar in all panels = 50 μm. (d) Quantification of NGF positive cells. (e) Schematic diagram of coronal brain section. The black rectangle in the ischemic ipsilateral parietal cortex of the penumbra represents the region selected for histology. Data are means ± SE ($n = 3$). $\Phi\Phi P < 0.01$ vs. the sham group; $^{**}P < 0.01$ vs. the vehicle-treated I/R group; $^{\#}P < 0.05$ vs. the UA-treated I/R group.

of MDA, protein carbonyls, and 8-OHDG were markedly decreased in rats with administration of UA. However, these changes could be largely blocked by the function of brusatol. Our results also showed that neuronal cells largely decreased with damaged morphology and the apoptotic cell death increased in the TUNEL assay in model rats. UA administration was able to improve histology changes and also attenuate TUNEL-positive cells. All these data support the view that UA treatment alleviates brain damage through reducing lipid, protein, and DNA peroxidation in cortical cells, subsequently reducing brain infarction.

Little is known about the mechanisms on how UA treatment protects neurons against oxidative stress. Evidences demonstrated that Nrf2 is a master regulator of the antioxidative defense responses [34]. Under basal conditions, Nrf2 largely localizes in the cytoplasm in an inactive form to maintain the expression of Nrf2-regulated genes in a low basal level. Under stressful conditions, Nrf2 translocates from the cytoplasm to the nucleus to bind ARE, which results in activation of transcription of multiple antioxidant and detoxifying genes [35, 36]. Our group and others have evidenced the Nrf2 pathway as therapeutic target of ischemic stroke [8, 37, 38]. Therefore, this study further detected

whether UA could activate the Nrf2 pathway. UA stimulation elevated Nrf2 protein expression in the nucleus and the binding activity of Nrf2 to AREs, with a corresponding decrease in the cytoplasm, suggesting that UA treatment induced nuclear translocation of Nrf2. The structure-activity relationship may account for one of the mechanisms that urate activates Nrf2. Structurally, UA displays ketoenol tautomeric forms and can react with cysteine residues in Kelch-like ECH-associated protein 1 (Keap1), which principally regulates the protein stability and transcriptional activity of Nrf2, through adduct formation and redox modifications as an electrophilic compound, triggering Nrf2 nuclear translocation. Simultaneously, UA promoted HO-1 expression. HO-1, which is regulated by Nrf2, has been recently considered to be important against ischemic brain injury [39]. It directly affects the antioxidative balance in the body, and it has antiapoptotic activities as well [40]. Importantly, the ability to promote Nrf2/HO-1 protein expression and Nrf2 nuclear translocation of UA was significantly blocked after preadministration of brusatol, suggesting that UA may regulate ARE-related gene expression through promoting Nrf2 activation to play antioxidative effects after FCI/R. In addition, brusatol treatment suppressed the antioxidative stress activities of UA and aggravated neuronal injury after FCI/R. These data strongly demonstrated that UA activated Nrf2 signaling pathway to perform its antioxidative and antiapoptotic activities as well as neuroprotective effects. However, while we have evidenced that the protein expression of HO-1 increased via UA treatment in this study, it is noteworthy that it does not implicate that HO-1 is the only factor involved in the protective effects of UA. An in vitro study proved that UA treatment increased mRNA levels of the modifier subunit of the γ-glutamyl cysteine ligase (GCL) and NAD(P)H:quinone oxidoreductase 1 (NQO1) and protein levels of GCLM in astrocyte cultures, whose inductions are governed by Nrf2, suggesting other antioxidants induced by Nrf2, may also contribute to the protective effects of UA [28]. Thus, the neuroprotective actions of UA may also be due to a wide spectrum of other Nrf2-regulated antioxidant genes potentially.

In addition, our study demonstrated that UA significantly increases the endogenous BDNF and NGF expressions. Several studies indicate that increased levels of neurotrophins have a protective role in experimental stroke studies [10]. The family of neurotrophins includes BDNF and NGF. Both animal and clinical studies have shown that BDNF has an effect to improve neurological recovery, prevent neuronal death, and support the survival of many types of neurons after cerebral ischemia [12, 13, 41]. NGF is also critical for neuronal survival, proliferation, and differentiation, and it has been reported that NGF is essential to improve neurological function after cerebral ischemia [12, 42]. By binding to tropomyosin receptor kinase (Trk) receptors, BDNF and NGF activate the downstream signaling pathways such as phosphatidylinositol 3-kinase (PI3K)/ protein kinase B (Akt) pathways and the mitogen-activated protein kinase (MAPK)/extracellular signal-regulated kinase (ERK) [43, 44]. Several lines of evidence reported that Nrf2 activation can be regulated via PI3K/Akt and MAPK/ERK pathways and thereby affects redox homeostasis [17, 19, 45–47]. Some studies suggested that BDNF can active antioxidant mechanisms constantly by inducing Nrf2 nuclear translocation [18]. Neurotrophic signaling pathway may be an upstream mechanism of the Nrf2 activation. Other studies have demonstrated that Nrf2 played a physiological role in the neuroprotective response to regulate BDNF and NGF expressions in a Nrf2-dependent manner which may confer neuroprotection by attenuating oxidative stress [48–50]. It is still difficult to propose the precise mechanisms that control Nrf2 translocation and how the Nrf2 antioxidant system talks to the neurotrophic signaling pathway. In the present study, the upregulation of BDNF and NGF expressions by UA was partially depressed by brusatol, suggesting that UA stimulates BDNF and NGF expressions through a Nrf2-mediated pathway. Although the precise mechanism of Nrf2-mediated induction of the BDNF and NGF expressions is still unclear, these findings implicate that augmenting the levels of neurotrophins via pharmacological strategies may be one of the factors contributing to the beneficial effects of UA, which may offer a powerful therapeutic target of oxidative damage. However, the exact events in the upregulation of neurotrophin expression by UA in the I/R rat brain need further exploration.

Our study has several limitations. First, it has been demonstrated that hyperemia at reperfusion can be a sign of worse I/R injury [51, 52]. Prior study has shown that the neuroprotective effect of UA is more marked in the rats that develop a hyperperfusion state after reperfusion [26]. However, the state of brain blood perfusion at early reperfusion was not detected in the current study. Second, sample sizes as 3-4 per group for immunochemistry and western blot detection methods are fairly small. The relatively small number of the samples often causes low statistical power, which is one of the factors related to low reproducibility of results from preclinical animal research. So sample sizes should be enlarged in the future investigation to validate our findings. And last, in the current study, 24 hours after transient FCI was chosen as the endpoint based on previous literature data as many studies reported neuroprotective effects of UA at this time point [23, 26]. The present study strengthens the concept that UA exhibits short-term antioxidant and neuroprotective effects. Further studies are essential to extend observation periods after transient FCI to detect the longer therapeutic effect of UA.

5. Conclusions

For the first time, this study demonstrates that UA confers neuroprotection against FCI/R-induced oxidative stress via Nrf2 pathway activation as well as BDNF and NGF expression upregulation. The protective effect of UA was blocked by Nrf2 inhibitor brusatol. Nonetheless, further study deserves to be done in the future to investigate whether other pathways or mechanisms participated in the neuroprotective effects of UA.

Authors' Contributions

Bai-liu Ya and Qian Liu contributed equally to this work.

Acknowledgments

This work was supported by the National Natural Science Foundation of China (nos. 81703490 and 81870948), the Natural Science Foundation of Shandong Province (nos. ZR2015HQ019 and ZR2017HQ056), the National Undergraduates Innovation Training Program (no. 201610443001), the Undergraduates Innovation Training Program and the Undergraduates Scientific Research Programs of Jining Medical University (nos. cx2016001, cx2017029, 2015, JYXS2017KJ011), the Jining Science and Technology Boost New Energy Conversion Plan (no. 2017SMNS004), the Teacher Scientific Research Support Fund of Jining Medical University (JY2017KJ021), and the International Cooperation Training Program of Outstanding Young Teachers of Shandong Province (2013).

References

[1] M. A. Moskowitz, E. H. Lo, and C. Iadecola, "The science of stroke: mechanisms in search of treatments," *Neuron*, vol. 67, no. 2, pp. 181–198, 2010.

[2] H. Chen, H. Yoshioka, G. S. Kim et al., "Oxidative stress in ischemic brain damage: mechanisms of cell death and potential molecular targets for neuroprotection," *Antioxidants & Redox Signaling*, vol. 14, no. 8, pp. 1505–1517, 2011.

[3] A. Janyou, P. Wicha, J. Jittiwat, A. Suksamrarn, C. Tocharus, and J. Tocharus, "Dihydrocapsaicin attenuates blood brain barrier and cerebral damage in focal cerebral ischemia/reperfusion via oxidative stress and inflammatory," *Scientific Reports*, vol. 7, no. 1, article 10556, 2017.

[4] S. Pundik, K. Xu, and S. Sundararajan, "Reperfusion brain injury: focus on cellular bioenergetics," *Neurology*, vol. 79, 13, Supplement 1, pp. S44–S51, 2012.

[5] T. Suzuki and M. Yamamoto, "Molecular basis of the Keap1-Nrf2 system," *Free Radical Biology & Medicine*, vol. 88, Part B, pp. 93–100, 2015.

[6] R. Zhang, M. Xu, Y. Wang, F. Xie, G. Zhang, and X. Qin, "Nrf2—a promising therapeutic target for defensing against oxidative stress in stroke," *Molecular Neurobiology*, vol. 54, no. 8, pp. 6006–6017, 2017.

[7] Y. Ding, M. Chen, M. Wang, Y. Li, and A. Wen, "Posttreatment with 11-keto-β-boswellic acid ameliorates cerebral ischemia–reperfusion injury: Nrf2/HO-1 pathway as a potential mechanism," *Molecular Neurobiology*, vol. 52, no. 3, pp. 1430–1439, 2015.

[8] B. Ya, H. Li, H. Wang et al., "5-HMF attenuates striatum oxidative damage via Nrf2/ARE signaling pathway following transient global cerebral ischemia," *Cell Stress and Chaperones*, vol. 22, no. 1, pp. 55–65, 2017.

[9] S. Otsuka, H. Sakakima, M. Sumizono, S. Takada, T. Terashi, and Y. Yoshida, "The neuroprotective effects of preconditioning exercise on brain damage and neurotrophic factors after focal brain ischemia in rats," *Behavioural Brain Research*, vol. 303, pp. 9–18, 2016.

[10] S. Lanfranconi, F. Locatelli, S. Corti et al., "Growth factors in ischemic stroke," *Journal of Cellular and Molecular Medicine*, vol. 15, no. 8, pp. 1645–1687, 2011.

[11] E. J. Huang and L. F. Reichardt, "Trk receptors: roles in neuronal signal transduction," *Annual Review of Biochemistry*, vol. 72, no. 1, pp. 609–642, 2003.

[12] Z. Kokaia, Q. Zhao, M. Kokaia et al., "Regulation of brain-derived neurotrophic factor gene expression after transient middle cerebral artery occlusion with and without brain damage," *Experimental Neurology*, vol. 136, no. 1, pp. 73–88, 1995.

[13] W. R. Schabitz, S. Schwab, M. Spranger, and W. Hacke, "Intraventricular brain-derived neurotrophic factor reduces infarct size after focal cerebral ischemia in rats," *Journal of Cerebral Blood Flow & Metabolism*, vol. 17, no. 5, pp. 500–506, 1997.

[14] M. P. Mattson, M. A. Lovell, K. Furukawa, and W. R. Markesbery, "Neurotrophic factors attenuate glutamate-induced accumulation of peroxides, elevation of intracellular Ca^{2+} concentration, and neurotoxicity and increase antioxidant enzyme activities in hippocampal neurons," *Journal of Neurochemistry*, vol. 65, no. 4, pp. 1740–1751, 1995.

[15] X. Y. Mao, H. H. Zhou, X. Li, and Z. Q. Liu, "Huperzine a alleviates oxidative glutamate toxicity in hippocampal HT22 cells via activating BDNF/TrkB-dependent PI3K/Akt/mTOR signaling pathway," *Cellular and Molecular Neurobiology*, vol. 36, no. 6, pp. 915–925, 2016.

[16] K. U. Tufekci, E. Civi Bayin, S. Genc, and K. Genc, "The Nrf2/ARE pathway: a promising target to counteract mitochondrial dysfunction in Parkinson's disease," *Parkinson's Disease*, vol. 2011, article 314082, 14 pages, 2011.

[17] T. Ishii, E. Warabi, and G. E. Mann, "Circadian control of BDNF-mediated Nrf2 activation in astrocytes protects dopaminergic neurons from ferroptosis," *Free Radical Biology & Medicine*, 2018.

[18] E. Bouvier, F. Brouillard, J. Molet et al., "Nrf2-dependent persistent oxidative stress results in stress-induced vulnerability to depression," *Molecular Psychiatry*, vol. 22, no. 12, p. 1795, 2017.

[19] O. Firuzi, F. Moosavi, R. Hosseini, and L. Saso, "Modulation of neurotrophic signaling pathways by polyphenols," *Drug Design, Development and Therapy*, vol. 10, pp. 23–42, 2015.

[20] B. F. Becker, "Towards the physiological function of uric acid," *Free Radical Biology and Medicine*, vol. 14, no. 6, pp. 615–631, 1993.

[21] G. L. Squadrito, R. Cueto, A. E. Splenser et al., "Reaction of uric acid with peroxynitrite and implications for the mechanism of neuroprotection by uric acid," *Archives of Biochemistry and Biophysics*, vol. 376, no. 2, pp. 333–337, 2000.

[22] G. R. Buettner, "The pecking order of free radicals and antioxidants: lipid peroxidation, α-tocopherol, and ascorbate," *Archives of Biochemistry and Biophysics*, vol. 300, no. 2, pp. 535–543, 1993.

[23] Y. H. Ma, N. Su, X. D. Chao et al., "Thioredoxin-1 attenuates post-ischemic neuronal apoptosis via reducing oxidative/nitrative stress," *Neurochemistry International*, vol. 60, no. 5, pp. 475–483, 2012.

[24] E. Romanos, A. M. Planas, S. Amaro, and A. Chamorro, "Uric acid reduces brain damage and improves the benefits of rt-PA in a rat model of thromboembolic stroke," *Journal of Cerebral Blood Flow & Metabolism*, vol. 27, no. 1, pp. 14–20, 2007.

[25] Z. F. Yu, A. J. Bruce-Keller, Y. Goodman, and M. P. Mattson, "Uric acid protects neurons against excitotoxic and metabolic insults in cell culture, and against focal ischemic brain injury in vivo," *Journal of Neuroscience Research*, vol. 53, no. 5, pp. 613–625, 1998.

[26] Y. Onetti, A. P. Dantas, B. Perez et al., "Middle cerebral artery remodeling following transient brain ischemia is linked to early postischemic hyperemia: a target of uric acid treatment," *American Journal of Physiology-Heart and Circulatory Physiology*, vol. 308, no. 8, pp. H862–H874, 2015.

[27] C. Justicia, A. Salas-Perdomo, I. Pérez-de-Puig et al., "Uric acid is protective after cerebral ischemia/reperfusion in hyperglycemic mice," *Translational Stroke Research*, vol. 8, no. 3, pp. 294–305, 2017.

[28] R. Bakshi, H. Zhang, R. Logan et al., "Neuroprotective effects of urate are mediated by augmenting astrocytic glutathione synthesis and release," *Neurobiology of Disease*, vol. 82, pp. 574–579, 2015.

[29] B. Ya, C. Li, L. Zhang, W. Wang, and L. Li, "Cornel iridoid glycoside inhibits inflammation and apoptosis in brains of rats with focal cerebral ischemia," *Neurochemical Research*, vol. 35, no. 5, pp. 773–781, 2010.

[30] B. Chen, H. Cao, L. Chen et al., "Rifampicin attenuated global cerebral ischemia injury via activating the nuclear factor

erythroid 2-related factor pathway," *Frontiers in Cellular Neuroscience*, vol. 10, p. 273, 2016.

[31] L. Belayev, O. F. Alonso, R. Busto, W. Zhao, and M. D. Ginsberg, "Middle cerebral artery occlusion in the rat by intraluminal suture. Neurological and pathological evaluation of an improved model," *Stroke*, vol. 27, no. 9, pp. 1616–1623, 1996, discussion 1623.

[32] T. Mokudai, I. A. Ayoub, Y. Sakakibara, E. J. Lee, C. S. Ogilvy, and K. I. Maynard, "Delayed treatment with nicotinamide (vitamin B₃) improves neurological outcome and reduces infarct volume after transient focal cerebral ischemia in Wistar rats," *Stroke*, vol. 31, no. 7, pp. 1679–1685, 2000.

[33] K. A. Conlon, D. O. Zharkov, and M. Berrios, "Immunofluorescent localization of the murine 8-oxoguanine DNA glycosylase (mOGG1) in cells growing under normal and nutrient deprivation conditions," *DNA Repair*, vol. 2, no. 12, pp. 1337–1352, 2003.

[34] J. W. Thompson, S. V. Narayanan, K. B. Koronowski, K. Morris-Blanco, K. R. Dave, and M. A. Perez-Pinzon, "Signaling pathways leading to ischemic mitochondrial neuroprotection," *Journal of Bioenergetics and Biomembranes*, vol. 47, no. 1-2, pp. 101–110, 2015.

[35] K. M. Kanninen, Y. Pomeshchik, H. Leinonen, T. Malm, J. Koistinaho, and A. L. Levonen, "Applications of the Keap1-Nrf2 system for gene and cell therapy," *Free Radical Biology & Medicine*, vol. 88, Part B, pp. 350–361, 2015.

[36] V. P. Nakka, P. Prakash-Babu, and R. Vemuganti, "Crosstalk between endoplasmic reticulum stress, oxidative stress, and autophagy: potential therapeutic targets for acute CNS injuries," *Molecular Neurobiology*, vol. 53, no. 1, pp. 532–544, 2016.

[37] Z. A. Shah, R. C. Li, A. S. Ahmad et al., "The flavanol (−)-epicatechin prevents stroke damage through the Nrf2/HO1 pathway," *Journal of Cerebral Blood Flow & Metabolism*, vol. 30, no. 12, pp. 1951–1961, 2010.

[38] A. Alfieri, S. Srivastava, R. C. M. Siow et al., "Sulforaphane preconditioning of the Nrf2/HO-1 defense pathway protects the cerebral vasculature against blood-brain barrier disruption and neurological deficits in stroke," *Free Radical Biology & Medicine*, vol. 65, pp. 1012–1022, 2013.

[39] Y. M. Kim, H. O. Pae, J. E. Park et al., "Heme oxygenase in the regulation of vascular biology: from molecular mechanisms to therapeutic opportunities," *Antioxidants & Redox Signaling*, vol. 14, no. 1, pp. 137–167, 2011.

[40] X. Fan and L. Mu, "The role of heme oxygenase-1 (HO-1) in the regulation of inflammatory reaction, neuronal cell proliferation and apoptosis in rats after intracerebral hemorrhage (ICH)," *Neuropsychiatric Disease and Treatment*, vol. 13, pp. 77–85, 2017.

[41] M. Ploughman, V. Windle, C. L. MacLellan, N. White, J. J. Dore, and D. Corbett, "Brain-derived neurotrophic factor contributes to recovery of skilled reaching after focal ischemia in rats," *Stroke*, vol. 40, no. 4, pp. 1490–1495, 2009.

[42] D. M. Holtzman, R. A. Sheldon, W. Jaffe, Y. Cheng, and D. M. Ferriero, "Nerve growth factor protects the neonatal brain against hypoxic-ischemic injury," *Annals of Neurology*, vol. 39, no. 1, pp. 114–122, 1996.

[43] A. Brunet, S. R. Datta, and M. E. Greenberg, "Transcription-dependent and -independent control of neuronal survival by the PI3K–Akt signaling pathway," *Current Opinion in Neurobiology*, vol. 11, no. 3, pp. 297–305, 2001.

[44] A. Bonni, A. Brunet, A. E. West, S. R. Datta, M. A. Takasu, and M. E. Greenberg, "Cell survival promoted by the Ras-MAPK signaling pathway by transcription-dependent and -independent mechanisms," *Science*, vol. 286, no. 5443, pp. 1358–1362, 1999.

[45] T. Chen, Y. Wu, Y. Wang et al., "Brain-derived neurotrophic factor increases synaptic protein levels via the MAPK/Erk signaling pathway and Nrf2/Trx Axis following the transplantation of neural stem cells in a rat model of traumatic brain injury," *Neurochemical Research*, vol. 42, no. 11, pp. 3073–3083, 2017.

[46] M. Chen, L. H. Dai, A. Fei, S. M. Pan, and H. R. Wang, "Isoquercetin activates the ERK1/2-Nrf2 pathway and protects against cerebral ischemia-reperfusion injury in vivo and in vitro," *Experimental and Therapeutic Medicine*, vol. 13, no. 4, pp. 1353–1359, 2017.

[47] B. Li, J. Sun, G. Lv et al., "Sevoflurane postconditioning attenuates cerebral ischemia-reperfusion injury via protein kinase B/nuclear factor-erythroid 2-related factor 2 pathway activation," *International Journal of Developmental Neuroscience*, vol. 38, pp. 79–86, 2014.

[48] J. Mimura, K. Kosaka, A. Maruyama et al., "Nrf2 regulates NGF mRNA induction by carnosic acid in T98G glioblastoma cells and normal human astrocytes," *The Journal of Biochemistry*, vol. 150, no. 2, pp. 209–217, 2011.

[49] Y. Y. Hsu, Y. T. Tseng, and Y. C. Lo, "Berberine, a natural antidiabetes drug, attenuates glucose neurotoxicity and promotes Nrf2-related neurite outgrowth," *Toxicology and Applied Pharmacology*, vol. 272, no. 3, pp. 787–796, 2013.

[50] A. Shi, J. Xiang, F. He et al., "The phenolic components of *Gastrodia elata* improve prognosis in rats after cerebral ischemia/reperfusion by enhancing the endogenous antioxidant mechanisms," *Oxidative Medicine and Cellular Longevity*, vol. 2018, Article ID 7642158, 16 pages, 2018.

[51] F. J. Pérez-Asensio, X. de la Rosa, F. Jiménez-Altayó et al., "Antioxidant CR-6 protects against reperfusion injury after a transient episode of focal brain ischemia in rats," *Journal of Cerebral Blood Flow & Metabolism*, vol. 30, no. 3, pp. 638–652, 2010.

[52] A. Tamura, T. Asano, and K. Sano, "Correlation between rCBF and histological changes following temporary middle cerebral artery occlusion," *Stroke*, vol. 11, no. 5, pp. 487–493, 1980.

15

Protective Effect of JXT Ethanol Extract on Radiation-Induced Hematopoietic Alteration and Oxidative Stress in the Liver

Xian-Zhe Dong,[1] Yu-Ning Wang,[2] Xiao Tan,[1] Ping Liu,[1] Dai-Hong Guo ⓘ,[1] and Can Yan ⓘ[3,4]

[1]*Center of Drug Security, General Hospital of Chinese PLA, Beijing 100853, China*
[2]*Department of Surgery, Chinese PLA General Hospital, Beijing 100853, China*
[3]*Department of Basic Theory of Chinese Medicine, School of Pre-Clinical Medicine, Guangzhou University of Chinese Medicine, Guangzhou 510060, China*
[4]*The Research Centre of Basic Integrative Medicine, Guangzhou University of Chinese Medicine, Guangzhou 510060, China*

Correspondence should be addressed to Dai-Hong Guo; guodh301@163.com and Can Yan; yancan999@sina.com

Academic Editor: Alexandros Georgakilas

This study aims at investigating the radioprotective effect of ethanol extract from Ji-Xue-Teng (JXT, *Spatholobus suberectus*) on radiation-induced hematopoietic alteration and oxidative stress in the liver. Mice were exposed to a single acute γ-radiation for the whole body at the dose of 6.0 Gy, then subjected to administration of amifostine (45 mg/kg) or JXT (40 g crude drug/kg) once a day for 28 consecutive days, respectively. Bone marrow cells and hemogram including white cells, red cells, platelet counts, and hemoglobin level were examined. The protein expression levels of pJAK2/JAK2, pSTAT5a/STAT5a, pSTAT5b/ STAT5b, and Bcl-2 in bone marrow tissue; levels of reactive oxygen species (ROS); and the activity of superoxide dismutase (SOD), malondialdehyde (MDA), and glutathione peroxidase (GSH-Px) in serum and liver tissue were determined. At the end of the experiment, the effect of JXT on cell viability and G-CSF and G-CSFR levels in NFS-60 cells were tested by CCK-8 assay, ELISA, and flow cytometry. The results showed that the mice exposed to γ-radiation alone exhibited a typical hematopoietic syndrome. In contrast, at the end of the 28-day experiment, irradiated mice subjected to oral administration of JXT showed an obvious improvement on blood profile with reduced leucopenia, thrombocytopenia (platelet counts), RBC, and hemoglobin levels, as well as bone marrow cells. The expression of pJAK2/JAK2, pSTAT5a/STAT5a, and Bcl-2 in bone marrow tissue was increased after JXT treatment. The elevation of ROS was due to radiation-induced toxicity, but JXT significantly reduced the ROS level in serum and liver tissue, elevated endogenous SOD and GSH-PX levels, and reduced the MDA level in the liver. JXT could also increase cell viability and G-CSFR level in NFS-60 cells, which was similar to exogenous G-CSF. Our findings suggested that oral administration of JXT effectively facilitated the recovery of hematopoietic bone marrow damage and oxidative stress of the mice induced by γ-radiation.

1. Introduction

Radiotherapy is widely used in cancer treatment. Although irradiation is targeted at malignant tissues, the surrounding normal tissues or organs are also affected [1–3]. Whole-body radiation may result in acute radiation syndrome with profound pathophysiological consequences characterized as severe suppressed hematopoiesis, gastrointestinal injury, cerebrovascular system, and neurological damage [4–7]. The

hematopoietic system is exceedingly sensitive to ionizing radiation, with an associated decrease in bone marrow cells (BMC) and circulating peripheral blood cells that may further cause anemia, bleeding, infection, and declined immune function [8, 9]. According to previous reports, oxidative damage to DNA can be a result from radiation-induced free radicals or ROS [10]. The ionizing radiation at a relatively high level can lead to changed gene expression pattern and mutation prevalence and blunt the repairing mechanisms of DNA damage [11, 12]. The development of efficacious radioprotectors to accelerate hematopoiesis recovery should be a valuable contribution to radiation oncology.

As a consequence, it is essential to search radioprotectors to control side effects in both planned exposure such as radiotherapy and unplanned exposure such as natural radiation [13]. Although synthetic compounds including thiols, baminothiols, thiadiazoles, or benzothiazoles reveal certain radioprotective effects, their side effects have also gained extensive attention [14]. Amifostine is the only agent approved so far by the Food and Drug Administration for treating radiation syndrome [15]. However, amifostine gives rise to significant adverse reactions in many cases; for example, a phase III clinical trial has found its adverse reactions in 41% of head and neck cancer patients, with symptoms including hypotension, hypocalcemia, nausea, vomiting, and allergy [16]. Therefore, it is a promising strategy to develop natural radioprotectors from plants and herbs [17, 18]. Herb-derived phytochemicals offer opportunities to develop efficacious radioprotective agents due to low toxicity and few side effects [19–21]. Recently, natural compounds such as genistein or ginsan from plant extracts have been extensively explored to have strong capacity to alleviate radiation-induced damage [2, 22].

Ji-Xue-Teng (JXT) is a traditional herb from the dry rattan of *Spatholobus suberectus* (*S. suberectus*) Dunn, recorded in Gang Mu Shi Yi as a holy drug of the blood, which can remove blood clot and produce fresh blood. Modern pharmacological researches have documented that JXT and its active components are widely used for improving blood circulation and executing anti-inflammation, antibacterial, neuroprotective, antioxidative, and anticancer effects [23–25]. According to our previous report, the bioactive components of JXT can promote the proliferation of hematopoietic progenitor cells (HPC) in bone marrow-depressed mice [26], but the impact and underlying molecule mechanism of JXT on irradiation-induced hematological toxicity and other organ injury are still unclear. In the present study, the effect of JXT on 6.0 Gy γ-radiation-induced myelosuppression and oxidative damage of the liver tissues in mice and the underlying hematopoietic mechanisms were explored.

2. Materials and Methods

2.1. Chemicals. JXT was purchased from Beijing Lvye Pharmaceutical Co. Ltd. (Beijing, China), Fujian (China) origin. JXT was cut into small pieces and soaked in 75% ethanol at 8 times volume overnight and then extracted 3 times with 1 h for each time. Finally, the filtrates were mixed and concentrated by a rotary evaporator with bath temperature lower than 40°C. Ethanol extract was lyophilized to powder.

The reagents and kits for determining enzyme activity were purchased from Nanjing Jiancheng Bioengineering Institute (NJBI, Nanjing, China). The antibodies for evaluating G-CSFR, Bcl-2, JAK2, pJAK2, STAT5a, pSTAT5a, STAT5b and pSTAT5b were purchased from Abcam (Abcam, USA). Amifostine was purchased from Dalian Merro Pharmaceutical Factory (Dalian, China); RPMI-1640

culture medium and fetal bovine serum (FBS) were purchased from HyClone (HyClone, USA). G-CSF ELISA kit was purchased from Shanghai Tongwei Biotech Co. Ltd. (Shanghai, China).

2.2. Animals. A total of 40 Chinese Kun Ming (KM) mice with the age of 6–8 weeks and inbred colony were purchased from the Laboratory Animal Breeding and Research Center in PLA General Hospital, Beijing, China, and maintained under controlled conditions of temperature ($23 \pm 2°C$) and light (12L : 12D). All mice were provided with standard chow diet and water ad libitum.

2.3. Irradiation and Administrations. Gamma radiation (γ-radiation) at the dose of 6 Gy was delivered in the Department of Radiotherapy and Oncology, the Military Medical Academy of Science. The mice were randomly divided into 4 groups including nonirradiation control, irradiation control, positive treatment control, and JXT treatment groups with 10 mice in each group. The mice from the positive treatment control group were administrated with amifostine at 43.6 mg/kg by tail vein injection [27], and the mice from the JXT treatment group were orally administrated with JXT ethanol extract at the dose of 40 g/kg based on the amount of crude drug. JXT was dissolved in sterile saline and orally administrated for 21 consecutive days after mouse irradiation.

2.4. Hematological Analysis. The effect of JXT extract on the peripheral blood of mice from each experiment group was analyzed. On day 21 after irradiation, hemoglobin (HGB) level, erythrocyte (RBC) count, total leukocyte (WBC) count, and platelet (PLT) count for each mouse were measured at 0 day (before irradiation) and 21 days postirradiation using an automated hematology analyzer (BC-2800vet; Mindray, China).

2.5. Antioxidant Activity. The ROS level in the serum and ROS, SOD, GSH-Px, and MDA levels in the liver tissue were analyzed, respectively, according to the instructions of the kits from the manufacturer.

2.6. Bone Marrow Cell Counting. Bone marrow cells were collected from both femurs of each mouse at day 10 after whole-body radiation at the dose of 6 Gy. The collected bone marrow cells were rinsed with PBS, and single-cell suspension was obtained. After the lysis of red blood cells, the bone marrow cells were suspended in RPMI-1640 with 10% fetal bovine serum (FBS) and 100 U/ml antibiotics. Then, the bone marrow cells were counted in a hemacytometer under an optical microscope to determine whether JXT extract can protect the bone marrow cells from the depletion induced by γ-radiation.

2.7. Western Blot. The preparation of bone marrow cells was the same as above. For western blot analysis, total protein was extracted first, and cells were washed twice with cold PBS and lysed in the radioimmunoprecipitation assay (RIPA) buffer (20 mM Tris-HCl, pH 7.5; 150 mM sodium chloride; 1% Triton; 1 mM EGTA; 1 mM EDTA; 2.5 mM sodium

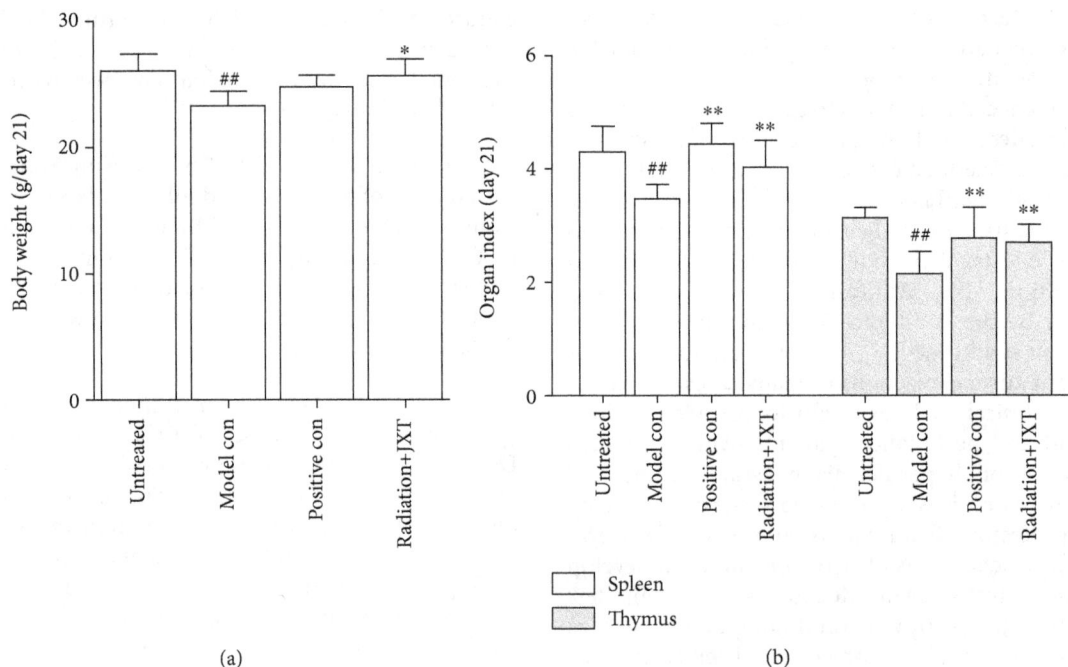

(a)   (b)

FIGURE 1: Effect of JXT on body weights of Co^{60}-irradiated mice. All data were expressed as mean $\pm$ SEM ($n = 10$). $^{\#}P < 0.05$; $^{\#\#}P < 0.01$ when compared with the untreated control group. $^{*}P < 0.05$; $^{**}P < 0.01$ when compared with the Co^{60}-irradiated group. (a) Body weight; (b) organ index.

pyrophosphate; 1 mM β-glycerophosphate; 1 mM sodium orthovanadate; 1 μg/ml leupeptin; and 1 mM PMSF) for 20 min on the ice. After centrifugation at 12000$\times g$ for 10 min, protein was then quantitated by using a bicinchoninic acid protein assay kit (Bioworld Technology, USA). After being heated at 95°C for 8 min, the samples were loaded on 12% SDS-polyacrylamide gel for electrophoresis and transferred to PVDF membrane (Millipore, Billerica, MA). The membrane was blocked for 2.5 h in TBS-T buffer (10 mM Tris, pH 8.0, 150 mM NaCl, and 0.1% Tween-20) containing 3% (w/v) bovine serum albumin (BSA; Sigma-Aldrich, USA) at room temperature and then probed with each primary antibody (1 : 500 dilution) at 4°C overnight. After washing with TBS-T for three times, the membrane was then incubated with appropriate horseradish peroxidase-labeled secondary antibody for 2 h at room temperature. For quantitative analysis of immunoblot bands, the densities of the bands were measured by scanning densitometry (Bio-Rad, Hercules, CA). All experiments were repeated at least three times.

2.8. Cell Culture.
NFS-60 cell line, derived from murine myeloid leukemia, is responsive to different growth factors including G-CSF. Cells were maintained in RPMI 1640 medium supplemented with 10% FBS, 50 U/ml penicillin, 50 μg/ml streptomycin, and 15 ng/ml G-CFS (Sigma, USA).

2.9. Cell Viability Detection by CCK-8 Assay.
NFS-60 cell viability after JXT treatment was evaluated with CCK-8 assay. Cells (3000 cells/well) were plated in 96-well plates. After 24 h culture, JXT at different final concentrations (1.6, 8, 40, and 200 g/ml) was added into the plates and detected after

24 h culture. Briefly, 20 μl of CCK-8 solution was added to the culture medium and incubated at 37°C for 4 h. Then, the OD was spectrophotometrically measured at 450 nm using a microplate spectrophotometer (1420 Victor^3, Perkin-Elmer, USA). Viability was expressed as the percentage of vehicle-treated (basal) culture that was set to 100%.

2.10. Enzyme-Linked Immunosorbent Assay.
Culture media were collected following treatments and promptly stored at -80°C until the future assay. The G-CSF level was measured using commercially available paired antibody quantitative ELISA kit according to the manufacturer's instructions. Data were expressed as 10^{-6} μg/ml. Dispensed antigen standards and samples were added to each well of 96-well plates precoated with primary antibodies. After adding biotin conjugate reagent and enzyme conjugate reagent into each well, the plates were incubated at 37°C for 30 min. Then, the plates were rinsed with distilled water for 5 times and measured using a microtiter plate reader (Perkin-Elmer, USA).

2.11. Flow Cytometric Detection of G-CSFR.
The G-CSFR level in cells was measured using flow cytometry. A total of 5×10^6 NFS-60 cells were plated in 6-well plates for each well. After treatment with JXT at different final concentrations (1.6, 8, 40, and 200 μg/ml) for 24 h, the cells were harvested and washed in PBS and then centrifuged at 1000$\times g$ for 5 min. The cell pellet was resuspended at the density of 5×10^6 cells/ml and incubated with G-CSFR antibody for 30 min at 37°C. Then, the cells were washed in PBS and incubated with IgG secondary antibody for 30 min at 37°C. The cells were then analyzed in a Becton Dickinson flow

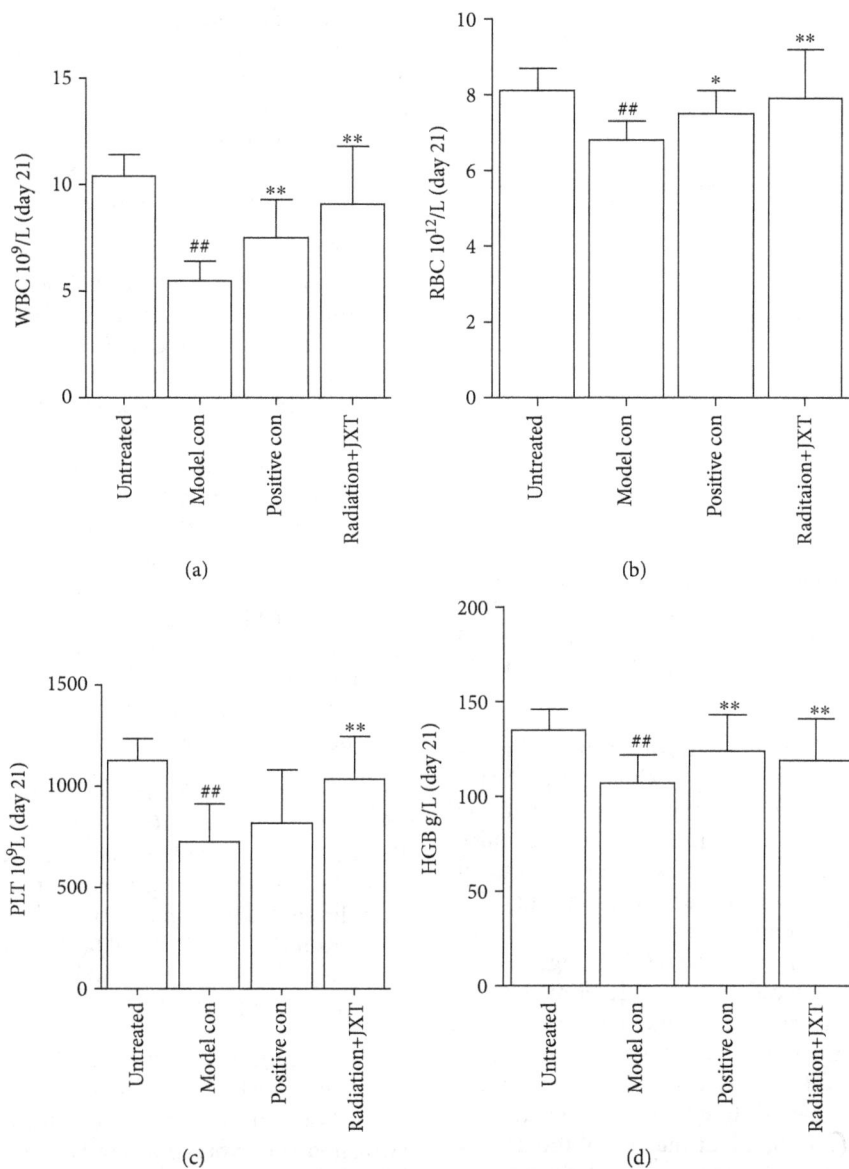

FIGURE 2: Effect of JXT on the number of circulating peripheral blood cells in Co^{60}-irradiated mice. All data were expressed as mean ± SEM ($n = 10$). $^{\#}P < 0.05$; $^{\#\#}P < 0.01$ when compared with the untreated control group. $^{*}P < 0.05$; $^{**}P < 0.01$ when compared with the Co^{60}-irradiated group. (a) White blood cell (WBC) number; (b) red blood cell (RBC) number; (c) platelet (PLT) number; (d) hemoglobin (HGB) level.

cytometer (Becton, Dickinson and Company, USA). Each sample was collected at the amount of ten thousand cells.

3. Statistical Analysis

All data were expressed as mean ± standard deviation (M ± SD). Statistical analysis was conducted by using SPSS 16.0 software. One-way analysis of variance (ANOVA) followed by Tukey's post hoc test was used for multiple group comparisons. The statistically significant difference was considered at $P < 0.05$.

4. Results

4.1. Effect of JXT Treatment on the Loss of Body Weights and Organ Indexes. Figure 1 demonstrated the changes of body weights, spleen index, and thymus index in each group at day 21. There was a profound loss in body weight, spleen index, and thymus index of the animals exposed to 6.0 Gy γ-radiation. The administration with JXT significantly increased the body weight ($P < 0.05$), spleen index, and thymus index ($P < 0.01$) when compared to the radiation group. The results suggested that JXT administration played a positive role in preventing radiation-induced loss of body weight, spleen index, and thymus index of the mice.

4.2. Effect of JXT Treatment on Peripheral Blood Cells. WBC counts of the mice before and after irradiation were shown in Figure 2(a). Total WBC counts in irradiated animals were determined to be significantly reduced at day 21 ($P < 0.01$) when compared with those in the control group. The administration with JXT and amifostine could attenuate the

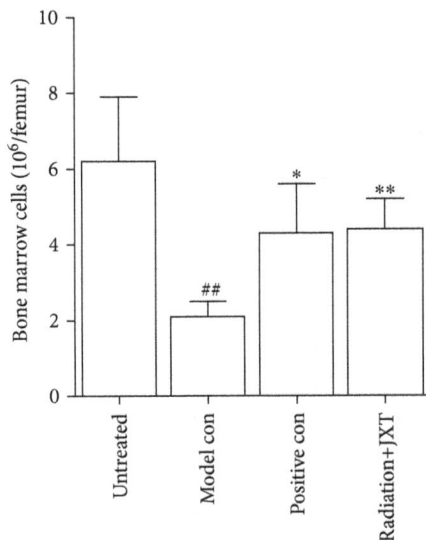

FIGURE 3: Effect of JXT on the number of bone marrow cells in Co^{60}-irradiated mice. All data were expressed as mean ± SEM ($n = 10$). $^{##}P < 0.01$ when compared with the untreated control group. $^{*}P < 0.05$; $^{**}P < 0.01$ when compared with the Co^{60}-irradiated group.

decrease in WBC counts. Figure 2(b) showed that irradiation reduced the RBC number at day 21, while a significant increase in the RBC number was observed on day 21 in the JXT-treated mice ($P < 0.01$) and amifostine-treated mice ($P < 0.05$). As shown in Figure 2(c), the number of peripheral PLT decreased markedly after irradiation, and the PLT decline was significantly attenuated by JXT on day 21 in comparison to the radiation group ($P < 0.01$). Figure 2(d) showed that irradiation reduced the HGB level at day 21; in contrast, a significant increase in the HGB level was observed on day 21 in the JXT- and amifostine-treated mice ($P < 0.01$ and 0.05). These results showed that the mice exposed to γ-radiation alone exhibited a typical hematopoietic syndrome. On the other hand, at the end of the 21-day experiment, irradiated mice receiving oral administration of JXT showed an improved blood profile with reduced leucopenia, thrombocytopenia (platelet counts), RBC, and hemoglobin levels.

4.3. Effect of JXT Treatment on the Depletion of Bone Marrow Cells. Subsequently, the potential of JXT to protect irradiation-induced damage of bone marrow cells was also investigated. The effect of JXT on hematopoietic tissue in irradiated mice was evaluated by HE staining in our previous study [28]. The marrow cellularity in the radiation group was decreased when compared with that in the naive group. Although the irradiation can result in a continuous increase in the number of adipocytes [29], JXT treatment could significantly increase the total number of bone marrow cells and ameliorate cellular contents of the bone marrow (Figure 3, $P < 0.01$).

4.4. Effect of JXT Treatment on the Expression of Proteins in JAK/STAT Signal Pathway. In order to identify whether JAK/STAT signal pathway can be activated by JXT, we

examined the phosphorylation of JAK2, STAT5a, and STAT5b in the bone marrow after JXT treatment. The expression of pJAK2/JAK2 and pSTAT5a/STAT5a in bone marrow tissue was decreased after radiation, and the expression of phosphor-JAK2 and phosphor-STAT5a was enhanced. But the expression of pSTAT5b/STAT5b was not changed after radiation and JXT treatment (Figure 4).

4.5. Effect of JXT Treatment on the Proliferation, G-CSF, and G-CSFR of NFS-60 Cells. The CCK-8 assay was used to evaluate the effect of JXT on the viability of NFS-60 cells. The cells treated with G-CSF (15 ng/ml) revealed an obvious increase in the percentage of viable cells when compared to the control group. After JXT treatment at different concentrations (6 μg/ml to 40 μg/ml), the viability of NFS-60 cells was increased in a concentration-dependent manner ($P < 0.05$ or $P < 0.01$). However, the viability of NFS-60 cells in the 200 μg/ml treatment group was suppressed (Figure 5(a)). At the same time, we measured the G-CSF level in the same conditioned media by ELISA. Only 15 ng/ml G-CSF could induce the release of G-CSF ($P < 0.01$), but no change in the JXT treatment groups (Figure 5(b)). Flow cytometry showed that JXT treatment at 6–200 μg/ml could also increase the G-CSFR level in NFS-60 cells (Figures 5(c)–5(i)).

4.6. Effect of JXT Treatment on ROS, SOD, GSH-Px, and MDA in the Serum and Liver. We next investigated whether JXT can regulate oxidative stress system in mice under radiation. JXT treatment significantly reduced the ROS level that was elevated due to radiation-induced toxicity in the liver and serum (Figures 6(a) and 6(b)) and improved endogenous SOD and GSH-Px levels, as well as reduced MDA level in the liver (Figures 6(c)–6(e)).

4.7. Effect of JXT Treatment on Bcl-2 Expression in the Bone Marrow. In order to explore the effect of JXT on the apoptosis of bone marrow cells from mice upon γ-radiation, we evaluated the expression levels of Bcl-2 protein before and after JXT treatment. As shown in Figure 7, the expression of Bcl-2 was significantly declined in the radiation-treated mice, and JXT could increase the expression of Bcl-2 in bone marrow tissue significantly ($P < 0.01$).

5. Discussion

The bone marrow is the most important hematopoietic organ with hematopoietic cells at different developmental stages. A high proliferation rate of bone marrow cells is highly susceptible to irradiation-induced injury [30]. Bone marrow injury can cause the suppression of hematopoiesis, thus resulting in the low number of circulating blood cells and undesirable side effects such as anemia, bleeding, and infection [31, 32]. We previously demonstrated the protection of bioactive components in JXT against radiation-induced bone marrow damage [26], and herein we have applied an irradiation-induced myelosuppressed mouse model to investigate the protection potential of ethanol extract from JXT on radiation-induced hematological toxicity. Results showed that the administration with JXT could ameliorate Co^{60}

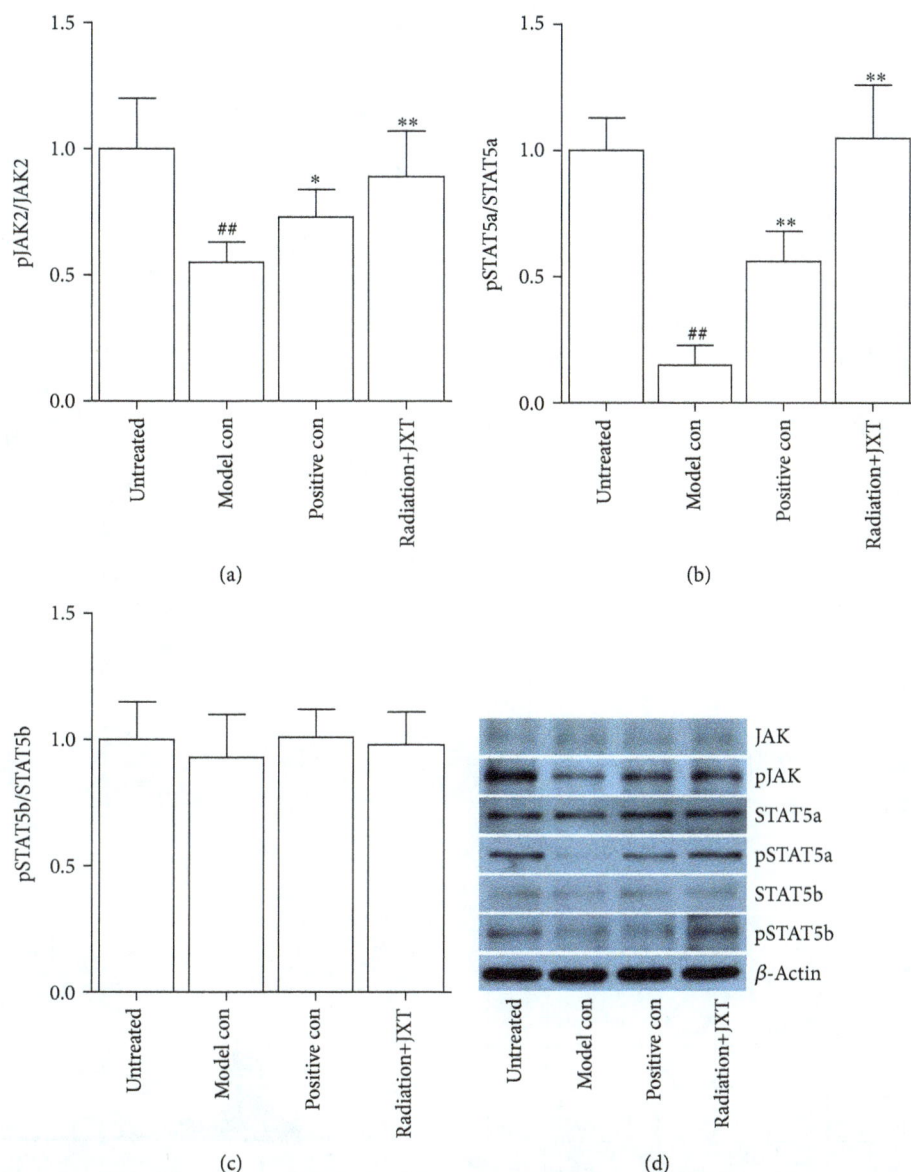

(a)

(b)

(c)

(d)

FIGURE 4: Effect of JXT on the phosphorylation of JAK2, STAT5a, and STAT5b in Co^{60}-irradiated mice. All data were expressed as mean ± SEM ($n = 10$). $^{##}P < 0.01$ when compared with the untreated control group. $^{*}P < 0.05$; $^{**}P < 0.01$ when compared with the Co^{60}-irradiated group.

irradiation-induced damage and significantly increase the number of peripheral blood cells (WBC, RBC, and PLT), body weight, spleen index, thymus index, and bone marrow cells. Together, these results confirm the enhancement of JXT on hematopoiesis.

Normally, the peripheral blood cell number maintains relative stability, depending on the hematopoietic function of the bone marrow [33]. Radiation exposure can cause injury in hematopoiesis and can result in peripheral blood cell cytopenia and the decrease in mature RBC in anemia. The decreased PLT can lead to bleeding, and the decreased WBC can result in infection [5]. Our results demonstrate that Co^{60} irradiation significantly reduced WBC and PLT counts in the peripheral blood of the mice; however, JXT administration can accelerate the recovery of peripheral blood cells. In order to investigate the effect of JXT treatment on bone

marrow injury, the analysis of BMC counts indicated that Co^{60} irradiation significantly decreased the BMC number, and JXT treatment attenuated this reduction, suggesting that JXT may accomplish the protection by improving the density of BMC and increasing the number of nucleated cells in the bone marrow of irradiated mice.

In the present study, we confirmed the radioprotective effect of JXT extract in the hematopoietic system *in vivo* and *in vitro*, and the alcohol extract of JXT can promote protein phosphorylation and the activation of JAK2-STAT5 signal pathway, thereby promoting hematopoiesis. The regulation of hematopoiesis involves multiple signal transduction pathways, in which the JAK-STAT signal pathway is an important signal pathway for the signal transduction of hematopoietic growth factors [34, 35]. Receptor dimerization induced by cytokine and receptor

(a)

(b)

(c)

(d)

(e)

(f)

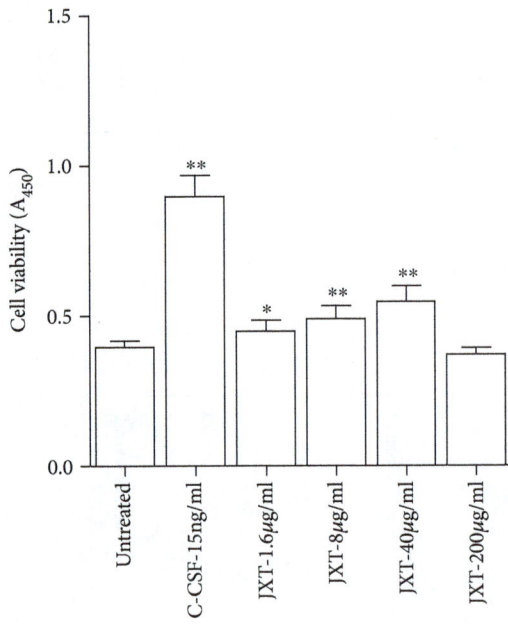

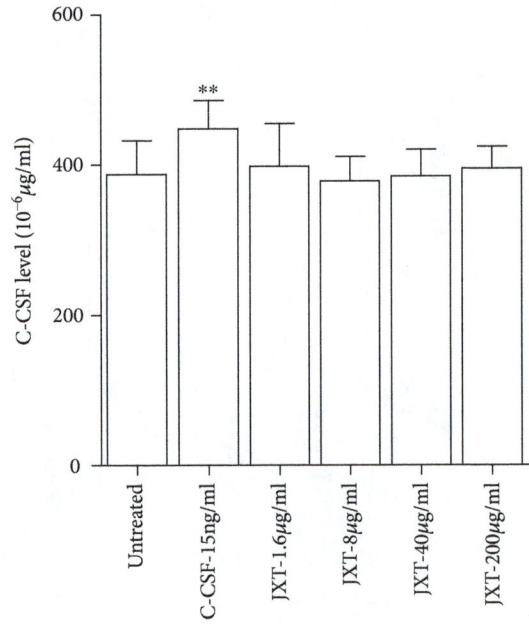

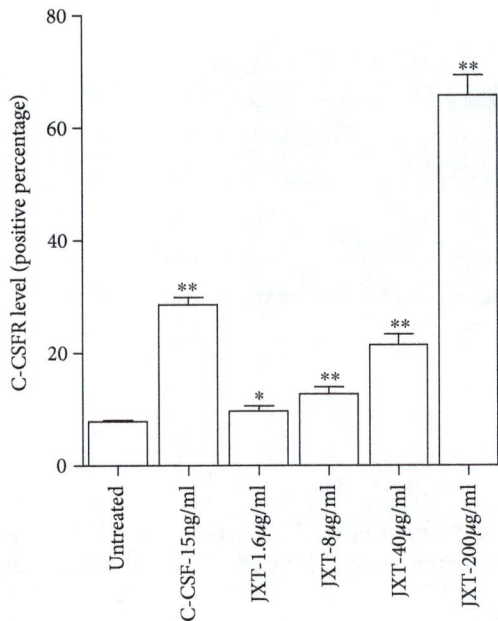

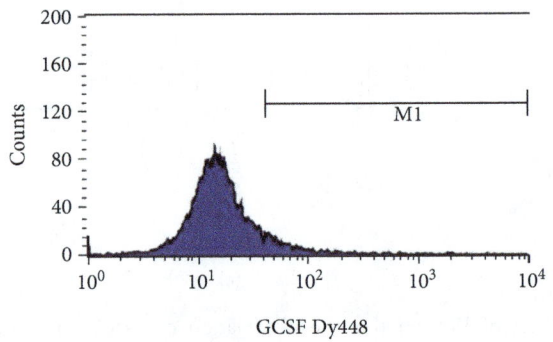

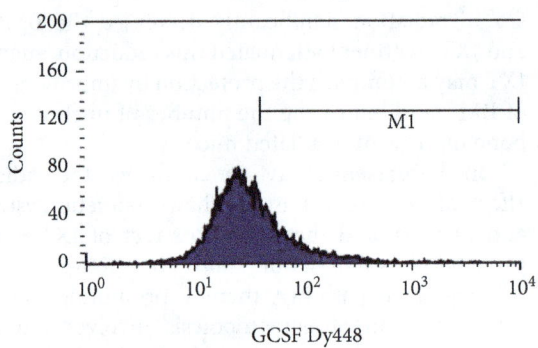

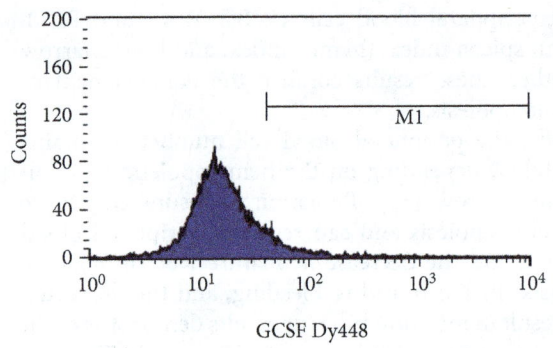

FIGURE 5: Continued.

(g)

(h)

(i)

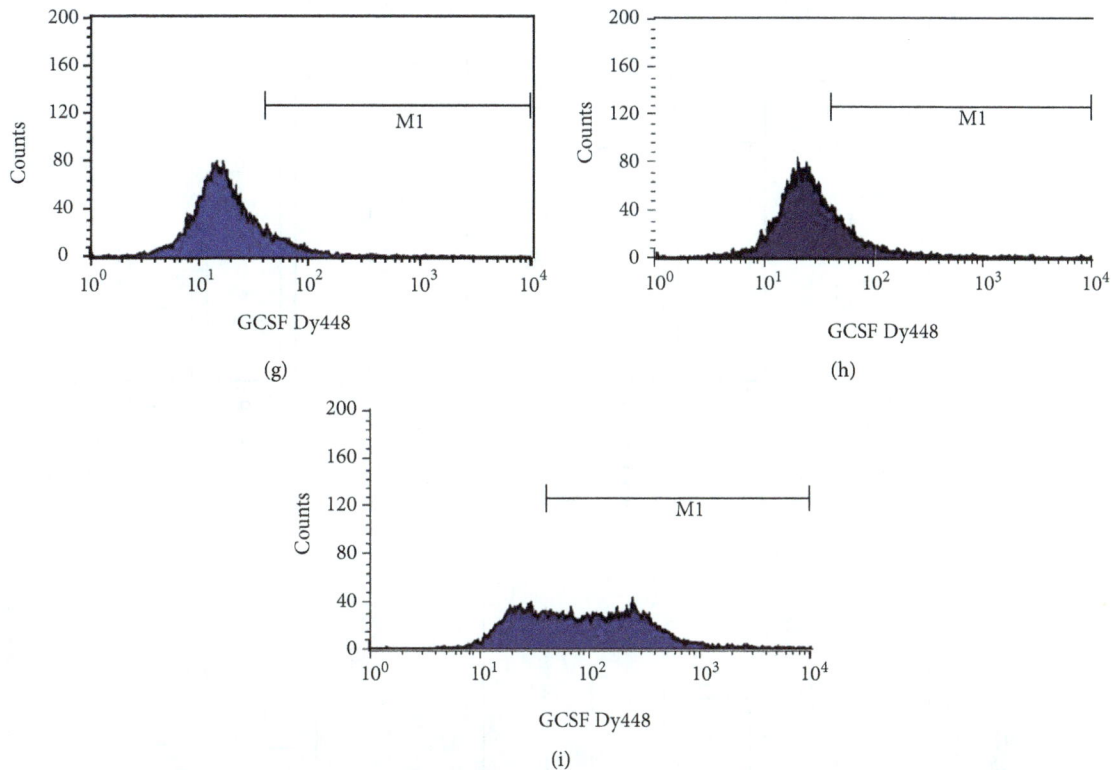

FIGURE 5: Effect of JXT on cell viability and G-CSF and G-CSFR levels in NSF-60 cells. All data were expressed as mean ± SEM ($n = 3$). $^{*}P < 0.05$; $^{**}P < 0.01$ when compared with the untreated control group.

binding can lead to JAK phosphorylation and initiate signal transduction. The activated JAK then catalyzes substrate proteins such as STAT, transmits the information to nuclei, and regulates gene expression, cell proliferation, and differentiation [36–38]. The signal transduction of G-CSF and GM-CSF receptors can be completed through the JAK2-STAT5 signal pathway [39].

In our studies, Bcl-2 was decreased after radiation treatment and increased in JXT-treated mice. The signal transducer and activator of transcription 5 (STAT5) are a critical regulator of normal and leukemic lymphomyeloid development through activating downstream early-acting cytokines, their receptors, and Janus kinases (JAKs) [40–43]. STAT5-mediated regulation of Bcl-2 in hematopoietic cells has been reported both in mouse [44] and in human hematopoietic cells [45]. STAT5ab$^{\Delta N/\Delta N}$ mast cells have a reduced level of Bcl-2 expression. Bcl-2 is a bona fide direct target of STAT5 so that STAT5 requires the N-domain for the suppression of miR15/16, induction of Bcl-2, and induction of survival signaling in mast cells and myeloproliferative neoplasms (MPNs) [46, 47]. The overexpression of Bcl-2 increases both stem cell number and repopulation potential [48–50]. Bcl-2 also has the antiapoptotic function so that the deficient survival function of BMC can be restored by adding Bcl-2 after JXT treatment.

Ionizing radiation can produce free radicals in cells, such as superanion, hydroxyl, and hydrogen peroxide free radicals [51]. The activity of free radicals can directly or indirectly damage the cell membrane and nucleic acid in the body, thus causing DNA strand breaks and the changes in tissue morphology and metabolism function, enzyme activity, and microcirculation. If free radicals are not timely removed, they could result in more serious physical or chemical injury [52, 53]. Radiation-induced liver injury often occurs in abdominal and pelvic tumors. The radiation-induced injury of the liver results in cell degeneration, apoptosis and necrosis, disordered enzyme activity, biofilm destruction, metabolic disorders, and severe functional failure of liver. Under normal circumstances, free radicals in the human body are in the dynamic balance of continuous production and scavenging. The scavenging of free radicals is mainly dependent on the action of antioxidant enzymes. SOD is a metal enzyme widely existed in organic organisms. It has super antioxidant function and can catalyze disproportionation of free radicals and scavenge free radicals, so as to protect damaged cells and maintain dynamic balance of oxidation and antioxidant reactions. MDA is the degradation product of lipid peroxide, and it has an attack on body cells. The content of MDA can reflect the extent of lipid peroxidation and indirectly reflect the damage of cells. The interaction of MDA and SOD has demonstrated that SOD activity can indirectly reflect scavenging capacity of oxygen free radicals. MDA content can indirectly reflect free radical-induced damage degree. In the present study, JXT could regulate the oxidative stress system of mice under radiation, suggesting that JXT can protect the liver from oxidative damage induced by radiation.

Many natural products and compounds have been found to have radioprotective effects. A novel lignin-derived polyphenolic composition with ammonium molybdate, BP-C2 mitigates radiation-induced damage in midlethal range of

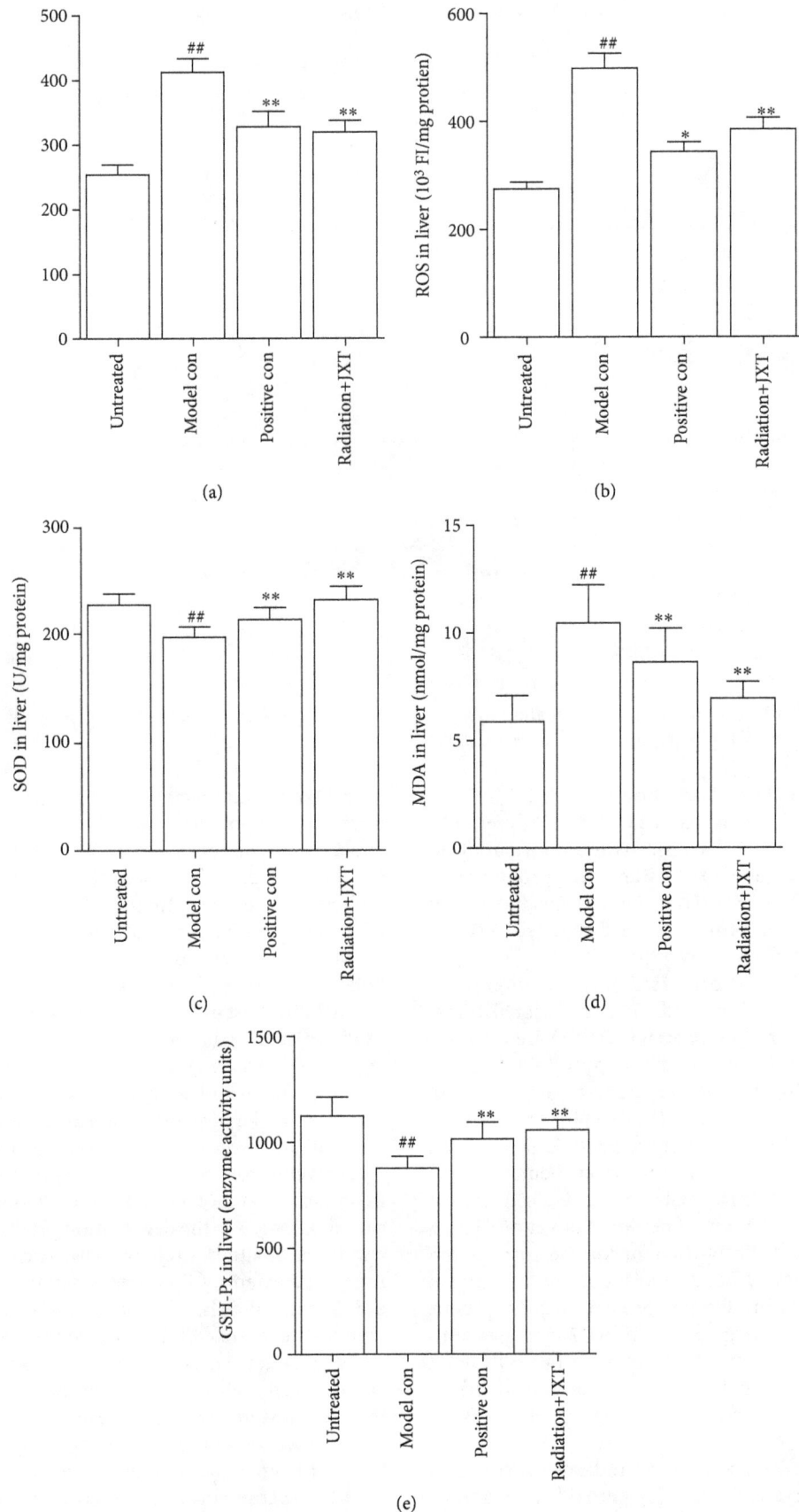

FIGURE 6: Effect of JXT on the levels of GSH-Px, SOD, and MDA in Co^{60}-irradiated mice. All data were expressed as mean ± SEM ($n = 10$). $^{##}P < 0.01$ when compared with the untreated control group. $^{*}P < 0.05$; $^{**}P < 0.01$ when compared with the Co^{60}-irradiated group.

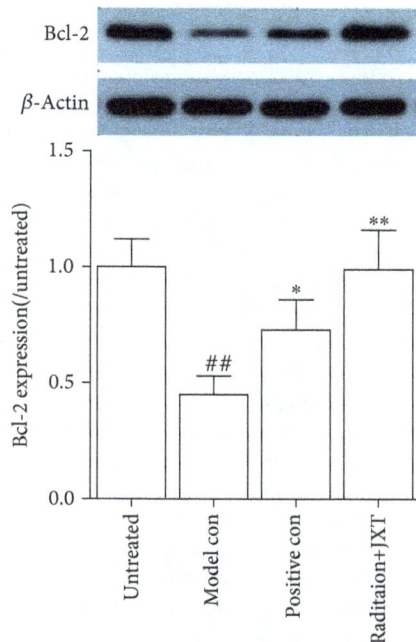

FIGURE 7: Effect of JXT on the expression of Bcl-2 in Co^{60}-irradiated mice. All data were expressed as mean ± SEM ($n = 10$). $^{##}P < 0.01$ when compared with the untreated control group. $^{*}P < 0.05$; $^{**}P < 0.01$ when compared with the Co^{60}-irradiated group.

radiation doses. Effects are mediated by the enhancement of extramedullar hematopoiesis in the spleen and a protective effect on the intestinal epithelium [54]. Tea polyphenols, particularly in the combination in TP50 as the radioprotector in mice, have antioxidant potential activity and can reduce inflammatory cytokines especially during the recovery of the hematopoietic system [55]. Beetroot has the potency to preserve bone marrow integrity and stimulate the differentiation of HSCs against ionizing radiation [56].

In our study, JXT has a protective function against hematopoietic dysfunction induced by Co^{60} radiation. JXT treatment can improve bone marrow damage and ameliorate cellular contents of the bone marrow through stimulating the JAK2/STAT5a signal pathway, thus increasing Bcl-2 expression and blocking bone marrow cell apoptosis in Co^{60}-irradiated mice. The antioxidant capacity of JXT in the liver can be attributed to the regulatory effect on SOD, GSH-Px, and MDA. Therefore, JXT may be a promising radioprotective agent for the suppression of hematopoiesis.

Authors' Contributions

Yu-Ning Wang and Xian-Zhe Dong contributed equally to this work.

Acknowledgments

This work was supported by a grant from the National Natural Science Foundation (no. 81373781).

References

[1] S. Khan, J. S. Adhikari, M. A. Rizvi, and N. K. Chaudhury, "Radioprotective potential of melatonin against ^{60}Co γ-ray-induced testicular injury in male C57BL/6 mice," *Journal of Biomedical Science*, vol. 22, no. 1, article 61, 2015.

[2] E. Park, I. Hwang, J. Y. Song, and Y. Jee, "Acidic polysaccharide of Panax ginseng as a defense against small intestinal damage by wholebody gamma irradiation of mice," *Acta Histochemica*, vol. 113, no. 1, pp. 19–23, 2011.

[3] J. F. Weiss, "Pharmacologic approaches to protection against radiation-induced lethality and other damage," *Environmental Health Perspectives*, vol. 105, Supplement 6, pp. 1473–1478, 1997.

[4] T. B. Elliott, N. E. Deutz, J. Gulani et al., "Gastrointestinal acute radiation syndrome in Göttingen minipigs (*Sus scrofa domestica*)," *Comparative Medicine*, vol. 64, no. 6, pp. 456–463, 2014.

[5] C. Liu, J. Liu, Y. Hao et al., "6, 7, $3',4'$-Tetrahydroxyisoflavone improves the survival of whole-body-irradiated mice via restoration of hematopoietic function," *International Journal of Radiation Biology*, vol. 93, no. 8, pp. 793–802, 2017.

[6] E. M. Rosen, R. Day, and V. K. Singh, "New approaches to radiation protection," *Frontiers in Oncology*, vol. 4, p. 381, 2015.

[7] L. Shao, Y. Luo, and D. Zhou, "Hematopoietic stem cell injury induced by ionizing radiation," *Antioxidants and Redox Signaling*, vol. 20, no. 9, pp. 1447–1462, 2014.

[8] T. A. Davis, T. K. Clarke, S. R. Mog, and M. R. Landauer, "Subcutaneous administration of genistein prior to lethal irradiation supports multilineage, hematopoietic progenitor cell recovery and survival," *International Journal of Radiation Biology*, vol. 83, no. 3, pp. 141–151, 2007.

[9] M. Liu, H. Tan, X. Zhang et al., "Hematopoietic effects and mechanisms of *Fufang E'jiao Jiang* on radiotherapy and chemotherapy-induced myelosuppressed mice," *Journal of Ethnopharmacology*, vol. 152, no. 3, pp. 575–584, 2014.

[10] D. Ewing and S. R. Jones, "Superoxide removal and radiation protection in bacteria," *Archives of Biochemistry and Biophysics*, vol. 254, no. 1, pp. 53–62, 1987.

[11] P. Cramers, E. E. Verhoeven, A. R. Filon et al., "Impaired repair of ionizing radiation-induced DNA damage in Cockayne syndrome cells," *Radiation Research*, vol. 175, no. 4, pp. 432–443, 2011.

[12] B. Mukherjee, N. Tomimatsu, K. Amancherla, C. V. Camacho, N. Pichamoorthy, and S. Burma, "The dual PI3K/mTOR inhibitor NVP-BEZ235 is a potent inhibitor of ATM- and DNA-PKCs-mediated DNA damage responses," *Neoplasia*, vol. 14, no. 1, pp. 34–IN8, 2012.

[13] C. K. Nair, D. K. Parida, and T. Nomura, "Radioprotectors in radiotherapy," *Journal of Radiation Research*, vol. 42, no. 1, pp. 21–37, 2001.

[14] R. R. Copp, D. D. Peebles, C. M. Soref, and W. E. Fahl, "Radioprotective efficacy and toxicity of a new family of aminothiol analogs," *International Journal of Radiation Biology*, vol. 89, no. 7, pp. 485–492, 2013.

[15] D. K. Maurya and C. K. Nair, "Preferential radioprotection to DNA of normal tissues by ferulic acid under *ex vivo* and *in vivo* conditions in tumor bearing mice," *Molecular and Cellular Biochemistry*, vol. 285, no. 1-2, pp. 181–190, 2006.

[16] D. Rades, F. Fehlauer, A. Bajrovic, B. Mahlmann, E. Richter, and W. Alberti, "Serious adverse effects of amifostine during radiotherapy in head and neck cancer patients," *Radiotherapy and Oncology*, vol. 70, no. 3, pp. 261–264, 2004.

[17] D. Citrin, A. P. Cotrime, F. Hyodo, B. J. Baum, M. C. Krishna, and J. B. Mitchell, "Radioprotectors and mitigators of radiation-induced normal tissue injury," *The Oncologist*, vol. 15, no. 4, pp. 360–371, 2010.

[18] S. Pal, C. Saha, and S. K. Dey, "Studies on black tea (Camellia sinensis) extract as a potential antioxidant and a probable radioprotector," *Radiation and Environmental Biophysics*, vol. 52, no. 2, pp. 269–278, 2013.

[19] Y. Chen, B. Zhu, L. Zhang, S. Yan, and J. Li, "Experimental study of the bone marrow protective effect of a traditional Chinese compound preparation," *Phytotherapy Research*, vol. 23, no. 6, pp. 823–826, 2009.

[20] R. Arora, D. Gupta, R. Chawla et al., "Radioprotection by plant products: present status and future prospects," *Phytotherapy Research*, vol. 19, no. 1, pp. 1–22, 2005.

[21] M. H. Whitnall, C. E. Inal, W. E. Jackson, V. L. Miner, V. Villa, and T. M. Seed, "*In vivo* radioprotection by 5-androstenediol: stimulation of the innate immune system," *Radiation Research*, vol. 156, no. 3, pp. 283–293, 2001.

[22] S. J. Bing, M. J. Kim, G. Ahn et al., "Acidic polysaccharide of Panax ginseng regulates the mitochondria/caspase-dependent apoptotic pathway in radiation-induced damage to the jejunum in mice," *Acta Histochemica*, vol. 116, no. 3, pp. 514–521, 2014.

[23] National Pharmacopoeia Committee, *Pharmacopoeia of the People's Republic of China, Part I*, China Medical Science Press, Beijing, 2010.

[24] Y. Zhang, L. Guo, L. Duan et al., "Simultaneous determination of 16 phenolic constituents in Spatholobi Caulis by high performance liquid chromatography/electrospray ionization triple quadrupole mass spectrometry," *Journal of Pharmaceutical and Biomedical Analysis*, vol. 102, pp. 110–118, 2015.

[25] T. Toyama, S. Wada-Takahashi, M. Takamichi et al., "Reactive oxygen species scavenging activity of Jixueteng evaluated by electron spin resonance (ESR) and photon emission," *Natural Product Communications*, vol. 9, no. 12, pp. 1755–1759, 2015.

[26] D. X. Wang, P. Liu, R. Y. Chen, M. L. Chen, and G. Y. Chen, "Effect of monomers extracted from Spatholobus suberectus Dunn on proliferation of hematopoietic progenitor cells in marrow-depressed mice," *Chinese Journal of Tissue Engineering Research*, vol. 12, no. 21, article 4166, 2008.

[27] Y. Hu, D. H. Guo, P. Liu et al., "Bioactive components from the tea polyphenols influence on endogenous antioxidant defense system and modulate inflammatory cytokines after total-body irradiation in mice," *Phytomedicine*, vol. 18, no. 11, pp. 970–975, 2011.

[28] X. Tan, X. Z. Dong, D. H. Guo et al., "Anti-radiation effect and mechanism studies of ethanol extracts from Spatholobus suberectus and its active component catechin," *China Journal of Chinese Materia Medica*, vol. 41, no. 9, pp. 1718–1724, 2014.

[29] Q. Zou, W. Hong, Y. Zhou et al., "Bone marrow stem cell dysfunction in radiation-induced abscopal bone loss," *Journal of Orthopaedic Surgery and Research*, vol. 11, no. 1, p. 3, 2016.

[30] S. M. Bentzen, "Preventing or reducing late side effects of radiation therapy: radiobiology meets molecular pathology," *Nature Reviews Cancer*, vol. 6, no. 9, pp. 702–713, 2006.

[31] Z. C. Ma, Q. Hong, Y. G. Wang et al., "Effects of ferulic acid on hematopoietic cell recovery in whole-body gamma irradiated mice," *International Journal of Radiation Biology*, vol. 87, no. 5, pp. 499–505, 2011.

[32] A. J. Simonnet, J. Nehmé, P. Vaigot, V. Barroca, P. Leboulch, and D. Tronik-le Roux, "Phenotypic and functional changes induced in hematopoietic stem/progenitor cells after gamma-ray radiation exposure," *Stem Cells*, vol. 27, no. 6, pp. 1400–1409, 2009.

[33] P. J. Carey, "Drug-induced myelosuppression: diagnosis and management," *Drug Safety*, vol. 26, no. 10, pp. 691–706, 2003.

[34] R. Gazit, H. Weissman, and D. J. Rossi, "Hematopoietic stem cells and the aging hematopoietic system," *Seminars in Hematology*, vol. 45, no. 4, pp. 218–224, 2008.

[35] H. J. Park, J. Li, R. Hannah et al., "Cytokine-induced mega-karyocytic differentiation is regulated by genome-wide loss of a uSTAT transcriptional program," *The EMBO Journal*, vol. 35, no. 6, pp. 580–594, 2016.

[36] S. Thomas, K. H. Fisher, J. A. Snowden, S. J. Danson, S. Brown, and M. P. Zeidler, "Methotrexate is a JAK/STAT pathway inhibitor," *PLoS One*, vol. 10, no. 7, article e0130078, 2015.

[37] C. Vitali, C. Bassani, C. Chiodoni et al., "SOCS2 controls proliferation and stemness of hematopoietic cells under stress conditions and its deregulation marks unfavorable acute leukemias," *Cancer Research*, vol. 75, no. 11, pp. 2387–2399, 2015.

[38] Z. Wang, G. Li, and K. D. Bunting, "STAT5 N-domain deleted isoforms are naturally occurring hypomorphs partially rescued in hematopoiesis by transgenic Bcl-2 expression," *American Journal of Blood Reserach*, vol. 4, no. 1, pp. 20–26, 2014.

[39] C. Leroy, N. V. Belkina, T. Long et al., "Caspase cleavages of the lymphocyte oriented kinase prevent ezrin, radixin, and moesin phosphorylation during apoptosis," *The Journal of Biological Chemistry*, vol. 291, no. 19, pp. 10148–10161, 2016.

[40] K. D. Bunting, H. L. Bradley, T. S. Hawley, R. Moriggl, B. P. Sorrentino, and J. N. Ihle, "Reduced lymphomyeloid repopulating activity from adult bone marrow and fetal liver of mice lacking expression of STAT5," *Blood*, vol. 99, no. 2, pp. 479–487, 2002.

[41] J. W. Snow, N. Abraham, M. C. Ma, N. W. Abbey, B. Herndier, and M. A. Goldsmith, "STAT5 promotes multilineage hemato-lymphoid development in vivo through effects on early hematopoietic progenitor cells," *Blood*, vol. 99, no. 1, pp. 95–101, 2002.

[42] H. Schepers, D. van Gosliga, A. T. Wierenga, B. J. L. Eggen, J. J. Schuringa, and E. Vellenga, "STAT5 is required for long-term maintenance of normal and leukemic human stem/progenitor cells," *Blood*, vol. 110, no. 8, pp. 2880–2888, 2007.

[43] A. T. Wierenga, E. Vellenga, and J. J. Schuringa, "Maximal STAT5-induced proliferation and self-renewal at intermediate STAT5 activity levels," *Molecular and Cellular Biology*, vol. 28, no. 21, pp. 6668–6680, 2008.

[44] A. T. Wierenga, H. Schepers, M. A. Moore, E. Vellenga, and J. J. Schuringa, "STAT5-induced self-renewal and impaired myelopoiesis of human hematopoietic stem/progenitor cells involves down-modulation of C/EBPalpha," *Blood*, vol. 107, no. 11, pp. 4326–4333, 2006.

[45] J. D. Lord, B. C. McIntosh, P. D. Greenberg, and B. H. Nelson, "The IL-2 receptor promotes lymphocyte proliferation and induction of the c-myc, bcl-2, and bcl-x genes through the

trans-activation domain of Stat5," *Journal of Immunology*, vol. 164, no. 5, pp. 2533–2541, 2000.

[46] M. Buitenhuis, B. Baltus, J. W. Lammers, P. J. Coffer, and L. Koenderman, "Signal transducer and activator of transcription 5a (STAT5a) is required for eosinophil differentiation of human cord blood–derived CD34$^+$ cells," *Blood*, vol. 101, no. 1, pp. 134–142, 2003.

[47] G. Li, K. L. Miskimen, Z. Wang et al., "STAT5 requires the N-domain for suppression of miR15/16, induction of bcl-2, and survival signaling in myeloproliferative disease," *Blood*, vol. 115, no. 7, pp. 1416–1424, 2010.

[48] H. Oguro and A. Iwama, "Life and death in hematopoietic stem cells," *Current Opinion in Immunology*, vol. 19, no. 5, pp. 503–509, 2007.

[49] J. Domen and I. L. Weissman, "Hematopoietic stem cells need two signals to prevent apoptosis; BCL-2 can provide one of these, Kitl/c-Kit signaling the other," *The Journal of Experimental Medicine*, vol. 192, no. 12, pp. 1707–1718, 2000.

[50] J. Domen, K. L. Gandy, and I. L. Weissman, "Systemic overexpression of BCL-2 in the hematopoietic system protects transgenic mice from the consequences of lethal irradiation," *Blood*, vol. 91, no. 7, pp. 2272–2282, 1998.

[51] K. Takeshita, K. Fujii, K. Anzai, and T. Ozawa, "In vivo monitoring of hydroxyl radical generation caused by X- ray irradiation of rats using the spin trapping/EPR technique," *Free Radical Biology & Medicine*, vol. 36, no. 9, pp. 1134–1143, 2004.

[52] L. F. Barbisan, C. Scolastici, M. Miyamoto et al., "Effects of crude extracts of Agaricus blazei on DNA damage and on rat liver carcinogenesis induced by diethylnitrosamine," *Genetics and Molecular Research*, vol. 2, no. 3, pp. 295–308, 2003.

[53] P. G. Wells, Y. Bhuller, C. S. Chen et al., "Molecular and biochemical mechanisms in teratogenesis involving reactive oxygen species," *Toxicology and Applied Pharmacology*, vol. 207, no. 2, pp. 354–366, 2005.

[54] V. N. Bykov, I. S. Drachev, S. Y. Kraev et al., "Radioprotective and radiomitigative effects of BP-C2, a novel lignin-derived polyphenolic composition with ammonium molybdate, in two mouse strains exposed to total body irradiation," *International Journal of Radiation Biology*, vol. 94, no. 2, pp. 114–123, 2018.

[55] Y. Hu, J. J. Cao, P. Liu et al., "Protective role of tea polyphenols in combination against radiation-induced haematopoietic and biochemical alterations in mice," vol. 25, pp. 1761–1769, 2011.

[56] J. Cho, S. J. Bing, A. Kim et al., "Beetroot (*Beta vulgaris*) rescues mice from γ-ray irradiation by accelerating hematopoiesis and curtailing immunosuppression," *Pharmaceutical Biology*, vol. 55, no. 1, pp. 306–316, 2017.

Permissions

All chapters in this book were first published in OMCL, by Hindawi Publishing Corporation; hereby published with permission under the Creative Commons Attribution License or equivalent. Every chapter published in this book has been scrutinized by our experts. Their significance has been extensively debated. The topics covered herein carry significant findings which will fuel the growth of the discipline. They may even be implemented as practical applications or may be referred to as a beginning point for another development.

The contributors of this book come from diverse backgrounds, making this book a truly international effort. This book will bring forth new frontiers with its revolutionizing research information and detailed analysis of the nascent developments around the world.

We would like to thank all the contributing authors for lending their expertise to make the book truly unique. They have played a crucial role in the development of this book. Without their invaluable contributions this book wouldn't have been possible. They have made vital efforts to compile up to date information on the varied aspects of this subject to make this book a valuable addition to the collection of many professionals and students.

This book was conceptualized with the vision of imparting up-to-date information and advanced data in this field. To ensure the same, a matchless editorial board was set up. Every individual on the board went through rigorous rounds of assessment to prove their worth. After which they invested a large part of their time researching and compiling the most relevant data for our readers.

The editorial board has been involved in producing this book since its inception. They have spent rigorous hours researching and exploring the diverse topics which have resulted in the successful publishing of this book. They have passed on their knowledge of decades through this book. To expedite this challenging task, the publisher supported the team at every step. A small team of assistant editors was also appointed to further simplify the editing procedure and attain best results for the readers.

Apart from the editorial board, the designing team has also invested a significant amount of their time in understanding the subject and creating the most relevant covers. They scrutinized every image to scout for the most suitable representation of the subject and create an appropriate cover for the book.

The publishing team has been an ardent support to the editorial, designing and production team. Their endless efforts to recruit the best for this project, has resulted in the accomplishment of this book. They are a veteran in the field of academics and their pool of knowledge is as vast as their experience in printing. Their expertise and guidance has proved useful at every step. Their uncompromising quality standards have made this book an exceptional effort. Their encouragement from time to time has been an inspiration for everyone.

The publisher and the editorial board hope that this book will prove to be a valuable piece of knowledge for researchers, students, practitioners and scholars across the globe.

List of Contributors

Camilo Rios and Verónica Barón-Flores
Departamento de Sistemas Biológicos, Universidad Autónoma Metropolitana Unidad Xochimilco Ciudad de México, Mexico

Iván Santander, Marcela Islas and Araceli Diaz-Ruiz
Departamento de Neuroquímica, Instituto Nacional de Neurología y Neurocirugía Manuel Velasco Suárez, Ciudad de México, Mexico

Marisela Méndez-Armenta and Concepción Nava-Ruiz
Laboratorio de Patología Experimental, Instituto Nacional de Neurología y Neurocirugía Manuel Velasco Suárez, Ciudad de México, Mexico

Sandra Orozco-Suárez
Unidad de Investigación Médica en Enfermedades Neurológicas, Hospital de Especialidades, Centro Médico Nacional Siglo XXI, Ciudad de México, Mexico

Miori Tanaka, Mizuho Sasaki and Akari Sato
Department of Food and Nutritional Sciences, Graduate School of Humanities and Sciences, Ochanomizu University, 2-1-1 Otsuka, Bunkyo-ku, Tokyo 112-8610, Japan

Yoshimi Kishimoto
Endowed Research Department "Food for Health", Ochanomizu University, 2-1-1 Otsuka, Bunkyo-ku, Tokyo 112-8610, Japan

Tomoyasu Kamiya
Research and Development Division, Toyo Shinyaku Co Ltd, 7-28 Yayoigaoka, Tosu-shi, Saga 841-0005, Japan

Kazuo Kondo
Endowed Research Department "Food for Health", Ochanomizu University, 2-1-1 Otsuka, Bunkyo-ku, Tokyo 112-8610, Japan
Institute of Life Innovation Studies, Toyo University, 1-1-1 Izumino, Itakura-machi, Ora-gun, Gunma 374-0193, Japan

Kaoruko Iida
Department of Food and Nutritional Sciences, Graduate School of Humanities and Sciences, Ochanomizu University, 2-1-1 Otsuka, Bunkyo-ku, Tokyo 112-8610, Japan
Institute for Human Life Innovation, Ochanomizu University, 2-1-1 Otsuka, Bunkyo-ku, Tokyo 112-8610, Japan

Gloria Lazzeri, Maria C. Scavuzzo and Paola Lenzi
Department of Translational Research and New Technologies in Medicine and Surgery, Human Anatomy, University of Pisa, Via Roma 55, Pisa 56126, Italy

Francesca Biagioni and Carla L. Busceti
I. R. C. C. S Neuromed, Via Atinense 18, Pozzilli 86077, Italy

Federica Fulceri, Chiara Ippolito and Alessandra Salvetti
Department of Clinical and Experimental Medicine, University of Pisa, Via Roma 55, Pisa 56126, Italy

Francesco Fornai
Department of Translational Research and New Technologies in Medicine and Surgery, Human Anatomy, University of Pisa, Via Roma 55, Pisa 56126, Italy
I.R.C.C.S Neuromed, Via Atinense 18, Pozzilli 86077, Italy

Serena De Matteis and Giorgia Marisi
Biosciences Laboratory, Istituto Scientifico Romagnolo per lo Studio e Cura dei Tumori (IRST) IRCCS, Meldola, Italy

Andrea Ragusa
Department of Engineering for Innovation, University of Salento, Lecce, Italy
CNR Nanotec, Institute of Nanotechnology, via Monteroni, 73100 Lecce, Italy

Stefania De Domenico
Italian National Research Council, Institute of Sciences of Food Production (ISPA), Lecce 73100, Italy

Andrea Casadei Gardini
Department of Medical Oncology, Istituto Scientifico Romagnolo per lo Studio e Cura dei Tumori (IRST) IRCCS, Meldola, Italy

Massimiliano Bonafè
Biosciences Laboratory, Istituto Scientifico Romagnolo per lo Studio e Cura dei Tumori (IRST) IRCCS, Meldola, Italy
Department of Experimental, Diagnostic and Specialty Medicine, Alma Mater Studiorum, University of Bologna, Bologna, Italy

Anna Maria Giudetti
Department of Biological and Environmental Sciences and Technologies, University of Salento, Lecce, Italy

C. Andreani, C. Bartolacci, A. Amici, C. Marchini and L. Tiano
University of Camerino, via Gentile III da Varano, 62032 Camerino, Italy

M. Guescini, M. Battistelli and V. Stocchi
University of Urbino, via Aurelio Saffi, 61029 Urbino, Italy

F. Orlando
Experimental Animal Models for Aging Unit Scientific Technological Area, IRCCS INRCA, via del Fossatello, 60127 Ancona, Italy

M. Provinciali
Experimental Animal Models for Aging Unit Scientific Technological Area, IRCCS INRCA, via del Fossatello, 60127 Ancona, Italy
Advanced Technological Center for Aging Research Scientific Technological Area, IRCCS INRCA, via Birarelli 8, 60121 Ancona, Italy
Polytechnic University of Marche, Department of Life and Environmental Sciences (DISVA), via Brecce Bianche, Ancona, Italy

P. Orlando
Polytechnic University of Marche, Department of Life and Environmental Sciences (DISVA), via Brecce Bianche, Ancona, Italy

S. Silvestri
Polytechnic University of Marche, Department of Life and Environmental Sciences (DISVA), via Brecce Bianche, Ancona, Italy
Biomedfood srl, Spinoff of Polytechnic University of Marche, via Brecce Bianche, 60131 Ancona, Italy

Weifeng Yao, Yihan Zhang, Jianqiang Guan, Mian Ge, Chaojin Chen, Shan Wu, Jiaxin Chen, Gangjian Luo, Pinjie Huang and Ziqing Hei
Department of Anesthesiology, Third Affiliated Hospital, Sun Yat-sen University, Guangzhou, Guangdong 510630, China

Xue Han
Department of Anesthesiology, Sun Yat-sen Memorial Hospital, Sun Yat-sen University, Guangzhou 510000, China

Hui Hua, Jiawei Cheng, Juan Liu, Weiwei Ma, Chenchen Si, Jie Wang, Bingrong Zhou and Dan Luo
Department of Dermatology, The First Affiliated Hospital of Nanjing Medical University, Nanjing 210029, China

Wenbo Bu
Institute of Dermatology, Chinese Academy of Medical Sciences (CAMS) and Peking Union Medical College (PUMC), Nanjing, Jiangsu, China

Mustafa S. Atta
Department of Physiology, Faculty of Veterinary Medicine, Kafrelsheikh University, Kafrelsheikh 33516, Egypt

Ali H. El-Far
Department of Biochemistry, Faculty of Veterinary Medicine, Damanhour University, Damanhour 22511, Egypt

Foad A. Farrag
Department of Anatomy and Embryology, Faculty of Veterinary Medicine, Kafrelsheikh University, Kafrelsheikh 33516, Egypt

Mohamed M. Abdel-Daim
Department of Pharmacology, Faculty of Veterinary Medicine, Suez Canal University, Ismailia 41522, Egypt

Soad K. Al Jaouni
Hematology/Pediatric Oncology, King Abdulaziz University Hospital and Scientific Chair of Yousef Abdullatif Jameel of Prophetic Medicine Application, Faculty of Medicine, King Abdulaziz University, Jaddah 21589, Saudi Arabia

Shaker A. Mousa
Pharmaceutical Research Institute, Albany College of Pharmacy and Health Sciences, Rensselaer, NY 12144, USA

I-Cheng Chen, Chih-Ying Chao, Yih-Ru Wu, Kuo-Hsuan Chang and Chiung-Mei Chen
Department of Neurology, Chang Gung Memorial Hospital, Chang Gung University College of Medicine, Taipei 10507, Taiwan

Te-Hsien Lin, Yu-Hsuan Hsieh and Guey-Jen Lee-Chen
Department of Life Science, National Taiwan Normal University, Taipei 11677, Taiwan

Ming-Chung Lee
Sun Ten Pharmaceutical Co. Ltd., New Taipei City 23143, Taiwan

Elba dos S. Ferreira, Anderson F. A. Diniz and Fernando R. Queiroga
Programa de Pós-graduação em Produtos Naturais e Sintéticos Bioativos, Centro de Ciências da Saúde, Universidade Federal da Paraíba, João Pessoa, PB, Brazil

Iara L. L. de Souza and Fabiana de A. Cavalcante
Programa de Pós-graduação em Produtos Naturais e Sintéticos Bioativos, Centro de Ciências da Saúde, Universidade Federal da Paraíba, João Pessoa, PB, Brazil

Departamento de Fisiologia e Patologia, Centro de Ciências da Saúde, Universidade Federal da Paraíba, João Pessoa, PB, Brazil

Maria Thaynan de L. Carvalho
Centro de Ciências da Saúde, Universidade Federal da Paraíba, João Pessoa, PB, Brazil

Lydiane T. Toscano and Alexandre S. Silva
Departamento de Educação Física, Centro de Ciências da Saúde, Universidade Federal da Paraíba, João Pessoa, PB, Brazil

Patrícia M. da Silva
Programa de Pós-graduação em Biologia Celular e Molecular, Centro de Ciências Exatas e da Natureza, Universidade Federal da Paraíba, João Pessoa, PB, Brazil

Bagnólia A. da Silva
Programa de Pós-graduação em Produtos Naturais e Sintéticos Bioativos, Centro de Ciências da Saúde, Universidade Federal da Paraíba, João Pessoa, PB, Brazil
Departamento de Ciências Farmacêuticas, Centro de Ciências da Saúde, Universidade Federal da Paraíba, João Pessoa, PB, Brazil

Joice Nascimento Barboza, Carlos da Silva Maia Bezerra Filho and Damião Pergentino de Sousa
Department of Pharmaceutical Sciences, Universidade Federal da Paraíba, 58051-970 João Pessoa, Paraíba, Brazil

Renan Oliveira Silva
Department of Biomedicine, University Center INTA-UNINTA, 62050-130 Sobral, Ceará, Brazil

Jand Venes R. Medeiros
Laboratory of Pharmacology of Inflammation and Gastrointestinal Disorders-LAFIDG, Federal University of Piauí, Parnaíba, Piauí, Brazil

G. Nannelli, E. Terzuoli, S. Donnini, P. Lupetti, A. Giachetti and M. Ziche
Department of Life Sciences, University of Siena, Siena, Italy

V. Giorgio and P. Bernardi
Department of Biomedical Sciences, University of Padua, Padua, Italy
Consiglio Nazionale delle Ricerche, Neuroscience Institute, Padua, Italy

Dimitrios Stagos, Dimitrios Balabanos, Salomi Savva, Zoi Skaperda, Alexandros Priftis, Efthalia Kerasioti and Demetrios Kouretas
Department of Biochemistry and Biotechnology, University of Thessaly, Viopolis, Larissa 41500, Greece

Eleni V. Mikropoulou, Konstantina Vougogiannopoulou, Sofia Mitakou and Maria Halabalaki
Division of Pharmacognosy and Natural Product Chemistry, Department of Pharmacy, University of Athens, Panepistimiopolis, Athens 15771, Greece

Bai-liu Ya, Hong-ju Cheng, Ting Yu, Wen-yan Liu and Bo Bai
Department of Physiology, Jining Medical University, Shandong 272067, China

Qian Liu
School of Clinical Medicine, Jining Medical University, Shandong 272067, China

Hong-fang Li
Department of Neurology, Affiliated Hospital of Jining Medical University, Shandong 272067, China

Lin Chen, You Wang and Li-li Yuan
School of Basic Medicine, Jining Medical University, Shandong 272067, China

Wen-juan Li
School of Forensic and Laboratory Medicine, Jining Medical University, Shandong 272067, China

Xian-Zhe Dong, Xiao Tan, Ping Liu and Dai-Hong Guo
Center of Drug Security, General Hospital of Chinese PLA, Beijing 100853, China

Yu-Ning Wang
Department of Surgery, Chinese PLA General Hospital, Beijing 100853, China

Can Yan
Department of Basic Theory of Chinese Medicine, School of Pre-Clinical Medicine, Guangzhou University of Chinese Medicine, Guangzhou 510060, China
The Research Centre of Basic Integrative Medicine, Guangzhou University of Chinese Medicine, Guangzhou 510060, China

Index